T0293061

Handbook of Multiple Sclerosis

Handbook of Multiple Sclerosis

Editor: Floyd Freemont

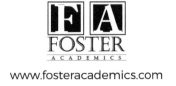

www.fosteracademics.com

www.fosteracademics.com

Cataloging-in-Publication Data

Handbook of multiple sclerosis / edited by Floyd Freemont.
    p. cm.
Includes bibliographical references and index.
ISBN 978-1-63242-730-4
1. Multiple sclerosis. 2. Myelin sheath--Diseases. 3. Virus diseases. 4. Neurology. I. Freemont, Floyd.
RC377 .H35 2019
616.834--dc23

Foster Academics,
118-35 Queens Blvd., Suite 400,
Forest Hills, NY 11375, USA

ISBN 978-1-63242-730-4 (Hardback)

Contents

Permissions

List of Contributors

Index

Preface

Multiple sclerosis (MS) is an immune-mediated disorder of the central nervous system caused by the systemic damage to the insulating covers of nerve cells. This disrupts the communication ability of the nervous system, resulting in signs and symptoms that are symptomatic of mental, physical and psychiatric issues. The underlying mechanism of the disease is generally attributed to the failure of the myelin-producing cells or destruction by the immune system, brought about by genetics or environmental factors. Multiple sclerosis is diagnosed on the basis of existing signs and symptoms, through medical imaging and lab testing. There is no cure of multiple sclerosis but several therapies allow a quality of care to patients. Such therapies strive to prevent new attacks, prevent disability and recuperate from an attack. This book aims to shed light on some of the unexplored aspects of multiple sclerosis and the recent researches in this disease. It strives to provide a fair idea about this condition and to help develop a better understanding of the latest advances in its management and treatment. The extensive content of this book provides the readers with a thorough understanding of the subject.

This book is a comprehensive compilation of works of different researchers from varied parts of the world. It includes valuable experiences of the researchers with the sole objective of providing the readers (learners) with a proper knowledge of the concerned field. This book will be beneficial in evoking inspiration and enhancing the knowledge of the interested readers.

In the end, I would like to extend my heartiest thanks to the authors who worked with great determination on their chapters. I also appreciate the publisher's support in the course of the book. I would also like to deeply acknowledge my family who stood by me as a source of inspiration during the project.

Editor

Neuroprotective therapies for multiple sclerosis and other demyelinating diseases

Pablo Villoslada[1,2]

Abstract

Damage to the Central Nervous Systems (CNS) in Multiple Sclerosis (MS) seems to be mainly due to chronic inflammation of the CNS with superimposed bouts of inflammatory activity by the adaptive immune system. The immune mediated damage can be amplified by neurodegenerative mechanisms in damaged axons including anterograde or retrograde axonal or transynaptic degeneration, synaptic pruning and neuronal or oligodendrocyte death. As such, it is highly unlikely that CNS damage can be prevented using only immunomodulatory drugs. For this reason, neuroprotection, aimed at preventing axonal, neuronal, myelin, and oligodendrocyte damage and cell death in the presence of this toxic microenvironment is highly pursued in MS and other demyelinating diseases. Neuroprotective strategies target different processes including oxidative stress, ionic imbalance (sodium, potassium or calcium), energy depletion, trophic factor support, metabolites balance, excitotoxicity, apoptosis, remyelination, etc. Although none of these strategies have translated into approved drugs to date, improvement in the understanding of underlying biology, in the design of clinical trials specific for assessing neuroprotection, and new technologies for developing novel therapies for neuroprotection suggest a new avenue for treating MS, Optic Neuritis or Neuromyelitis Optica (NMO). Several of these therapies are now entering clinical phases and if successful, such strategies would improve patients' quality of life, and will be even more critical for patients with progressive MS. In the event that such therapies target natural repair mechanisms rather than disease specific processes, they can potentially be useful for other brain diseases such as stroke, neurodegenerative diseases, brain trauma or epilepsy.

Keywords: Multiple sclerosis, Neuromyelitis optica, Demyelinating diseases, Neuroprotection, Trophic factors, Axonal damage, Remyelination

Background
The central nervous system is highly sensitive to damage: the role of neuroprotection

The Central Nervous System (CNS) is especially sensitive to damage compared to other tissues because of its highly specialized structure and function; it is composed of billions of neurons making both long and short-range connections, requires high energy and metabolite consumption, and has significant post-damage repair restrictions. Brain connections are made in a highly complex and synchronized process during development and are refined with training [1]. Once defined, brain connectivity is fixed by myelination and other processes in order to preserve memory and function [1, 2]. For this reason,

there are significant limitations for promoting neuronal network regeneration in adults after damage (e.g. presence of axonal growth inhibitory molecules such as neurite outgrowth inhibitor A (Nogo-A)). Nevertheless, even if regenerative therapy for the CNS is highly sought after, an intermediate, longer-term promising alternative approach is neuroprotection [3].

After insults such as ischemia, inflammation or excitotoxicity, neurons and axons may suffer significant damage, resulting in oxidative damage of DNA and proteins, reduced energy production, imbalance of ionic homeostasis and ion channel functioning, endoplasmic reticulum impairment and protein folding degradation or microtubule mediated axonal transport impairment. Due to the high level energetic and functional requirements that neurons have for maintaining long-distance nerve conduction (with axons up to 0.5 m long in the corticospinal

Correspondence: pvilloslada@clinic.ub.es
[1]Center of Neuroimmunology, Institut d'Investigacions Biomèdiques August Pi i Sunyer (IDIBAPS), Centre Cellex 3A, Casanova 145, Barcelona 08036, Spain
[2]Department of Neurology, University of California, San Francisco, USA

tract), neuronal malfunction can trigger self-destruction processes such as apoptosis, autophagia, synaptic pruning and many other forms of neuronal cell death [4–6]. Furthermore, damaged axons can trigger an active process of axonal degeneration regulated by levels of nicotinamide adenine dinucleotide (NAD). Axonal degeneration is a process different from apoptosis, which results in acute axonal transection and chronic anterograde (Wallerian) or retrograde degeneration. This process is regulated by several key molecules such as nicotinamide nucleotide adenylyltransferase 2 (NMNAT2), Sterile Alpha And TIR Motif Containing 1 (Sarm1) and phosphate starvation response 1 (PHR1) which regulates levels of NAD, or downstream steps regulated by c-Jun N-terminal kinases (JNK), glycogen synthase kinase 3 (GSK3) or inhibitor of kappa B kinase (IKK) converging in mitochondria and energy dysfunction and calpains activation leading to calcium imbalance [7, 8]. Additionally, myelin is highly susceptible to damage in the white matter because oligodendrocytes are also high-energy demanding cells (myelin turn-over is around one month) but the blood supply prioritizes grey over white matter [6]. Moreover, lipid structures such as myelin are highly susceptible to damage by immune mediators and oxidative stress [9]. In this context, inflammatory, ischemic or degenerative insults can induce either direct damage of the neurons (e.g. necrosis) or delayed degenerative processes that are triggered once surviving neurons identify they can no longer maintain their function and initiate different forms of cell death, axonal degeneration or synaptic pruning [10]. Another feature to take into account when managing neurological damage is the plastic and redundant nature of the CNS, which explain why damage of many CNS regions are not eloquent at the clinical level. This implies that CNS damage need to surpass a given threshold of damage in order to translate to clinical symptoms, which prevents close monitoring of CNS damage by clinical assessment and cause delayed diagnosis or disability monitoring. All these facts, including sensitivity of neural networks to damage, poor regenerative ability, and late diagnosis of CNS damage, support neuroprotection as an important therapeutic strategy for decreasing the burden of neurological diseases.

Neuroprotective strategies

Almost every mechanism of damage identified in brain diseases has been proposed as a therapeutic target for neuroprotection (Fig. 1). Several biological processes specific to the CNS (e.g. trophic factor signaling, axonal guidance, myelin formation) or critical for neurons (e.g. apoptosis, energetic supply, ionic balance) have been mimicked with experimental therapies [3, 11]. In addition, several regenerative therapies, such as stem cells, may provide some benefits via neuroprotective effects, including

the release of trophic factors, suppressing local inflammation or promoting a microenvironment supporting the survival of neurons, axons and oligodendrocytes [12]. Finally, secondary neuroprotection can be achieved by the reduction of the insult such as restoring blood supply in ischemia, decreasing excitotoxicity by reducing epileptogenic activity in seizures or decreasing CNS inflammation with the use of immunomodulatory drugs (e.g. glatiramer acetate, fingolimod, dimethyl-fumarate or laquinimod) in the case of MS [13–16].

Table 1 displays a list of several therapeutic strategies being pursued for neuroprotection. In the pursuit for neuroprotective strategies, trophic factors are proposed as the Holy Grail [17, 18]. Rather than coding for all neuronal connections during development, evolution developed the trophic factor strategy, which regulates neuronal survival and connection maintenance with the release of trophic factors from the target cell to the projecting neuron. For this reason, trophic factors activate a set of signaling pathways in neurons, such as Phosphoinositide 3-kinase (PI3K), Mitogen-activated protein kinase kinase (MAPKK), Nuclear factor-κB (NFKB) and others that stop apoptosis, promote cell survival and differentiation and trigger other beneficial effects such as decreasing oxidative stress, regulating ion channels, etc. [19]. Several growth factors have been tested in animal models or clinical trials including neurotrophins (nerve growth factor, brain-derived nerve factor, neurotrophin-3), insulin-growth factor (IGF-1), neurocytokines (cilliary-neurotrophic factor, leukemia inhibitor factor, interleukin-6), and glial-derived nerve factor family (erythropoietin, etc.) [20, 21]. They were tested in trials of peripheral neuropathy (diabetes or adquired immunodeficiency syndrome) or neurodegenerative diseases (Alzheimer disease, Parkinson disease, Huntington disease, Amyotrophic Lateral Sclerosis (ALS)) using human recombinant proteins delivered intravenously, intrathecaly or using engineered cells or gene therapy vectors [22–25]. Lack of success to date for the use of trophic factors to prevent CNS damage does not preclude the usefulness of trophic factors as a therapeutic target. Lack of efficacy was attributed to poor pharmacological properties of the recombinant proteins to enter the CNS and reach the target neurons, inadequate clinical trial design, such as testing patients in late stages when neuronal death is massive and using insensitive clinical or imaging outcomes, or side effects that limited dosing and patient exposition [26, 27]. However, the trophic factor pathways are at the core of cellular processes promoting neuronal and oligodendrocyte survival and for this reason are worth pursuing to see if activation of these pathways using different strategies might prevent permanent CNS damage.

Energy depletion and mitochondria dysfunction are another key factor in promoting neuronal degeneration

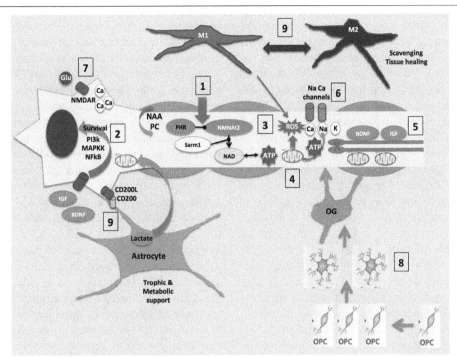

Fig. 1 Proposed targets for neuroprotective therapies. The pathways involved in neuroprotection include 1) Active axonal degeneration pathway activation (mediated by depletion of NAD levels by NMNAT2, PHR1 and Sarm1 activation); 2) trophic factor signaling (PI3K, MAPKK, NFkB); 3) oxidative stress (induced by inflammatory cells and mitochondria dysfunction); 4) energy depletion (due to mitochondria impairment and increased demand from Ca channels); 5) axonal transport blockade (failing to deliver mitochondria, signaling and molecular complexes to soma, nodes of Ranvier or synpasis); 6) ionic imbalance (due to ion channel redistribution and changes in activity, leading to increase of intracellular calcium); 7) Excitotoxicity (mediated by excess of glutamate signaling through the NMDA receptors); 8) remyelination (from OPC repopulation of demyelinated areas to myelination of denuded axons by mature oligodendrocytes (OG), which provide metabolic support to the axon (NAA or PC); 9) protective effects of astrocytes (providing trophic factors such as IGF-1 or BDNF, metabolic substrates such as lactate, or pro-survival signals such as CD200-CD200L) and M2 microglia (with scavenger and tissue healing activity)

Table 1 Molecules and pathways targeted in neuroprotection

Pathway	Molecule	Candidate drugs
Trophic factors	BDNF, IGF-1, CNTF, etc.	rhBNDF, rhIGF-1, rhCNTF, etc., CERE-110 (AAV2-NGF)
Mitochondria dysfunction and energy depletion	Cytochrome C, ATP	Resveratrol, Rosiglitazone, Pioglitazone, Troglitazone, Bezafibrate (PPARγ activator)
Ion channel	Sodium, Potassium or Calcium channels, Acid-Sensing Ion Channels	Phenitoin, Lamotrigin, Amiloride
Oxidative stress	iNOS, Nerf2	Dimethyl-Fumarate, Resveratrol, Vitamin E, Vitamin C, Melatonin, Carnosine, Coenzyme-Q, Idebenone, Carotenoids
Excitotoxicity	Glutamate	Memantine, Riluzole
Demyelination	MOG, Lingo-1	BIIB003, Clemastine benztropine, miconazole and clobetasol
Axonal transport	Dynamin, kinesin, microtubules	Epothilone B
Inhibitory molecules axonal growth and myelination	Lingo-1, Nogo-A	BIIB003, GSK1223249
Apoptosis	Bcl2, Bim, Bax, Cytochrome C, Caspase-3	Caspase or calpain inhibitors, Mynocycline
Microglia M2 mediated neuroprotection	CD200, trophic factors (BDNF), anti-inflammatory cytokines (IL-4, IL-10, TGFß)	Interferon-beta, Glatiramer acetate, Fumarate, Dimethyl-Fumarate, Mesenchymal stem cells
Astrocyte mediated neuroprotection	Trophic factors, NAA, pyruvate, lactate	Pentamidine, Methylthioadenosine, Fingolimod

BDNF brain-derived nerve factor, *IGF-1* insulin growth factor, *CNTF* cilliary neurotrophic factor, *NGF* Nerve growth factor, *rh* recombinant human, *iNOS* inducible nitric oxide synthase, *ATP* adenosine triphosphate, *MOG* myelin oligodendrocyte glycoprotein, *NAA* N-Acetyl aspartate

[4, 28, 29]. The CNS consumes 20 % of the overall oxygen and energy of the body and neurons require the support of astrocytes for maintaining their metabolic activity [6]. Neurons use lactate as a substrate for the Krebs cycle, which is provided by astrocytes. Neurons are very sensitive to adenosine triphosphate (ATP) depletion and mitochondrial damage due to their high-energy consumption needed to maintain the intensive protein systems supporting their connections as well as the ion channels in charge of maintaining the electrical impulse. This is particularly true for axons, because they are long and tiny structures receiving support from the soma as well as from the axon-myelin unit [4]. Energy depletion, mitochondria function impairment and axonal transport deficits are common in CNS diseases and for this reason targeting energy supply to the CNS has been pursued as well. Studies began by providing additional sugar supplies or decreasing metabolic rate (e.g. hypothermia) but now other strategies such as administering metabolite precursors, or preserving mitochondria functioning have also been tested in trials [29–31]. There is now a strong interest in understanding the early molecular events in mitochondria damage during neuronal and axonal damage in order to prevent energetic failure [4, 7, 32].

Ion channels are key for neuronal homeostasis and for maintaining the electrical impulse. Due to the highly specialized neuronal design, ion channel activity is highly prominent in the axonal initial segment as well as at the node of Ranvier [33]. This creates specific sites where ion fluxes are modulated and energy is required for axon functioning. Ion channel modulators have been explored as neuroprotective therapies in addition to their known beneficial effects in epilepsy or pain, including sodium channel modulators phenytoin, carbamacepin, lamotrigine, amiloride; and potassium channel modulators, aminopyridine or diazoxide (Table 2) [33]. Although benefits has been observed in animal models and small clinical trials, the challenge is determining how to maintain their beneficial effects in the long-term and understanding to which degree their effects are just maintaining the electrical impulse (symptomatic effects) versus promoting long-term neuronal or axonal survival (neuroprotection effects) [34].

Oxidative stress is another hot topic in neuroprotection [35]. The concept that free radicals degrade DNA and proteins suggest that anti-oxidative strategies would prevent cell death. There is ample evidence of the presence of increased oxidative stress in the damaged CNS in MS, neurodegenerative diseases, stroke and epilepsy [36–38]. However, oxidation in mitochondria and other organelles is a complex process required for energy production and other metabolic activities (e.g. signaling by nitric oxide (NO)) and for this reason is very difficult

to modulate without inducing further damage. However, several approved therapies reduce oxidative stress induced by the insult such as the immunomodulatory drug dimethyl-fumarate (through activation of nuclear factor (erythroid-derived 2)-like 2 (Nerf2)) [39], and mesenchymal stem cells [40], which decrease reactive oxygen species induced by inflammation.

Excitotoxicity is postulated as the prime mechanism of damage in epilepsy and it has also been associated with neurodegenerative diseases as well with MS [41, 42]. By over-activating the excitatory glutamate receptors, neurons experience high levels of electrical and energetic activity, inducing ion imbalance and promoting neuronal death. Although there is clear evidence about the role of this process in animal models, its involvement in MS and other brain diseases has not been clarified in detail. Riluzole is an approved drug inhibiting N-methyl-D-aspartate (NMDA) receptors, in addition to modulating sodium channels, but its efficacy in ALS is modest and trials in MS failed to show benefits [43]. Memantine is approved for Alzheimer's disease and was shown to modulate glutamate excitatory activation [44], but it was found to transiently worsen symptoms in patients with MS, reproducing pseudoexacerbations [45, 46].

Demyelination is the most prominent feature in MS. Promoting myelin recovery through remyelination is a natural strategy for treating demyelinating diseases. It is important to keep in mind that myelin is one of the most important elements for protecting axons, the myelin-axon unit [9]. Myelin is active not only in promoting saltatory conduction (which increases electrical conduction speed and reduces energy needs), but also in providing metabolic support to axons (e.g. N-Acetyl-Aspartate (NAA), phosphatidylcholine (PC), etc.) [47]. For this reason, preventing demyelination and promoting remyelination is one of the most important neuroprotective strategies for MS [48]. There are several drugs being tested at present to promote remyelination by blocking leucine rich repeat and immunoglobin-like domain-containing protein 1 (Lingo-1) using anti-Lingo-1 monoclonal antibody, or repurposing drugs such as clemastine or guanabenz (Table 2). The main challenge will be to probe in humans whether such drugs are able to induce remyelination of the CNS and whether this biological activity translates to clinical benefits. Quantifying demyelination and remyelination in the living human CNS still remains a challenge at the clinical level due to technological limitations (e.g. lack of specificity of MRI sequences such as magnetic transfer ratio) [49].

Axonal transport is a key process in the homeostasis of neurons and their long connections. Axons need to transport to the synapsis most of the protein synthesis machinery as well as providing energy supply to the nodes of Ranvier and synapsis. In addition trophic factor

Table 2 Neuroprotective drugs in clinical development for MS

Drug	Company	Type of compound	MoA summary	Route of administration	Phase	CT.org
KPT-350	Karyopharm Therapeutic	Small molecule - Selective Inhibitor of Nuclear Export (SINE)	Antioxidant Neuroprotection	Oral	Preclinical	N/A
NDC-1308	ENDECE Neural	Small molecule Estradiol analog	Neuroprotection Remyelination	N/A	Preclinical	N/A
Methylthioadenosine	Digna Biotech	Metabolite	Methyltransferases modulator Neuroprotection Remyelination	Oral	Preclinical	N/A
NRP2945	CuroNZ	Peptide	Neuroprotection	N/A	Preclinical	N/A
ER agonist	Karo Bio AB	Smal chemicals	Estrogen Receptor beta agonist Neuroprotection	N/A	Preclinical	N/A
VX15/2503	Vaccinex	mAb - anti-semaphorin 4D	Anti-SEMA4D Neuroprotection Remyelination	Intravenous	Phase 1	NCT01764737
RNS60	Revalesio	Physically-Modified Saline	Immunomodulation Neuroprotection	Intravenous	Phase 2	NCT01714089
GNbAC1	GeNeuro	mAb First-in-Class	Immunomodulation Remyelination	Intravenous	Phase 2a	NCT01639300
TRO19622 Olesoxime	Trophos SA	Small chemical	Antioxidant	Oral	Phase 1	NCT01808885
BIIB0033 - Anti-LINGO1	Biogen Idec	mAb	LINGO-1 antagonist Remyelination Neuroprotection	Intravenous	Phase 2 / Phase 2	NCT01864148 / NCT01721161
rHIgM22	Acorda Therapeutics	mAb - Recombinant human IgM	Remyelination	Intravenous	Phase 1	NCT01803867
MN-166 Ibudilast	MediciNova	Small molecule	Immunomodulation Neuroprotection	Oral	Phase 2	NCT01982942
RGN-352	RegeneRx	Peptide	Neuroprotection Remyelination	N/A	N/A	N/A
EGCG - Epigallocatechin-gallate	Generic	Green tea extract (Polyphenon E)	Anti-oxidant	Oral	Phase 2	NCT00525668 / NCT01451723
Lamotrigine	GlaxoSmithKline	Small chemical	Sodium channel modulator Neuroprotection	Oral	Oral	NCT01879527
Phenitoin	Generic	Small chemical	Sodium channel modulator Neuroprotection	Oral	Phase 2	NCT01451593
MRF-008 Guanabenz	Myelin Repair Foundation	Small chemical	Alpha agonist of the alpha-2 adrenergic receptor Remyelination	Oral	Phase 1	NCT02423083
Clemastine	Generic	Small chemical	Remyelination	Oral	Phase 2	NCT02040298
BAF312	Novartis	Small chemical - Siponimod	S1P1 antagonist Neuroprotection	Oral	Phase 2 RRMS Phase 3 SPMS	NCT00879658
Amiloride	Generic	Small chemical	Sodium channel modulator	Oral	Phase 2	NCT01910259
BN201	Bionure	Small chemical	Neurotrophin agonist Neuroprotection	Intravenous	Phase 1	N/A
Erythropietin	Generic	Human recombinant protein	Trophic factor Neuroprotection	Intravenous	Phase 3	NCT01962571
GSK1223249 – Ozanezumab	GlaxoSmithKline	mAb	Anti-Nogo-A Axonal regeneration	Intravenous	Phase 2	NCT01435993
Diazoxide	Generic	Small chemical	Potassium channel opener & mitochondrial channel modulator	Oral	Phase 2	NCT01428726
Minocycline	Generic	Small chemical	Anti-apoptotic & anti-oxidant	Oral	Phase 2	NCT01073813
Riluzole	Generic	Small chemical	Sodium channel and NMDA modulator	Oral	Phase 2	NCT00501943

Table 2 Neuroprotective drugs in clinical development for MS *(Continued)*

	Generic				
MD1003 - Biotin	Vitamin	Carboxylases coenzyme (acetylCoA carboxylase) Remyelination	Oral	Phase 3	NCT02220933
BG12 - Dimethyl Fumarate	Biogen Idec	Metabolite	Anti-oxidant hydroxycarboxylic acid receptor 2 agonist	Oral	Approved	NCT00420212
FTY720 - Fingolimod	Novartis	Small chemical	S1P1 and S1P5 antagonist neuroprotection	Oral	Approved	NCT00355134

transportation (e.g. brain-derived neurotrophic factor (BDNF)) from synapsis to the soma is also critical for neuronal survival [29]. This requires efficient transport through the axons based on intraxonal fluxes but mainly driven by microtubules transporting organelles to and from the soma using the dynein and kinesin systems respectively. Such molecular transporters are very sensitive to protein denaturation, lack of energy, inflammation and other types of damage [32, 50]. Also, it is known that mitochondria accumulate in the nodes of Ranvier (stationary sites) in order to provide extra ATP to sites rich in ion channels, and they are also transported to synapses to provide energy and are retrogradely transported for degradation. Inflammation, ischemia and other processes severely impair axonal transportation, including mitochondria delivery at nodes of Ranvier, contributing to energy and metabolite depletion and axonal damage [32, 51]. Recently, it has been shown that tubuline targeting drugs may preserve microtubule function and protect axons from degradation in models of spinal cord injury [52]. In addition, neurofilaments are in charge of keeping the 3D axonal structure and after damage, neurofilaments become hyperphosphorylated, losing their function and inducing the collapse of axons [53]. Therefore, preserving axonal structure and function is an important strategy for promoting neuroprotection.

For more than a century, since Cajal seminal studies, it has been known that the brain inhibits axonal regrowth, which prevents CNS regeneration. The identification that myelin was the main inhibitor of axonal growth was followed by the identification of several proteins such as Lingo-1 and Nogo-A that prevent axonal growth signaling through the nerve growth factor (NGF) receptor p75^{NGF} receptor [54]. This mechanism is important for avoiding the formation of aberrant connections and preserving brain connectivity, at the cost of decreasing the regenerative capacity of the CNS. The discovery of the molecules responsible for such processes has been followed by the development of monoclonal antibodies (mAb) targeting these pathways in order to promote axonal regeneration. There are several clinical trials in MS testing such approaches including the use of mAb against Lingo-1 and Nogo-A (Table 2). The main concern is the pharmacological restrictions that mAb has in order to reach high levels in the CNS as well as the timing for this therapeutic intervention after injury.

Finally, it is well known that glia, including astrocytes and microglia, can display neuroprotective activities, although many of them are poorly understood [12, 55]. For example, healthy neurons express CD200, which interacts with CD200L promoting survival signals [56]. Also, both microglia and astrocytes can release trophic factors and provide metabolic support to neuronal function [57]. The neuroprotective phenotype of microglia,

also termed M2, is associated with suppressing inflammation and the creation of a supportive microenvironment supporting neuronal survival [12]. Furthermore, astrocytes, as the main supporters of neuronal function, display a wide array of positive functions for promoting neuronal survival. Moreover, stem cell therapy may show beneficial effects above and beyond just replacing cells by creating a supportive microenvironment and suppressing inflammation [12, 40]. Identification of the different mechanisms involved will provide new targets for developing neuroprotective strategies.

Unmet needs for neuroprotection in MS and demyelinating diseases

In MS, CNS damage is produced by a complex inflammatory process. Although in the past it was believed that in the relapsing-remitting phase CNS damage was due only to the presence of inflammatory infiltrates within the MS plaques, in the last decade it has been clearly shown that MS is a diffuse disease with inflammation, demyelination and axonal loss both in the grey and white matter [58, 59]. This diffuse inflammation, also termed trapped inflammation, is mainly drive by activated microglia, although cells of the adaptive immune system may be also present. Therefore, myelin and axons are acutely damaged by inflammatory infiltrates and chronically damaged by chronic microglia activation; both processes being present in relapsing and progressive MS to different extent and dynamics [36]. However, in progressive MS, relapses due to new inflammatory infiltrates tend to decrease or disappear because less tissue is available for damage. Also, in parallel to the inflammatory process, axonal degeneration takes place in CNS areas already damaged long time ago because of the lack of myelin support, presence of an aggressive microenvironment, retrograde axonal degeneration or transynaptic degeneration [60]. Moreover, after one decade of damage and recovery during the relapsing-remittig phase, oligodendrocytes fail to produce new myelin and ultimately die; with time, the capacity of oligodendrocyte precursors to replace lost oligodendrocytes also decreases, leading to large areas of demyelination [61]. In this scenario, it is clear that MS patients require therapies aimed at stopping the degenerative process and preventing new CNS damage, on top of the immunomodulatory strategy aimed at preventing inflammation [62].

Current immunomodulatory drugs are not completely effective and drugs with high efficacy may induce severe adverse-events. We must also take into account patient heterogeneity as well as the difficulty for predicting disease activity at the time of defining the immunomodulatory therapy. For this reason, at present is not possible to guarantee that treated patients are going to be free of disease activity and CNS damage induced by the autoimmune attack. And even in the best scenario, damaged tissue is still at risk of developing degenerative processes in the long-term. Considering that regenerative therapies are still far from being applied in clinical practice, protecting the brain against chronic inflammation (not significantly modulated by current immunotherapy), and preventing neurodegeneration in the long-term, is being pursued as the main strategy in the medium term for decreasing disability accumulation in patients with MS. This is true both for patients with relapsing MS as well as in the case of patients with progressive MS, in which inflammation is still present until the end and degenerative processes [55, 59].

In the case of other demyelinating diseases such as NMO, the need for neuroprotection is also present but for different reasons [63]. In NMO there is no evidence of progressive course of the disease or presence of chronic trapped inflammation in the CNS. For this reason, all CNS damage and clinical disability observed in NMO is attributed to the damage induced during acute relapses, which are significantly more tissue destructive than in MS [64]. The necrotic characteristic of the NMO lesions has parallelism with stroke-induced damage, a prototypic model for neuroprotection in which is critical preventing severe CNS damage in order to reduce disability. The good news is that the inflammatory-induced damage in NMO may operate over longer periods of time than brain ischemia, providing a wider therapeutic window for intervention (from minutes to days). Recurrent Idiopatic Optic Neuritis, Relapsing Optic Neuritis or Transverse Myelitis are also other less common types of demyelinating diseases that would follow the NMO paradigm for neuroprotection, decreasing CNS damage due to relapses.

Neuroprotective therapies under development for MS and other demyelinating diseases

Neuroprotection is a well-accepted concept in the therapeutic strategy of neurologists, but in order to be useful at the clinical level, efficacy must be demonstrated in randomized clinical trials [65, 66]. At present there is a growing list of new drugs and repurposing of drugs being tested from phase 1 to phase 3 trials (Table 2). One of the most active areas of research are remyelinating therapies, which can be categorized either as regenerative therapy (aimed to restore myelin) or neuroprotective therapy (aimed to protect axons and restore nerve conduction) [67]. A recent trial testing the mAb blocking Lingo-1 (BIIB033) has shown improvement in the latencies of the visual evoked potentials in patients with optic neuritis, suggesting an improvement of nerve conduction typically associated with remyelination (NCT01721161). Another mAb promoting remyelination is rHIgM22, which was discovered as part of the natural antibody repertoire in

humans with remyelinating potential [68] and it is now being tested in clinical trials in MS patients (NCT01803867, NCT02398461). Regarding small chemicals, two approved drugs that are being explored for their effect on remyelination are clemastine and guanabenz after having shown a remyelinating effect in vitro and animal models [69].

Other strategies in clinical phases include the use of trophic factor compounds (eritropoietin, BN201), antioxidant compounds (the green tea extract epigallocatechin-3-gallate, ginkgo biloba extracts, biotin, dimethyl-fumarate, olexosime), modulating estrogen receptors, metabolites (dimethyl-fumarate, methyltioadenosine), blocking semaphorins (VX15/2503), and ion channels modulators (carbamacepin, phenytoin, lamotrigin, amiloride, riluzole) (Table 2) [21, 70]. All these drugs still need to show their efficacy in phase 3 trials and then define how they would be integrated in the MS armamentarium, probably as a combination therapy with immunomodulators for relapsing MS or perhaps in combination with different agents for progressive MS.

In addition to drugs being tested as neuroprotectants, we must also consider stem cells as another approach to neuroprotection in MS [71]. At present, the most tested stem cells are mesenchymal stem cells, which have shown immunomodulatory and neuroprotective properties in vitro and in animal models [72]. Recent trials in patients with relapsing and progressive MS have shown some beneficial effects in terms of decreasing relapse rate or disability [73–75], but without clarifying whether these effects are due to its immunomodulatory or neuroprotective effects. A large multicentric randomized trial (MESEMS trial; NCT02403947) is ongoing to evaluate its efficacy in MS. In addition, phase 1 and 2 trials are ongoing or being planned to test the efficacy of other stem cells such as oligodendrocyte or olfactory ensheeting glial cells and probably neural cells in the near future.

Challenges for developing neuroprotective therapies

Lack of approved neuroprotective drugs is due to both poor understanding of the mechanisms of damage and the low recovery ability of the CNS (as discussed above) as well as the limitations of clinical trials for probing the efficacy of such drugs. First, probing the efficacy of a neuroprotective drug requires selecting the right indication, stage of the disease and group of patients in which such intervention can translate to a biological benefit as well as to a clinical benefit. For example, treating patients in the very late stages of the disease, when damage of the CNS is very severe and few neurons and axons can be rescued, may not translate to clinical benefits. This late diagnosis is one of the greatest limitations to date in other neurodegenerative diseases such as Alzheimer or Parkinson disease and probably in progressive MS.

Second, pharmacological properties of the drug should be good enough to be sure to deliver the signal in the right site of the CNS and with enough intensity to obtain positive outcomes. This is one of the limitations of mAb, stem cells and some other drugs. Also, dose selection and defining the therapeutic window based in efficacy-toxicity balance as well as in the timing of the intervention from the onset of damage is critical as well. Previous studies with recombinant trophic factors may have failed because poor pharmacokinetic properties as well as toxicity of the recombinant proteins prevented the use of efficacious doses [27]. Also, we must keep in mind that patients with MS are young and the disease evolves slowly over years, and for this reason MS patients are not likely to accept the risk of side-effects.

Third, biomarkers are envisioned as a key strategy for moving new drugs from preclinical stages to phase 1 and 2 trials, helping to select the best therapeutic regimen and dose, identify the best patient subgroups to be tested (avoiding non-responders) and match surrogate with clinical endpoints in order to optimize trials results [76]. Also, systems medicine is going to help in the integration of biological and clinical knowledge in a more comprehensive understanding of the disease and patients' heterogeneity, which will pay off by improving our accuracy for transition from preclinical to clinical stages of drug development [77, 78].

Finally, in order to probe efficacy of neuroprotective drugs in clinical trials, we need sensitive surrogate and clinical endpoints for the mechanism of action and the level of damage. Again, this is critical because many drugs may have failed not due to a lack of efficacy, but because the incapacity to measure such effects with the proposed end-points. The most common proposed surrogate endpoints is imaging. In the case of MRI, the most validated marker for MS is presence of new lesions (either contrast enhancing lesions or new lesions in T2), but this marker is useful for immunomodulatory drugs, not for neuroprotective drugs. Alternatively, brain atrophy is the best correlate of disability in MS, but brain atrophy is difficult to measure requiring advanced imaging methods, prone to high variability between scanners and techniques and with low sensitivity to changes [79]. For this reason, other approaches such as optical coherence tomography offer the opportunity to quantify with high accuracy retina atrophy [80] and is now being added to phase 2 and 3 clinical trials [81]. Regarding clinical endpoints, clinical scales such as the Expanded Disability Status Scale (EDSS) are complex, with high variability and subjectivity and with low sensitivity to meaningful clinical changes associated with neuroprotection. For this reason, several new clinical outcomes such as low contrast visual acuity [82] or activity levels measured with accelerometers [83] are promising avenues for evaluating neuroprotective drugs.

Conclusions

Relapsing MS and other demyelinating diseases have benefited significantly from the advancements of new immunomodulatory therapies, but the challenge of protecting CNS from damage remains one of the top priorities for all demyelinating diseases as well as neurodegenerative diseases or acute brain damage by trauma or stroke. Novel discoveries in neurobiology provide new therapeutic targets, and new imaging modalities provide the opportunity to evaluate the efficacy of these new neuroprotective drugs. Because several of the mechanisms being targeted by neuroprotective therapies are common between diseases, some of the biomarkers and therapeutics strategies may be useful for different type of diseases, although medicine use to tell us that any single therapeutic approach fitting all CNS diseases is highly unlikely.

We will hopefully soon have effective neuroprotective therapies ready to use in patients, which combined with immunomodulatory drugs, will help to prevent CNS damage, decrease neurological disability and improve MS patients' quality of life. Although several therapeutic regimens can be proposed, neuroprotective therapy is envisioned as combination therapy with other disease modifying drugs targeting the pathogenic cascade, such as immunomodulatory therapy in MS. Neuroprotective therapies should be started early in the course of the disease, because axonal damage start to accumulate from the beginning of the disease. And such therapies may extent for the whole life and for almost all types of disease, from clinically isolated syndromes to progressive MS. In addition to the use of neuroprotective therapies for preventing chronic damage in MS, these therapies would be used for acute neuroprotection at the time patients suffer an acute relapse of MS, NMO or Optic Neuritis. However, we need to learn which neuroprotective therapy is more required for each subgroup of patients to be more effective. To this aim, it is required development of biomarkers of CNS damage processes, to be used to select the right drugs at each stage of the disease process. This may also help to identify MS subtypes with different involvement of CNS damage mechanisms operating at a given time. Such subtypes may overlap with MS pathological subtypes or with genetic risks, which is unknown at present. Tailoring combination therapy with immunotherapies using biomarkers would be one of the next challenges for MS therapeutics in the medium term that hopefully is going to improve the quality of life of people with MS.

Abbreviations

ALS: amiotrophic lateral sclerosis; ATP: adenosin tri-phosphate; BDNF: brain derived nerve factor; CNS: central nervous system; EDSS: expanded disability status scale; GSK3: glycogen synthase kinase 3; IKK: inhibitor of kappa B kinase; JNK: c-Jun N-terminal kinases; Lingo-1: leucine rich repeat and immunoglobin-like domain-containing protein 1; mAb: monoclonal antibody; MAPKK: mitogen-activated protein kinase kinase; Nerf2: nuclear factor (erythroid-derived 2)-like 2; NMDA: N-methyl-D-aspartate; MS: multiple sclerosis; NMO: neuromyelitis optica; NO: nitric oxide; MRI: magnetic resonance imaging; NAA: N-Acetyl- Aspartate; NAD: nicotinamide adenine dinucleotide; NFKB: nuclear factor-κB; Nogo-A: neurite outgrowth inhibitor A; NMNAT2: nicotinamide nucleotide adenylyltransferase 2; PC: phosphatidilcholine; PI3K: phosphoinositide 3-kinase; PHR1: phosphate starvation response 1; Sarm1: Sterile Alpha And TIR Motif Containing 1.

Competing interests

PV has received consultancy fees from Roche, Novartis and Digna Biotech. He is founder and advisor of Bionure Inc. and holds patent rights for the use of Methylthioadenosine and BN201 for the treatment of MS and other neurological diseases.

Acknowledgement

I would like to thanks Erika Lampert for the English review of the manuscript. This work was supported by the Instituto de Salud Carlos III, Spain (FIS: PI12/01823) to PV.

References

1. Hagmann P, Sporns O, Madan N, Cammoun L, Pienaar R, Wedeen VJ, et al. White matter maturation reshapes structural connectivity in the late developing human brain. Proc Natl Acad Sci U S A. 2010;107(44):19067–72.
2. Nave KA, Werner HB. Myelination of the nervous system: mechanisms and functions. Annu Rev Cell Dev Biol. 2014;30:503–33.
3. Franklin RJ, ffrench-Constant C, Edgar JM, Smith KJ. Neuroprotection and repair in multiple sclerosis. Nat Rev Neurol. 2012;8(11):624–34.
4. Court FA, Coleman MP. Mitochondria as a central sensor for axonal degenerative stimuli. Trends Neurosci. 2012;35(6):364–72.
5. Lassmann H. Axonal and neuronal pathology in multiple sclerosis: what have we learnt from animal models. Exp Neurol. 2010;225(1):2–8.
6. Harris JJ, Attwell D. The energetics of CNS white matter. J Neurosci. 2012;32(1):356–71.
7. Conforti L, Gilley J, Coleman MP. Wallerian degeneration: an emerging axon death pathway linking injury and disease. Nat Rev Neurosci. 2014;15(6):394–409.
8. Adalbert R, Coleman MP. Review: Axon pathology in age-related neurodegenerative disorders. Neuropathol Appl Neurobiol. 2013;39(2):90–108.
9. Nave KA. Myelination and support of axonal integrity by glia. Nature. 2010;468(7321):244–52.
10. Jurgens T, Jafari M, Kreutzfeldt M, Bahn E, Bruck W, Kerschensteiner M, et al. Reconstruction of single cortical projection neurons reveals primary spine loss in multiple sclerosis. Brain. 2015.;139(Pt 1):39–46
11. Lipton SA. Pathologically activated therapeutics for neuroprotection. Nat Rev Neurosci. 2007;8(10):803–8.
12. Giunti D, Parodi B, Cordano C, Uccelli A, Kerlero de Rosbo N. Can we switch microglia's phenotype to foster neuroprotection? Focus on multiple sclerosis. Immunology. 2014;141(3):328–39.
13. Colombo E, Di Dario M, Capitolo E, Chaabane L, Newcombe J, Martino G, et al. Fingolimod may support neuroprotection via blockade of astrocyte nitric oxide. Ann Neurol. 2014;76(3):325–37.
14. Reick C, Ellrichmann G, Thone J, Scannevin RH, Saft C, Linker RA, et al. Neuroprotective dimethyl fumarate synergizes with immunomodulatory interferon beta to provide enhanced axon protection in autoimmune neuroinflammation. Exp Neurol. 2014;257:50–6.
15. Ruffini F, Rossi S, Bergamaschi A, Brambilla E, Finardi A, Motta C, et al. Laquinimod prevents inflammation-induced synaptic alterations occurring in experimental autoimmune encephalomyelitis. Mult Scler. 2013;19(8):1084–94.
16. Aharoni R. Immunomodulation neuroprotection and remyelination - the fundamental therapeutic effects of glatiramer acetate: a critical review. J Autoimmun. 2014;54:81–92.
17. Loeb JA. Neuroprotection and repair by neurotrophic and gliotrophic factors in multiple sclerosis. Neurology. 2007;68(22 Suppl 3):S38–42. discussion S3-54.
18. Villoslada P, Genain CP. Role of nerve growth factor and other trophic factors in brain inflammation. Prog Brain Res. 2004;146:403–14.
19. Segal RA. Selectivity in neurotrophin signaling: theme and variations. Annu Rev Neurosci. 2003;26:299–330.
20. Villoslada P, Hauser SL, Bartke I, Unger J, Heald N, Rosenberg D, et al. Human nerve growth factor protects common marmosets against autoimmune encephalomyelitis by switching the balance of T helper cell type 1 and 2 cytokines within the central nervous system. J Exp Med. 2000;191(10):1799–806.
21. Colafrancesco V, Villoslada P. Targeting NGF pathway for developing neuroprotective therapies for multiple sclerosis and other neurological diseases. Arch Ital Biol. 2011;149(2):183–92.
22. The BDNF Study Group (Phase III). A controlled trial of recombinant methionyl human BDNF in ALS: Neurology. 1999;52(7):1427–33.
23. ALS CNTF Treatment Study Group. A double-blind placebo-controlled clinical trial of subcutaneous recombinant human ciliary neurotrophic factor (rHCNTF) in amyotrophic lateral sclerosis. Neurology. 1996;46(5):1244–9.
24. Sorenson EJ, Windbank AJ, Mandrekar JN, Bamlet WR, Appel SH, Armon C, et al. Subcutaneous IGF-1 is not beneficial in 2-year ALS trial. Neurology. 2008;71(22):1770–5.
25. Tuszynski MH, Thal L, Pay M, Salmon DP, U HS, Bakay R, et al. A phase 1 clinical trial of nerve growth factor gene therapy for Alzheimer disease. Nat Med. 2005;11(5):551–5.
26. Cudkowicz ME, Katz J, Moore DH, O'Neill G, Glass JD, Mitsumoto H, et al. Toward more efficient clinical trials for amyotrophic lateral sclerosis. Amyotroph Lateral Scler. 2010;11(3):259–65.
27. Apfel SC. Nerve growth factor for the treatment of diabetic neuropathy: what went wrong, what went right, and what does the future hold? Int Rev Neurobiol. 2002;50:393–413.
28. Beal MF. Mitochondria take center stage in aging and neurodegeneration. Ann Neurol. 2005;58(4):495–505.
29. Schapira AH, Olanow CW, Greenamyre JT, Bezard E. Slowing of neurodegeneration in Parkinson's disease and Huntington's disease: future therapeutic perspectives. Lancet. 2014;384(9942):545–55.
30. Tiwari SK, Chaturvedi RK. Peptide therapeutics in neurodegenerative disorders. Curr Med Chem. 2014;21(23):2610–31.
31. Ries V, Oertel WH, Hoglinger GU. Mitochondrial dysfunction as a therapeutic target in progressive supranuclear palsy. J Mol Neurosci. 2011;45(3):684–9.
32. Errea O, B M, Gonzalez-Franquesa A, Garcia-Roves P, Villoslada P. The disruption of mitochondrial axonal transport is an early event in neuroinflammation. J Neuroinflammation. 2015;12:152–167.
33. Waxman SG. Axonal conduction and injury in multiple sclerosis: the role of sodium channels. Nat Rev Neurosci. 2006;7(12):932–41.
34. Waxman SG. Mechanisms of disease: sodium channels and neuroprotection in multiple sclerosis-current status. Nat Clin Pract Neurol. 2008;4(3):159–69.
35. Sureda FX, Junyent F, Verdaguer E, Auladell C, Pelegri C, Vilaplana J, et al. Antiapoptotic drugs: a therapautic strategy for the prevention of neurodegenerative diseases. Curr Pharm Des. 2011;17(3):230–45.
36. Lassmann H. Multiple sclerosis: Lessons from molecular neuropathology. Exp Neurol. 2014;262PA:2–7.
37. Haider L, Fischer MT, Frischer JM, Bauer J, Hoftberger R, Botond G, et al. Oxidative damage in multiple sclerosis lesions. Brain. 2011;134(Pt 7):1914–24.
38. Niedzielska E, Smaga I, Gawlik M, Moniczewski A, Stankowicz P, Pera J, et al. Oxidative Stress in Neurodegenerative Diseases. Mol Neurobiol. 2015. in press.
39. Linker RA, Lee DH, Ryan S, van Dam AM, Conrad R, Bista P, et al. Fumaric acid esters exert neuroprotective effects in neuroinflammation via activation of the Nrf2 antioxidant pathway. Brain. 2011;134(Pt 3):678–92.
40. Lanza C, Morando S, Voci A, Canesi L, Principato MC, Serpero LD, et al. Neuroprotective mesenchymal stem cells are endowed with a potent antioxidant effect in vivo. J Neurochem. 2009;110(5):1674–84.
41. Fern RF, Matute C, Stys PK. White matter injury: Ischemic and nonischemic. Glia. 2014;62(11):1780–9.
42. Kostic M, Zivkovic N, Stojanovic I. Multiple sclerosis and glutamate excitotoxicity. Rev Neurosci. 2013;24(1):71–88.
43. Mitsumoto H. Riluzole-what is its impact in our treatment and understanding of amyotrophic lateral sclerosis? Ann Pharmacother. 1997;31(6):779–81.
44. Lipton SA. Paradigm shift in neuroprotection by NMDA receptor blockade: Memantine and beyond. Nat Rev Drug Discov. 2006;1–11.
45. Villoslada P, Arrondo G, Sepulcre J, Alegre M, Artieda J. Memantine induces reversible neurologic impairment in patients with MS. Neurology. 2008;72(19):1630–3.
46. Green AJ. Understanding pseudo: the symptoms are real, the cause is unclear. Neurology. 2009;72(19):1626–7.

47. Nave KA, Trapp BD. Axon-glial signaling and the glial support of axon function. Annu Rev Neurosci. 2008;31:535–61.

48. DeLuca GC, Williams K, Evangelou N, Ebers GC, Esiri MM. The contribution of demyelination to axonal loss in multiple sclerosis. Brain. 2006;129(Pt 6):1507–16.

49. van den Elskamp IJ, Knol DL, Vrenken H, Karas G, Meijerman A, Filippi M, et al. Lesional magnetization transfer ratio: a feasible outcome for remyelinating treatment trials in multiple sclerosis. Mult Scler. 2010;16(6):660–9.

50. De Vos KJ, Grierson AJ, Ackerley S, Miller CC. Role of axonal transport in neurodegenerative diseases. Annu Rev Neurosci. 2008;31:151–73.

51. Sorbara CD, Wagner NE, Ladwig A, Nikic I, Merkler D, Kleele T, et al. Pervasive axonal transport deficits in multiple sclerosis models. Neuron. 2014;84(6):1183–90.

52. Ruschel J, Hellal F, Flynn KC, Dupraz S, Elliott DA, Tedeschi A, et al. Axonal regeneration. Systemic administration of epothilone B promotes axon regeneration after spinal cord injury. Science. 2015;348(6232):347–52.

53. Kim S, Chang R, Teunissen C, Gebremichael Y, Petzold A. Neurofilament stoichiometry simulations during neurodegeneration suggest a remarkable self-sufficient and stable in vivo protein structure. J Neurol Sci. 2011;307(1–2):132–8.

54. Llorens F, Gil V, del Rio JA. Emerging functions of myelin-associated proteins during development, neuronal plasticity, and neurodegeneration. FASEB J. 2011;25(2):463–75.

55. Rottlaender A, Kuerten S. Stepchild or Prodigy? Neuroprotection in Multiple Sclerosis (MS) Research. Int J Mol Sci. 2015;16(7):14850–65.

56. Hernangomez M, Mestre L, Correa FG, Loria F, Mecha M, Inigo PM, et al. CD200-CD200R1 interaction contributes to neuroprotective effects of anandamide on experimentally induced inflammation. Glia. 2012;60(9):1437–50.

57. Vecino E, Rodriguez FD, Ruzafa N, Pereiro X, Sharma S. Glia-neuron interactions in the mammalian retina. Prog Retin Eye Res. 2015;51:1–40.

58. Ransohoff RM, Hafler DA, Lucchinetti CF. Multiple sclerosis-a quiet revolution. Nat Rev Neurol. 2015;11(3):134–42.

59. Mahad DH, Trapp BD, Lassmann H. Pathological mechanisms in progressive multiple sclerosis. Lancet Neurol. 2015;14(2):183–93.

60. Lassmann H. Pathology and disease mechanisms in different stages of multiple sclerosis. J Neurol Sci. 2013;333(1–2):1–4.

61. Piaton G, Gould RM, Lubetzki C. Axon-oligodendrocyte interactions during developmental myelination, demyelination and repair. J Neurochem. 2010;114(5):1243–60.

62. Mullard A. Success of immunomodulators in MS shifts discovery focus to neuroprotection. Nat Rev Drug Discov. 2011;10(12):885–7.

63. Weinshenker BG, Barron G, Behne JM, Bennett JL, Chin PS, Cree BA, et al. Challenges and opportunities in designing clinical trials for neuromyelitis optica. Neurology. 2015;84(17):1805–15.

64. Pittock SJ, Lucchinetti CF. Neuromyelitis optica and the evolving spectrum of autoimmune aquaporin-4 channelopathies: a decade later. Ann N Y Acad Sci. 2015.in press.

65. Maghzi AH, Minagar A, Waubant E. Neuroprotection in multiple sclerosis: a therapeutic approach. CNS Drugs. 2013;27(10):799–815.

66. Aktas O, Kieseier B, Hartung HP. Neuroprotection, regeneration and immunomodulation: broadening the therapeutic repertoire in multiple sclerosis. Trends Neurosci. 2010;33(3):140–52.

67. Luessi F, Kuhlmann T, Zipp F. Remyelinating strategies in multiple sclerosis. Expert Rev Neurother. 2014;14(11):1315–34.

68. Mitsunaga Y, Ciric B, Van Keulen V, Warrington AE, Paz Soldan M, Bieber AJ, et al. Direct evidence that a human antibody derived from patient serum can promote myelin repair in a mouse model of chronic-progressive demyelinating disease. FASEB J. 2002;16(10):1325–7.

69. Mei F, Fancy SP, Shen YA, Niu J, Zhao C, Presley B, et al. Micropillar arrays as a high-throughput screening platform for therapeutics in multiple sclerosis. Nat Med. 2014;20(8):954–60.

70. Raftopoulos RE, Kapoor R. Neuroprotection for acute optic neuritis-Can it work? Mult Scler Relat Disord. 2013;2(4):307–11.

71. Payne N, Siatskas C, Barnard A, Bernard CC. The prospect of stem cells as multi-faceted purveyors of immune modulation, repair and regeneration in multiple sclerosis. Curr Stem Cell Res Ther. 2011;6(1):50–62.

72. Uccelli A, Moretta L, Pistoia V. Mesenchymal stem cells in health and disease. Nat Rev Immunol. 2008;8(9):726–36.

73. Llufriu S, Sepulveda M, Blanco Y, Marin P, Moreno B, Berenguer J, et al. Randomized placebo-controlled phase II trial of autologous mesenchymal stem cells in multiple sclerosis. PLoS One. 2014;9(12), e113936.

74. Connick P, Kolappan M, Crawley C, Webber DJ, Patani R, Michell AW, et al. Autologous mesenchymal stem cells for the treatment of secondary progressive multiple sclerosis: an open-label phase 2a proof-of-concept study. Lancet Neurol. 2012;11(2):150–6.

75. Karussis D, Karageorgiou C, Vaknin-Dembinsky A, Gowda-Kurkalli B, Gomori JM, Kassis I, et al. Safety and immunological effects of mesenchymal stem cell transplantation in patients with multiple sclerosis and amyotrophic lateral sclerosis. Arch Neurol. 2010;67(10):1187–94.

76. Villoslada P. Biomarkers for multiple sclerosis. Drug News Perspect. 2010;23(9):585–95.

77. Villoslada P, Steinman L, Baranzini SE. Systems biology and its application to the understanding of neurological diseases. Ann Neurol. 2009;65(2):124–39.

78. Villoslada P, Baranzini S. Data integration and systems biology approaches for biomarker discovery: Challenges and opportunities for multiple sclerosis. J Neuroimmunol. 2012;248(1–2):58–65.

79. Barkhof F, Calabresi PA, Miller DH, Reingold SC. Imaging outcomes for neuroprotection and repair in multiple sclerosis trials. Nat Rev Neurol. 2009;5(5):256–66.

80. Martinez-Lapiscina E, Sanchez-Dalmau B, Fraga-Pumar E, Ortiz-Perez S, Tercero-Uribe A, Torres-Torres R, et al. The visual pathway as a model to understand brain damage in multiple sclerosis. Mult Scler. 2014;20(13):1678–85.

81. Zarbin MA, Jampol LM, Jager RD, Reder AT, Francis G, Collins W, et al. Ophthalmic evaluations in clinical studies of fingolimod (FTY720) in multiple sclerosis. Ophthalmology. 2013;120(7):1432–9.

82. Balcer LJ. Clinical trials to clinical use: using vision as a model for multiple sclerosis and beyond. J Neuroophthalmol. 2014;34(Suppl):S18–23.

83. Sola-Valls N, Blanco Y, Sepulveda M, Llufriu S, Martinez-Lapiscina EH, La Puma D, et al. Walking function in clinical monitoring of multiple sclerosis by telemedicine. J Neurol. 2015;262(7):1706–13.

Methylthioadenosine promotes remyelination by inducing oligodendrocyte differentiation

Beatriz Moreno[1,2], Gemma Vila[1], Begoña Fernandez-Diez[1], Raquel Vázquez[1], Alessandra di Penta[1,3], Oihana Errea[1], Nagore Escala[1], Andrés Miguez[4], Jordi Alberch[4] and Pablo Villoslada[1,5,6*] (iD)

Abstract

Background: Methylthioadenosine is a metabolite of the polyamine pathway that modulates methyltransferase activity, thereby influencing DNA and protein methylation. Since methylthioadenosine produces neuroprotection in models of inflammation, ischemia and epilepsy, we set out to evaluate the role of methylthioadenosine in promoting remyelination, a process that will protect axons in demyelinating diseases and that will aid functional recovery.

Methods: The effect of methylthioadenosine in promoting remyelination was tested in mouse cerebellum organotypic cultures that were exposed to lipopolysaccharide to induce neuroinflammation, or lysolecithin to induce chemical demyelination. In addition methylthioadenosine administration was also tested in vivo, using the cuprizone model of demyelination. The molecular pathways involved in this methylthioadenosine activity were evaluated in primary cortical mouse astrocytes.

Results: In models of neuroinflammation or chemical demyelination, methylthioadenosine prevented the loss of myelin and promoted remyelination in vitro by increasing the number of mature myelinating oligodendrocytes. Methylthioadenosine enhanced myelin production in the cuprizone model, in conjunction with a clinical improvement. Methylthioadenosine enhanced STAT-3 phosphorylation in astrocytes in vitro, and the production of ciliary neurotrophic factor (CNTF), a trophic factor known to promote oligodendrocyte maturation and differentiation, as well as remyelination.

Conclusions: The remyelination promoted by methylthioadenosine suggests a role for the polyamine pathway in oligodendrocyte maturation and survival, paving the way for new therapeutic strategies to promote regeneration in Multiple Sclerosis and other demyelinating diseases.

Keywords: Methylthioadenosine, Remyelination, Oligodendrocyte, Neuroprotection, Multiple sclerosis, Demyelinating diseases, Therapy

Background

Multiple Sclerosis (MS) is an autoimmune disease characterized by Central Nervous System (CNS) demyelination, oligodendrocyte damage and axonal loss [1]. Current treatments have focused on preventing inflammation and they have limited efficacy on the progressive phase. Remyelination is considered to be a promising way to protect neurons and restore functionality, a therapeutic strategy for MS that

is being actively pursued [2, 3]. The myelin-axon unit is critical to maintain the trophism of long axons, and for the exchange of metabolites and macromolecules like lactate, N-acetyl Aspartate or lipids [4]. This metabolic relationship further reinforces the attractiveness of remyelination as a therapeutic strategy to preventing axon loss in the later stages of the disease [5]. Yet even if remyelination would have been efficient in the early stages of MS its effects might be limited in the long term, particularly given the resistance of adult oligodendrocyte precursor cells (OPCs) to differentiate into myelinating oligodendrocytes (OLs) [6] and the molecular changes in demyelinated axons that lead to the rejection of myelin (e.g. PSA-NCAM re-expression) [7].

---

* Correspondence: pvilloslada@clinic.ub.es; Pablo.VillosladaDiaz@ucsf.edu
[1]Center of Neuroimmunology, Institut d'Investigacions Biomediques August
Pi Sunyer (IDIBAPS), Barcelona, Spain
[5]University of California, San Francisco, USA
Full list of author information is available at the end of the article

Methylthioadenosine is a natural metabolite of the polyamine pathway and it serves many functions in cell metabolism: driving the regeneration of adenosine and methionine stocks; modulating gene expression (e.g. activating serine-threonine phosphatase 1 that leads to the dephosphorylation of SR proteins), proliferation, differentiation and apoptosis; or inhibiting protein and DNA methylation by competing with S-adenosylmethionine for methyltransferases [8, 9]. Methylthioadenosine is a selective inhibitor of protein arginine methyltransferase 5 (PRMT5) activity [10, 11], which in turn dampens cRAF methylation and degradation; this cRAF being responsible for increasing MEK1-2 and STAT3 phosphorylation [12]. Methylthioadenosine also exhibits immunomodulatory activity by suppressing the production of pro-inflammatory cytokines and enhancing the production of anti-inflammatory cytokines through an interaction with the nuclear factor kappa B (NFkB) pathway. Interestingly, such activity produces benefits in models of autoimmune diseases like MS [13, 14]. Finally, methylthioadenosine displays neuroprotective activity, preventing neuronal damage in models of ischemia, epilepsy and Parkinson's disease [15].

In light of these protective effects of methylthioadenosine, we set out to evaluate the role of methylthioadenosine in promoting OPC maturation and OL myelination in vitro and in vivo using different models of demyelination. We found that this metabolite increases the number of mature myelinating OLs. Thus, methylthioadenosine may prove to be beneficial as a therapeutic agent to manage demyelinating diseases.

Methods

In vivo studies

Animals

All animals handling was carried out in accordance with the European Council Directive (2010/63/EU) and the Spanish regulations for the procurement and care of experimental animals (1201 RD/2005, October 10). The animal protocols used were approved by the Ethical Committee on Animal Research at the University of Barcelona.

Treatments

Methylthioadenosine (Sigma) was dissolved in phosphate buffered saline (PBS) at a concentration of 12 mg/ml and mice received a daily intraperitoneal (i.p.) injection at a dose of 60mg/kg. Placebo animals were injected daily with PBS alone i.p.

Cuprizone demyelinating mouse model

We fed 2-month-old C57BL/6J mice of either sex with 0.2% (wt/wt) cuprizone (Sigma Aldrich) for 4, 5 or 6 weeks (Additional file 1: Figure S1). The animals were then allowed to recover for 7, 8 or 9 weeks before methylthioadenosine (60mg/kg) or the placebo were injected daily (ip) as preventive or curative treatments. Methylthioadenosine dose was selected from previous animal studies in experimental autoimmune encephalomyelitis [14].

Sensory motor behavior testing

Animals were trained in the rotarod using constant speed (18rpm) 3x per day during 8 days with a rest of 5 min between each trial. Animals were tested during the remyelination phase after cuprizone treatment twice a week.

In vitro studies

Primary cortical mouse astrocytes

Cortical astrocytes were obtained from P3 C57BL6 wild-type mouse pups (of either sex) after dissection of the cortex and removal of the meninges. The tissue obtained was dissociated, plated in 75 cm^2 flasks in NM-15 conditioned medium (MEM 1X, Gibco; 15% fetal bovine serum –FBS-, Gibco; 90 mM D-glucose, Sigma) and maintained in an incubator at 37°C in an atmosphere of 5% CO_2. After 5 days in vitro (DIV), the cells were purified by agitating in an orbital shaker for 16–18h at 250 rpm, discarding the detached cells and incubating the adherent cells for a further two DIV in fresh medium. Astroglial cells were replated into 6-well plates and cultured to confluence. Prior to performing the experiments, NM-15 medium was replaced with DMEM/F12 (Gibco) serum free medium and the cells were left for 48 h. The cells were then treated with Lipopolysaccharide (LPS) (10 µg/ml, L4391; Sigma) overnight and methylthioadenosine (192µM) or placebo was added the following day for the ELISA and PCR studies (24 h), or it was maintained over the next 5 days for xMAP phosphorylation assays (samples collected 15, 30 min or 1 h after the last treatment was added).

Cerebellar organotypic mouse cultures

Cerebellar organotypic cultures were established as described previously [16]. Parasagittal slices (300 µm) of the postnatal day 7 (P7) C57BL/6 mouse cerebellum (of either sex) were obtained with a tissue slicer (McIIwain), the slices were placed in medium on collagen-coated Millicell-CM culture semiporous inserts (0.4 µm; Millipore, Bedford, MA, USA) and they were kept for up to 3 weeks in an atmosphere of 5% CO_2 at 37°C in 50% basal medium containing: Earle's salts (GIBCO), 25% Hank's balanced salt solution (GIBCO), 25% heat inactivated horse serum, 5 mg/ml glucose, 0.25 mM L-glutamine, and 25 µg/ml penicillin/streptomycin. To induce neuro-inflammation, LPS (15 µg/ml, L4391; Sigma) was added to the organotypic cultures 7 days after preparing the inserts. Methylthioadenosine or a placebo were added 24 h before LPS and the samples were collected 24 h after LPS addition for Myelin Basic Protein (MBP) and Neurofilament (NFL) staining, and 0, 1, 3, 6, 12, 24, 48, 72 and 96 h after the addition of LPS for IL-1β, TNF-α, iNOS and CNPase detection. For chemical demyelination, lysolecithin (0.5 mg/ml, L4129; Sigma) was added 7 days after insert preparation and the cultures were incubated overnight (14 h.) at 37°C. Subsequently, the medium containing lysolecithin was replaced with fresh medium and methylthioadenosine or saline were added the next day and every 2 days thereafter until the tissue was analyzed after 9, 13, 17 and 21 DIV. All control cultures analyzed were time matched with the treated cultures and LLL12 (partial and reversible inhibitor of STAT3 phosphorylation, Ref: 1792–5 Deltaclon) was used at 2.5 μM and 5 μM.

Western blotting

Expression of inducible nitric oxide synthase (iNOS) and 2′,3′-cyclic-nucleotide 3′-phosphodiesterase (CNPase) was assessed in Western blots of mouse cerebellum organotypic slices pre-treated with methylthioadenosine (48 μM or 192 μM) or the placebo, and stimulated with LPS (15 μg/ml) at different time points (0, 1, 3, 6, 12, 24, 48, 72 and 96 h), as described previously [16]. The Western blots were probed with a mouse antibody against CNPase (Abcam) and a rabbit antibody against iNOS (BD Bioscience).

Enzyme-linked immunosorbent assay (ELISA)

Cerebellar organotypic cultures were pre-treated with methylthioadenosine (48 μM or 192 μM) or a placebo at seven DIV and they were then stimulated with LPS (15 μg/ml) at different time points (0, 1, 3, 6, 12, 24, 48, 72 and 96 h). The culture supernatants were collected to quantify interleukin 1β (IL-1β), tumor necrosis factor (TNF-α) and CNTF using mouse enzyme-linked immunosorbent assay (ELISA) kits according to the manufacturer's instructions (eBioscience, San Diego, CA, USA).

Immunostaining

Immunostaining was performed as previously published [16]. After fixation with 4% paraformaldehyde, cerebellar slices were removed gently from the inserts and they were blocked for 2–4 h at room temperature in PBS + 10% goat serum + 1% bovine serum albumin (BSA) + 0.2% Triton X-100. The sections were incubated overnight at 4°C with the primary and secondary antibodies diluted in PBS + 1% goat serum + 1% BSA + 0.2% Triton X-100. After each overnight incubation, the slices were washed at room temperature three times in PBS + 0.05% Triton X-100, each wash lasting 1 h. Finally, the slices were mounted on slides, coverslipped and analyzed on a confocal microscope (LSM 510; Zeiss). Primary

antibodies against the following proteins were used for immunostaining: myelin basic protein (MBP, Rat anti-MBP 82–87 antibody; Serotec), Neurofilament light (NF-L, anti-NF-L C28E10; Cell Signaling), glial fibrillary acidic protein (GFAP, rabbit anti-GFAP; DakoCytomation), oligodendrocyte transcription factor 2 (Olig 2, rabbit anti-Olig 2; Santa Cruz Biotechnology) and CNTF (rabbit polyclonal anti-CNTF; Abcam). The secondary antibodies used were: Cy2-linked mouse immunoglobulin G (IgG), Cy3-linked rabbit IgG (from goat, 1:200; GE Healthcare, Freiburg, Germany) and Fluor 488 Goat anti-Rat IgG Alexa (1:200; Molecular Probes, Eugene, OR, USA).

Image analysis

A confocal microscope (Laser Scanning Confocal Microscope Leica SP2) was used to obtain stacks of photographs of MBP and NFH immunolabelling at 1 μm intervals in the organotypic cultures × 40 magnification. Slices thinned after culture to approximately 30μm thickness (depending on the number of days in culture). Myelinated fibers are best observed between a depth of 5 to 20 μm from the upper surface and this is the reason why our results were taken from this level. Myelinated neurofilaments were quantified as the percentage of axons stained with NfL with MBP surrounding sheaths respect to the total number of axons (without MBP sheaths).

Percentage of the area immunoreactive for Olig2 or MBP antibodies was measured in × 40 magnification images acquired by confocal microscopy. The range of the slice was determined using Z-stack imaging at 1-μm intervals and a series of images derived from Z-stack imaging were analyzed. Briefly, binary masks were defined using the same cut-off intensity threshold value for each region of interest, which corresponds to each cell immunostained, defined as the minimum intensity because of specific staining above background values. Then, the percentage of the area occupied by Olig2 or MBP was measured automatically using ImageJ software in each cerebellum organotypic tissue. Results are given by averaging values determined in at least four separate microscopic fields from six different slices. MBP immunoreactivity of the brain stained sections was quantified after obtaining the integrated densities of the midline corpus callosum from the different animals ($n = 6$ per group).

Electron microscopy

Cerebellar slices were fixed for 24 h in 2% paraformaldehyde and 2.5% glutaraldehyde in 0.1 M PBS at 4°C, and they were then washed in 0.1 M PBS for 12 h and post-fixed in 2% osmium tetroxide in 0.1 M PBS for 1 h at 4 °C, dehydrated and included in EPON. Ultra-thin sections were stained in a 1% uranyl acetate and lead citrate solution, and visualized with a Tecnai SPIRIT Transmission Electron Microscope (FEI Company, Eindhoven,

The Netherlands) working at an acceleration voltage of 120 KV. Electron micrographs were taken from similar regions in the slices. Images were acquired with a Megaview III camera and digitized with the iTEM software (Soft Imaging System). Myelin measurements were obtained with the same program and the g-ratio was determined (axon circumference to myelin circumference). More than 50 randomly selected axons were analyzed per slice, in 3–4 slices per treatment.

Intracellular protein phosphorylation assays by xMAP technology

The phosphorylation state of different intracellular proteins was evaluated in xMAP assays (Luminex). Mouse cerebellar organotypic cultures were collected in lysis buffer and tested with different antibodies against: total Akt/PKB, total p38/SAPK, total STAT3, total extracellular signal-regulated kinase (ERK)/MAPK, total P70 S6Kinase, total JNK/SAPK1, total activating transcription factor-2 (ATF-2), phosphorylated Akt/PKB (Ser473), phosphorylated Akt/PKB (Thr 308), phosphorylated p38/SAPK (Thr180/Tyr182), phosphorylated STAT3 (Tyr705/Ser727), phosphorylated ERK/MAPK (Thr185/Tyr187), phosphorylated P70 S6Kinase (Thr412), phosphorylated JNK/SAPK1 (Thr183/Tyr185) and phosphorylated ATF-2 (Thr69/71). Control beads were used to verify calibration and optical integrity of the system. Moreover, a positive and negative antibody control was used in each experiment.

Real-time PCR

RNA was extracted from the mouse cerebellar organotypic slices after different treatment times using the RNeasy kit, according to the manufacturer's instructions (Qiagen). Using the RNA (1 μg) as a template, cDNAs were synthesized (Applied Biosystems) and the following genes were assayed by real-time PCR (Applied Biosystems): Brain derived neurotrophic factor (BDNF), Neurotrophin 3 (NT3), leukemia inhibitory factor (LIF), hairy and enhancer of split 5 (Hes5), CNTF, fibroblast growth factor 2 (FGF-2), mammalian target of rapamycin (mTOR), and nerve growth factor (NGF). To quantify gene expression the comparative CT method was used where the ΔCT value was obtained by subtracting the CT value of an endogenous gene (GAPDH for mouse samples, 18S for human samples) from the CT value of the gene of interest, in each case using a mean value of three reactions.

Data analysis

The data is expressed as the mean ± SEM and statistical analyses were performed with SPSS 20.0 software. The data were tested using the paired sample Student t-test or with an one-way analysis of variance (ANOVA) and the Bonferroni's t-test for multiple comparisons. The relevant statistical results are indicated in the figure legends.

Results

Methylthioadenosine promotes remyelination in organotypic cerebellar cultures

Neuroinflammation is a common process in several neurological diseases, including MS where it leads to demyelination and axonal damage. To assess how methylthioadenosine might affect demyelination/remyelination under inflammatory conditions, we used an in vitro model of neuroinflammation, which was provoked in mouse cerebellar organotypic cultures by stimulation with LPS [16]. We found that the LPS challenge induced microglial/astrocytes activation through the release of the pro-inflammatory cytokines TNF-α and IL-1ß, and the production of iNOS, consequently provoking demyelination and axonal damage (axonal swelling and end bulbs: Fig. 1A, panels b, e, h and j, and B). However, when cultures were pre-treated with methylthioadenosine (48 or 192 μM), there was significantly less demyelination and no axonal abnormalities were observed (Fig. 1A, panels c, f, i, j). We also observed a significant decrease in IL-1β, TNF-α and iNOS expression in methylthioadenosine pretreated cultures (Fig. 1B), as described previously [16], as well as the persistence of CNPase detected in Western blots (Fig. 1B). These results indicate that methylthioadenosine dampened the effects of neuroinflammation, which contributed to the preservation of myelin. However, because the immunomodulatory effects of methylthioadenosine [13], we cannot discriminate in this model whether the preservation of myelin was due to a reduction in inflammatory damage either on microglia or astrocytes activation, or to a direct effect on OLs.

In order to assess the direct effects of methylthioadenosine on remyelination, we used organotypic cerebellar cultures that were challenged with lysolecithin [17]. Following a 7d recovery post-isolation, the slices were treated with lysolecithin (0.5 mg/ml) for 14 h to induce demyelination with minimal axonal injury and neuronal damage [17]. Quantification of the g-ratio demonstrated widespread demyelination in the cultures (Fig. 2) and when these demyelinated cultures were treated with methylthioadenosine (192 μM), significant remyelination was observed relative to the placebo (saline) treated cultures at all the time points tested (9, 13, 17 and 21 days in vitro). Changes in the g-ratio were observed for nearly all axons, although they were most pronounced for smaller-caliber axons (Fig. 2, panel c).

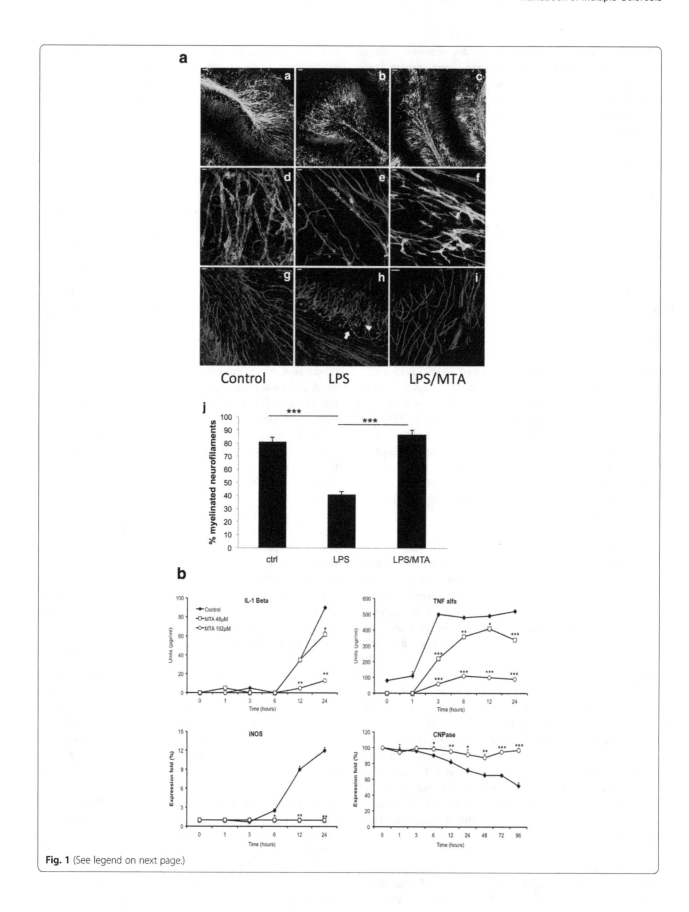

Fig. 1 (See legend on next page.)

Fig. 1 Methylthioadenosine (MTA) dampens neuroinflammation, and prevents demyelination and axonal loss in mouse cerebellar cultures. **A** Organotypic cultures were treated with MTA (192 μM) or the placebo for 24 h at seven DIV and thereafter, they were stimulated with LPS (15 μg/ml) for 24 h. Immunofluorescent staining for NFL (*red*) and MBP (*green*) was analyzed in the slices, and in time-matched untreated control slices (*arrow*, axonal swelling; *arrowhead*, end bulb). Panels *a*, *b* and *c* scale bars: 50 μm. Panels *d-i* scale bar: 5 μm. Panel *j* shows the percentage of myelinated neurofilaments. **B** Cerebellar organotypic cultures at seven DIV were pre-treated with MTA (48 μM and 192 μM) or the placebo and stimulated with LPS (15 μg/ml) at different time points (0, 1, 3, 6, 12, 24, 48, 72 and 96 h). IL-1β and TNF-α production was measured by ELISA and the cytokine release into the medium is expressed in pg/ml. The expression of iNOS and CNPase was measured in Western blots. Results are the mean of three independent experiments. *$P < 0.05$, **$P < 0.01$ and ***$P < 0.001$

Methylthioadenosine increases the number of mature myelinating oligodendrocytes in cerebellar organotypic cultures

Mouse cerebellar organotypic cultures exposed to lysolecithin demyelination contained more mature OLs (Olig2 + MBP + cells) when they were exposed to methylthioadenosine 1 day after demyelination was induced and when treated with methylthioadenosine in a preventive manner (overnight prior to lysolecithin challenge: Fig. 3a-b). These results indicate that methylthioadenosine promoted OLs

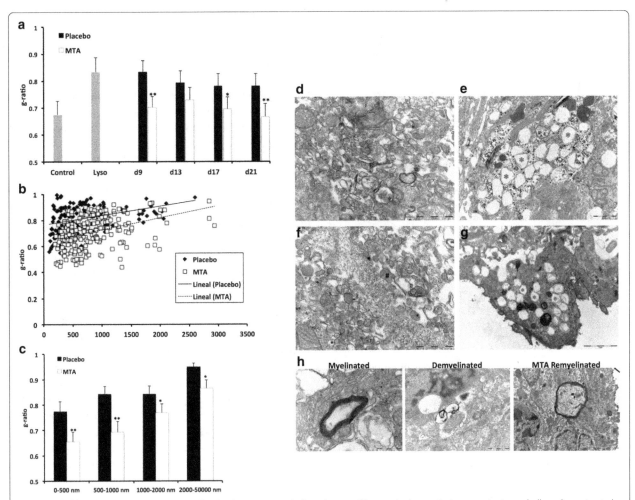

Fig. 2 Methylthioadenosine promotes remyelination in mouse cerebellar cultures. **a** Changes in the g-ratio in organotypic cerebellar cultures treated with methylthioadenosine (MTA, 192μM, *white*) or the placebo (*black*) at different time points after lysolecithin demyelination. **b** The scatter plot displays the g-ratios of individual axons in function of the respective axon diameter. **c** Changes in the g-ratio clustering in samples relative to the respective axonal diameter. Electron microscopy images are shown from mouse cerebellar organotypic cultures showing normal myelinated axons in control tissue (**d**), nude axons in lysolecithin cultures not treated or treated with placebo (**e, g**) while remyelinated axons are shown in MTA-treated slices (**f**). Zoom images of myelinated, demyelinated and MTA treated remyelinated axons (**h**). Results are the mean of three independent experiments with six slices per condition. Between four and seven animals were used in each experiment being the slices per condition randomly selected from different animals. *demyelinated axons. # remyelinated axons.*$P < 0.05$, **$P < 0.01$. Scale bars: 1–2 μm

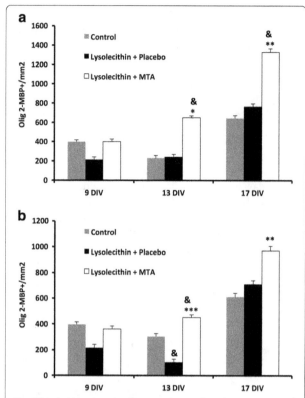

Fig. 3 Methylthioadenosine increases the number of mature myelinating OLs in mouse cerebellar cultures. **a** Effect of methylthioadenosine (MTA, 192μM) treatment before lysolecithin induced demyelination. Olig2/MBP staining was used as a marker of mature OLs: *Grey*, control tissue (no lysolecithin); *White*, lysolecithin challenged tissue treated with MTA at different time points (9, 13 and 17 DIV); *Black*, lysolecithin challenged tissue treated with the placebo. **b** Effect of MTA (192μM) on mature myelinating OLs after lysolecithin induced demyelination: *Grey*, control tissue without lysolecithin; *White*, lysolecithin tissue treated with MTA; *Black*, lysolecithin tissue treated with placebo at different time points (9, 13 and 17 DIV). Results are the mean of three independent experiments with six slices per condition in each experiment. * $p \leq 0.05$; **$p \leq 0.01$ and ***$p \leq 0.001$ with respect to the placebo; & $p \leq 0.01$ relative to the controls

survival and differentiation, therefore preventing demyelination and stimulating remyelination.

Methylthioadenosine induces remyelination and functional recovery in vivo in the cuprizone model

We used the cuprizone model of demyelination in mice to assess the effect of methylthioadenosine on remyelination in vivo. We induced demyelination in C57BL6 mice through 4, 5 and 6 weeks of cuprizone intoxication [18]. We followed the remyelination process for 4 weeks after cuprizone removal, administering methylthioadenosine either as a preventive therapy from the same day the mice began to receive cuprizone or as a curative therapy from the 5th week after cuprizone administration had commenced. As expected 4, 5 or 6 weeks of cuprizone treatment significantly diminished the area of

MBP staining in the corpus callosum (Fig. 4a). MBP staining was significantly more extensive at weeks 5 and 6 in animals pretreated with methylthioadenosine (preventive therapy group) than in those that received the vehicle alone (Fig. 4a). In addition, there was stronger MBP staining in animals that received methylthioadenosine (curative therapy group) 2 weeks after cuprizone removal compared to the control animals and those that received the vehicle alone (Fig. 4b). However, there were no differences in MBP staining by weeks 8 and 9 due to the spontaneous remyelination in this model. To assess functional repair, mice were subjected to the rotarod test twice a week from week 5 (upon cessation of the cuprizone supplement) to week 8. We found significative differences in the motor coordination and balance by week 7 to 8 between methylthioadenosine and vehicle treated animals (Fig. 4c), which corresponds to the time of MBP analysis in the corpus callosum of these animals. We also saw differences at weeks 6 and 7 tested between methylthioadenosine treated animals and cuprizone animals (Fig. 4c).

Methylthioadenosine promotes STAT-3 phosphorylation and CNTF release in cerebellar cultures

In order to gain insight as to how methylthioadenosine might promote remyelination, we assessed the phosphorylation of key signaling pathways in the mouse cerebellar organotypic model of chemical demyelination with lysolecithin. In this model, the JNK/SAPK pathway normally associated with activation of apoptotic signaling in OLs is activated by the lysolecithin challenge [17]. However, methylthioadenosine dampened the phosphorylation of JNK/SAPK at 13 and 17 DIV, while enhancing the phosphorylation of STAT3 and ERK1/2 compared to that in the slices that received the placebo (Fig. 5a–c). In addition, phosphorylation of the Activating Transcription Factor 2 (ATF2), a transcription factor involved in protection against oxidative stress [19], was also significantly enhanced in cultures exposed to methylthioadenosine after demyelination (Fig. 5d). We did not observe phosphorylation of other relevant kinases such as AKT/PKB, p38/SAPK or the p70S6 Kinase (data not shown).

A physiological response of the CNS to damage is the release of trophic factors that promote cell survival and restore the CNS microenvironment [20]. For this reason, we performed real-time PCR to measure the expression of genes encoding different trophic factors that could protect OPCs or OLs against damage when the mouse cerebellar slices were challenged with lysolecithin. Of the trophic factors associated with myelin maintenance tested (CNTF, LIF, BDNF, NT3, NGF and FGF-2), only CNTF expression had increased significantly in methylthioadenosine treated slices by day 17 DIV. We also quantified Hes5 expression, a transcription factor associated with the Notch/Jagged pathway that is implicated in the inhibition of remyelination, and

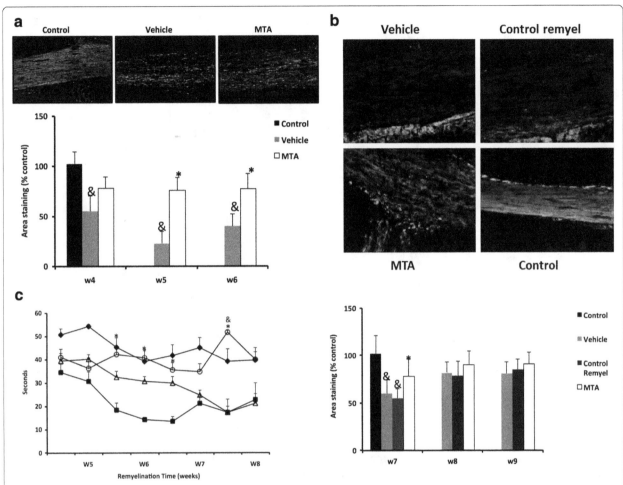

Fig. 4 Methylthioadenosine promotes remyelination in the mouse cuprizone model. **a** Preventive trial. *Top*: representative images of MBP immunostaining in the corpus callosum of mice fed with a normal diet (control) or with a cuprizone supplement for 4, 5 or 6 weeks and injected intraperitoneally daily with methylthioadenosine (MTA, 60mg/kg/day) or the vehicle alone (saline) for 6 weeks (treatments started the same day as cuprizone supplementation). *Bottom*: quantification of the area of MBP staining shown as the mean ± standard error of the mean ($n = 6$ per group). **b** Curative trial. *Top*: representative images of MBP immunostaining in the corpus callosum of mice fed with normal diet (control) or with a cuprizone supplement for 5 weeks, after which the animals received a normal diet and a daily intraperitoneal injection of the vehicle alone, MTA (60mg/kg/day) or a placebo for 7, 8 or 9 weeks. Each treatment started after the cessation of cuprizone supplementation at week 5. *Bottom*: quantification of the area stained for MBP. The values shown are the means ± standard error of the mean ($n = 6$ per group): & $p \leq 0.05$ respect to control; *$p \leq 0.05$ respect to vehicle. **c** Clinical score in cuprizone model. Motor coordination and balance were evaluated twice a week from week 5 to week 9 using the rotarod test and expressed as seconds mice stay in the rotarod. *Black diamonds*, control with no cuprizone; *black squares*, cuprizone-fed mice; *white triangles*, cuprizone-fed vehicle treated mice; and *white circles*, cuprizone-fed and MTA treated mice. The graph represents the average time spent by mice on the rotarod at 18 rpm constant speed. * $p \leq 0.05$ respect to cuprizone fed animals. & $p \leq 0.05$ respect to vehicle cuprizone fed animals

mTOR, a serine-protein kinase that regulates several pathways involved in cell growth, and survival. We found that neither Hes5 nor mTOR expression changed significantly in cultures exposed to methylthioadenosine (Additional file 2: Figure S2).

To confirm the increase in STAT-3 phosphorylation in the organotypic cultures and study the sequence of events implicated in remyelination induced by methylthioadenosine, we exposed cerebellar cultures challenged with lysolecithin to the inhibitor of STAT-3 phosphorylation, LLL12. This inhibitor partially inhibited STAT-3

phosphorylation in these cultures, an effect that was reversed by methylthioadenosine (Fig. 6a). When we assessed the expression of the CNTF gene when STAT3 phosphorylation was blocked, there was a significant decrease in CNTF expression in cultures that received LLL12 but not in those that were also administered methylthioadenosine (Fig. 6b). In summary, the effects of methylthioadenosine in cerebellar cultures were associated with the phosphorylation of STAT3 and other kinases, and with the expression of CNTF.

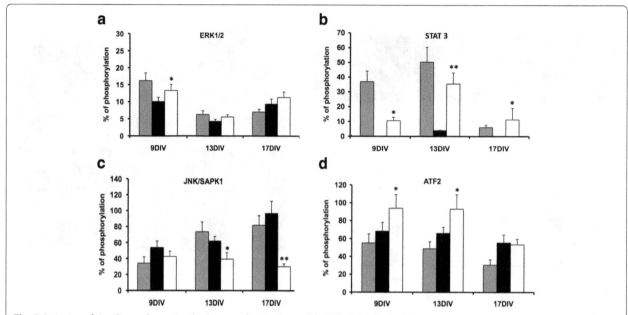

Fig. 5 Activation of signaling pathways involved in remyelination. Intracellular ERK1/2 (**a**), STAT3 (**b**), JNK/SAPK1 (**c**) and ATF2 (**d**) phosphoproteins measured in xMAP assays (Luminex) of mouse cerebellum cultures exposed to lysolecithin (0.5 mg/ml) and treated with methylthioadenosine (MTA, 192 μM) or the placebo at 9, 13 and 17 DIV. Samples for the phosphorylation assay were obtained 30 min after the last administration of MTA or the placebo. Results are the mean of three independent experiments with 10 slices per condition in each experiment. *Gray*, Control samples without lysolecithin; *Black*, Lysolecithin samples treated with placebo; *White*, Lysolecithin samples treated with MTA; * $p < 0.05$ and ** $p < 0.01$ with respect to the samples that received the placebo

Role of astrocytes in Methylthioadenosine mediated remyelination

In order to identify the source of CNTF promoted by MTA, we performed immunohistochemistry on the mouse cerebellum slices. We observed a co-localization of GFAP with CNTF, suggesting that astrocytes are the main producers of CNTF in these cultures (Fig. 6c). We also used mouse primary cortical astrocyte cultures stimulated with LPS to validate the role of methylthioadenosine in promoting the expression of CNTF by astrocytes. Astrocytes exposed to methylthioadenosine for 24h produced significantly more CNTF RNA (Fig. 7a) and protein (Fig. 7b). Moreover, STAT-3 phosphorylation in mouse astrocyte cultures challenged with LPS increased significantly 30 min and 1 h after methylthioadenosine treatment (Fig. 7c).

Discussion

In this study, we evaluated the ability of methylthioadenosine, a natural metabolite, to promote remyelination and protect against demyelination in models of inflammatory and chemical demyelination. Intermediate metabolism plays a critical role in maintaining cell homeostasis and in the response to stress. For example, an intermediate metabolite of the Kreb's cycle, fumarate acid, displays antioxidant properties by increasing the expression of Nrf2, a transcription factor that induces the expression of antioxidant enzymes [21]. Kynurenines or the methylthioadenosine precursor S-Adenosyl-Methionine are other

examples, both able to modulate cell proliferation and survival in different pathological situations [22–24]. In this study we provide in vitro and in vivo evidence that methylthioadenosine promotes remyelination and protects against demyelination in two different model of demyelination. First, methylthioadenosine promotes remyelination and prevents demyelination in mouse cerebellar cultures exposed to LPS (a model of inflammatory demyelination) and promotes remyelination when exposed to lysolecithin (a model of chemical demyelination), increasing the number of mature myelinating OLs. In the in vivo model of demyelination with cuprizone, methylthioadenosine was able to prevent demyelination and also enhanced remyelination 2 weeks after starting the treatment, as reflected by a clinical improvement in locomotion in this period of time. In this study we did not use the experimental autoimmune encephalitis model because the immunomodulatory activity of methylthioadenosine would prevent the emergence of its effect in demyelination/remyelination.

In mediating these effects on myelination, methylthioadenosine appears to employ a complex and pleiotropic mechanism of action, even though it is a well-documented antioxidant [9, 13, 25]. In this study, we show that methylthioadenosine dampens the expression of iNOS and it enhances the phosphorylation of ATF2, a factor that protects against oxidative stress [19]. Indeed, this finding agrees with previous studies showing that methylthioadenosine can counteract oxidative stress in other cell types and settings [9,

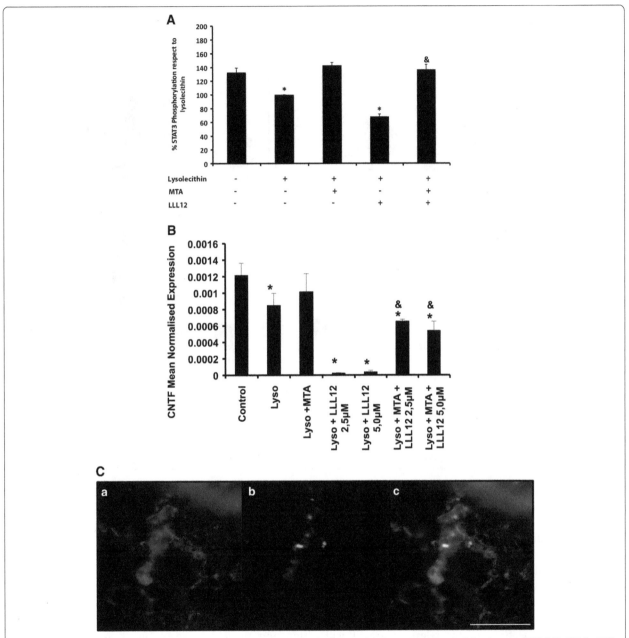

Fig. 6 Modulation of signaling pathways associated with remyelination and cell survival. **A** Proportion of intracellular phospho-STAT-3 (Tyr705/Ser727) measured in xMAP assays of cerebellar cultures exposed to lysolecithin (0.5 mg/ml) and treated with MTA (192 µM) or the STAT3 inhibitor LLL12 (5 µM) for 4 days. The cells were processed 30 min after MTA or LLL12 exposure on the last day of experiment: *$P < 0.05$, statistical differences respect to control without lysolecithin; $P < 0.05$, statistical differences respect to Lysolecithin + LLL12 (no MTA). **B** CNTF gene expression in cerebellar organotypic cultures exposed to lysolecithin (0.5 mg/ml) and treated with MTA (192 µM) or LLL12 (2.5µM or 5µM): *$P < 0.05$, statistical differences relative to the control without lysolecithin; & $P < 0.05$, statistical differences relative to Lysolecithin + LLL12 (no MTA). **C** Immunohistochemistry for GFAP (*red*) and CNTF (*green*) in mouse cerebellar organotypic cultures exposed to lysolecithin and treated with MTA (192 µM) 4 d after treatment. Scale bar: 50 µm. Results are the mean of three independent experiments with 10 slices per condition in each experiment

13, 25]. Here, we also show that methylthioadenosine can down-regulate microglia/astrocytes activation, inhibiting the release of pro-inflammatory cytokines like TNF-α and IL-1β. Microglia/astrocytes activation apparently plays a critical role in amplifying brain damage and has been considered an interesting therapeutic strategy in many brain diseases [26].

Methylthioadenosine also promotes STAT-3 phosphorylation in the mouse cerebellum organotypic cultures exposed to lysolecithin, a signaling protein previously associated with neurite outgrowth [27], axonal regeneration and survival [28]. It should be noted that STAT-3 expression and activation in the CNS is very specific

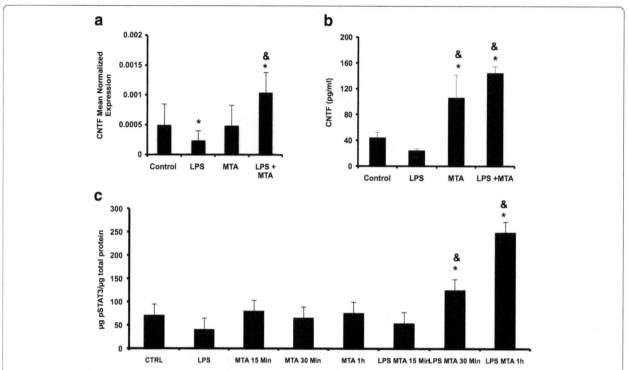

Fig. 7 Role of methylthioadenosine in CNTF production and STAT-3 phosphorylation in astrocytes. **a** CNTF gene expression in primary cortical mouse astrocytes exposed to LPS (10 µg/ml) overnight and treated for 24 h with methylthioadenosine (MTA, 192µM) or the placebo on the following day. **b** CNTF protein measured by ELISA in supernatants of primary cortical mouse astrocytes exposed to LPS (10 µg/ml) overnight and treated for 24 h with MTA (192µM) or placebo the following day. **c** Intracellular phospho-STAT-3 (Tyr705/Ser727) levels measured in xMAP assays carried out on primary cortical mouse astrocytes exposed to LPS (10 µg/ml) overnight and treated with MTA (192µM) or placebo for the next 5 days (samples collected 15, 30 min or 1 h after the last treatment was given): * $p < 0.05$, statistical differences relative to the controls that did not receive LPS; $p < 0.05$, statistical differences relative to the cells that received LPS but not MTA. Results are the mean of two independent experiments

given that it can fulfill a number of different roles both in the developing and adult brain, many related to neuroprotection [29]. The enhanced STAT-3 phosphorylation induced by methylthioadenosine in the CNS was associated with the release of CNTF by astrocytes, as demonstrated using a partial and reversible chemical inhibitor of STAT3 phosphorylation in organotypic cultures. However, understanding the mechanisms by which methylthioadenosine promotes STAT-3 phosphorylation and the release of CNTF will require further studies.

CNTF promotes remyelination and it enhances the survival and differentiation of CNS-derived oligodendroglia [30–33]. The identification of pathways that control OPC differentiation and myelination has paved the way for the development of new approaches to achieve remyelination [34]. CNTF is produced by microglia and astrocytes following brain injury [35, 36], and it enhances the survival and differentiation of OLs [30–33]. Finally, methylthioadenosine is signalling through adenosine receptors [37], and activation of adenosine receptor in OPCs promote myelination [38]. Therefore, methylthioadenosine might contribute to myelin repair through

activation of adenosine pathway as well. Further studies are required to understand the role of each pathway involved in the remyelinating activity we have observed.

Conclusion

Based on these results, we propose that methylthioadenosine may offer a natural means to obtain cell protection and to achieve repair in circumstances of CNS damage. Methylthioadenosine therapy may recapitulate such responses and also provides benefits by limiting brain damage in neuroinflammation. The results of this study provide the opportunity to test methylthioadenosine as a regenerative therapy for neuroinflammatory diseases like MS. Accordingly, methylthioadenosine could be integrated in a combination therapy for MS taking advantage of the immunomodulatory activity of current drugs along with methylthioadenosine's immunomodulatory and regenerative effects. Indeed, methylthioadenosine has already proven to be safe in previous phase I studies [39], a critical consideration when developing combination therapies for autoimmune diseases.

Additional files

> **Additional file 1: Figure S1.** Experimental design cuprizone model. Cuprizone induced demyelination was induced by feeding mice with cuprizone from week 0 to week 6. MTA was tested in as preventive therapy in order to decrease demyelination (from week 0 to week 6) or as curative therapy in order to promote remyelination (from week 5 until week 9). Placebo animals were also feed with cuprizone and were treated with placebo (Plac); control animals did not received cuprizone.
>
> **Additional file 2: Figure S2.** Expression of trophic factors after in vitro demyelination in cerebellar organotypic cultures. The expression of genes encoding trophic factors such as LIF, Hes5, BDNF, NT3, CNTF, NGF, mTOR and FGF-2 was assessed in mouse cerebellum cultures exposed to lysolecithin (0.5 mg/ml) and treated with MTA (192 μM) or the placebo at 9, 13, 17 and 21 DIV by real-time PCR. The data represent the increase relative to the housekeeping gene GAPDH. Results are the mean of three independent experiments with 10 slices per condition in each experiment. * $p < 0.05$.

Abbreviations

ANOVA: One-way analysis of variance; BDNF: Brain derived neurotrophic factor; BSA: Bovine serum albumin; CNPase: 2′,3′-cyclic-nucleotide 3′-phosphodiesterase; CNS: Central Nervous System; CNTF: Ciliary neurotrophic factor; DIV: Days in vitro; FGF-2: Fibroblast growth factor 2; GFAP: Glial fibrillary acidic protein; Hes5: Hairy and enhancer of split 5; iNOS: Inducible nitric oxide synthase; ip: Intraperitoneal; LIF: Leukemia inhibitory factor; LPS: Lipopolysaccharide; MBP: Myelin basic protein; MS: Multiple sclerosis; mTOR: Mammalian target of rapamycin; NFkB: Nuclear factor kappa B; NFL: Neurofilament; NGF: Nerve growth factor; NT3: Neurotrophin 3; OLs: Oligodendrocytes; OPCs: Oligodendrocyte precursor cells; PRMT5: Protein arginine methyltransferase 5

Acknowledgement

We would like to thank Mark Sefton for the English revision.

Funding

This work was supported by grants PI12/01823 and RD07/60/001 to PV from the Instituto de Salud Carlos III, Spanish Ministry of Economy and Competitivity (Spain) and CERCA Programme / Generalitat de Catalunya. Funding agency has no role in the design, analysis and writing of the article.

Author's contributions

PV and BM designed the research plan, analyzed the results and wrote the manuscript. BM, AdP, GV, RV, OE, NE and BF performed the organotypic culture assays, and the mechanism of action studies. AM and JA performed the astrocyte assays. All authors read and approved the final manuscript.

Competing interests

PV and BM hold patent rights on the use of methylthioadenosine for the treatment of MS and other neurological diseases. PV has received consultancy honoraria from Digna Biotech (Pamplona, Spain).

Ethics approval

The animal protocols used were approved by the Ethical Committee on Animal Research at the University of Barcelona.

Author details

[1]Center of Neuroimmunology, Institut d'Investigacions Biomediques August Pi Sunyer (IDIBAPS), Barcelona, Spain. [2]Department of Basic Sciences. Facultad de Medicina i Ciències de la Salut, Universitat International de Catalunya (UIC), Sant Cugat del Vallés, Spain. [3]Neurogenomiks, University of Basque Country, Leioa, Spain. [4]University of Barcelona, Barcelona, Spain. [5]University of California, San Francisco, USA. [6]Centre Cellex 3A, Casanova 145, 08036 Barcelona, Spain.

References

1. Ransohoff RM, Hafler DA, Lucchinetti CF. Multiple sclerosis-a quiet revolution. Nat Rev Neurol. 2015;11(3):134–42.
2. Hauser SL, Chan JR, Oksenberg JR. Multiple sclerosis: prospects and promise. Ann Neurol. 2013;74(3):317–27.
3. Lubetzki C, Stankoff B. Demyelination in multiple sclerosis. Handb Clin Neurol. 2014;122:89–99.
4. Nave KA, Werner HB. Myelination of the nervous system: mechanisms and functions. Annu Rev Cell Dev Biol. 2014;30:503–33.
5. Luessi F, Kuhlmann T, Zipp F. Remyelinating strategies in multiple sclerosis. Expert Rev Neurother. 2014;14(11):1315–34.
6. Franklin RJ, ffrench-Constant C, Edgar JM, Smith KJ. Neuroprotection and repair in multiple sclerosis. Nat Rev Neurol. 2012;8(11):624–34.
7. Charles P, Reynolds R, Seilhean D, Rougon G, Aigrot MS, Niezgoda A, et al. Re-expression of PSA-NCAM by demyelinated axons: an inhibitor of remyelination in multiple sclerosis? Brain. 2002;125(Pt 9):1972–9.
8. Williams-Ashman HG, Seidenfeld J, Galletti P. Trends in the biochemical pharmacology of 5′-deoxy-5′-methylthioadenosine. Biochem Pharmacol. 1982;31(3):277–88.
9. Avila MA, Garcia-Trevijano ER, Lu SC, Corrales FJ, Mato JM. Methylthioadenosine. Int J Biochem Cell Biol. 2004;36(11):2125–30.
10. Mavrakis KJ, McDonald 3rd ER, Schlabach MR, Billy E, Hoffman GR, deWeck A, et al. Disordered methionine metabolism in MTAP/CDKN2A-deleted cancers leads to dependence on PRMT5. Science. 2016;351(6278):1208–13.
11. Kryukov GV, Wilson FH, Ruth JR, Paulk J, Tsherniak A, Marlow SE, et al. MTAP deletion confers enhanced dependency on the PRMT5 arginine methyltransferase in cancer cells. Science. 2016;351(6278):1214–8.
12. Andreu-Perez P, Esteve-Puig R, de Torre-Minguela C, Lopez-Fauqued M, Bech-Serra JJ, Tenbaum S, et al. Protein arginine methyltransferase 5 regulates ERK1/2 signal transduction amplitude and cell fate through CRAF. Sci Signal. 2011;4(190):ra58.
13. Moreno B, Hevia H, Santamaria M, Sepulcre J, Munoz J, Garcia-Trevijano ER, et al. Methylthioadenosine reverses brain autoimmune disease. Ann Neurol. 2006;60:323–34.
14. Moreno B, Fernandez-Diez B, Di Penta A, Villoslada P. Preclinical studies of methylthioadenosine for the treatment of multiple sclerosis. Mult Scler. 2010;16(9):1102–8.
15. Moreno B, Lopez I, Fernandez-Diez B, Gottlieb M, Matute C, Sanchez-Gomez MV, et al. Differential neuroprotective effects of 5′-deoxy-5′-methylthioadenosine. PLoS One. 2014;9(3):e90671.
16. Di Penta A, Moreno B, Reix S, Fernandez-Diez B, Villanueva M, Errea O, et al. Oxidative stress and proinflammatory cytokines contribute to demyelination and axonal damage in a cerebellar culture model of neuroinflammation. PloSONE. 2013;8(2):e54722.
17. Birgbauer E, Rao TS, Webb M. Lysolecithin induces demyelination in vitro in a cerebellar slice culture system. J Neurosci Res. 2004;78(2):157–66.
18. Liebetanz D, Merkler D. Effects of commissural de- and remyelination on motor skill behaviour in the cuprizone mouse model of multiple sclerosis. Exp Neurol. 2006;202(1):217–24.
19. Kiryu-Seo S, Ohno N, Kidd GJ, Komuro H, Trapp BD. Demyelination increases axonal stationary mitochondrial size and the speed of axonal mitochondrial transport. J Neurosci. 2010;30(19):6658–66.
20. Villoslada P, Genain CP. Role of nerve growth factor and other trophic factors in brain inflammation. Prog Brain Res. 2004;146:403–14.
21. Linker RA, Lee DH, Ryan S, van Dam AM, Conrad R, Bista P, et al. Fumaric acid esters exert neuroprotective effects in neuroinflammation via activation of the Nrf2 antioxidant pathway. Brain. 2011;134(Pt 3):678–92.
22. Lu SC, Ramani K, Ou X, Lin M, Yu V, Ko K, et al. S-adenosylmethionine in the chemoprevention and treatment of hepatocellular carcinoma in a rat model. Hepatology. 2009;50(2):462–71.
23. Luo J, Li YN, Wang F, Zhang WM, Geng X. S-adenosylmethionine inhibits the growth of cancer cells by reversing the hypomethylation status of c-

myc and H-ras in human gastric cancer and colon cancer. Int J Biol Sci. 2010;6(7):784–95.

24. Sahin M, Sahin E, Gumuslu S, Erdogan A, Gultekin M. Inhibition of angiogenesis by S-adenosylmethionine. Biochem Biophys Res Commun. 2011;408(1):145–8.

25. Simile MM, Banni S, Angioni E, Carta G, De Miglio MR, Muroni MR, et al. 5'-Methylthioadenosine administration prevents lipid peroxidation and fibrogenesis induced in rat liver by carbon-tetrachloride intoxication. J Hepatol. 2001;34(3):386–94.

26. Moreno B, Jukes JP, Vergara-Irigaray N, Errea O, Villoslada P, Perry VH, et al. Systemic inflammation induces axon injury during brain inflammation. Ann Neurol. 2011;70(6):932–42.

27. He JC, Gomes I, Nguyen T, Jayaram G, Ram PT, Devi LA, et al. The G alpha(o/i)-coupled cannabinoid receptor-mediated neurite outgrowth involves Rap regulation of Src and Stat3. J Biol Chem. 2005;280(39):33426–34.

28. Sun F, Park KK, Belin S, Wang D, Lu T, Chen G, et al. Sustained axon regeneration induced by co-deletion of PTEN and SOCS3. Nature. 2011;480(7377):372–5.

29. Dziennis S, Alkayed NJ. Role of signal transducer and activator of transcription 3 in neuronal survival and regeneration. Rev Neurosci. 2008;19(4–5):341–61.

30. Barres BA, Hart IK, Coles HS, Burne JF, Voyvodic JT, Richardson WD, et al. Cell death and control of cell survival in the oligodendrocyte lineage. Cell. 1992;70(1):31–46.

31. Barres BA, Schmid R, Sendnter M, Raff MC. Multiple extracellular signals are required for long-term oligodendrocyte survival. Development. 1993;118(1):283–95.

32. Louis JC, Magal E, Takayama S, Varon S. CNTF protection of oligodendrocytes against natural and tumor necrosis factor-induced death. Science. 1993;259(5095):689–92.

33. D'Souza SD, Alinauskas KA, Antel JP. Ciliary neurotrophic factor selectively protects human oligodendrocytes from tumor necrosis factor-mediated injury. J Neurosci Res. 1996;43(3):289–98.

34. Chari DM. Remyelination in multiple sclerosis. Int Rev Neurobiol. 2007;79:589–620.

35. Moore CS, Abdullah SL, Brown A, Arulpragasam A, Crocker SJ. How factors secreted from astrocytes impact myelin repair. J Neurosci Res. 2011;89(1):13–21.

36. Tanaka T, Murakami K, Bando Y, Yoshida S. Minocycline reduces remyelination by suppressing ciliary neurotrophic factor expression after cuprizone-induced demyelination. J Neurochem. 2013;127(2):259–70.

37. Keyel PA, Romero M, Wu W, Kwak DH, Zhu Q, Liu X, et al. Methylthioadenosine reprograms macrophage activation through adenosine receptor stimulation. PLoS One. 2014;9(8):e104210.

38. Stevens B, Porta S, Haak LL, Gallo V, Fields RD. Adenosine: a neuron-glial transmitter promoting myelination in the CNS in response to action potentials. Neuron. 2002;36(5):855–68.

39. Stramentinoli G, Gennari F, inventors; Adenosine derivatives of anti-inflammatory and analgesic activity, and therapeutic compositions which contain them as their active principle. US patent 4,454,122. 1984 1984.

3

Hands on Alemtuzumab-experience from clinical practice: whom and how to treat

Lina Hassoun, Judith Eisele, Katja Thomas and Tjalf Ziemssen[*]

Abstract

Alemtuzumab is a monoclonal antibody, which was recently approved for the treatment of active relapsing remitting multiple sclerosis. Its main mechanism of action is based on targeting CD52, an antigen of unknown function which is found on B and T lymphocytes, leading to depletion followed by repopulation of these cells. The high efficacy of Alemtuzumab in controlling relapsing remitting MS has been shown in several clinical trials. This new therapy approach is associated with a specific side effects profile requiring regular longterm monitoring. The most important side effects are infusion-associated reactions, a slight increase of infections as well as autoimmune events in almost one third of treated patients.

Based on two years of clinical experience in Germany, this review covers the first steps with the careful patient selection to be treated with Alemtuzumab over the preparation steps and the infusion courses up to the longterm monitoring after Alemtuzumab treatment.

Background

In September 2013, Alemtuzumab was approved in Europe as an additional therapeutic option for active relapsing-remitting Multiple Sclerosis (RRMS). Since its synthesis in the early eighties as the first humanized monoclonal antibody, Alemtuzumab therapeutic potentials were explored for many diseases (eg. Graft versus host disease, transplantation, vasculitis, rheumatoid arthritis, immunologically mediated cytopenia) [1, 2]; it is the first depleting monoclonal antibody which was licensed for the treatment of RRMS. The mechanism of Alemtuzumab differs from immunmodulating and other immunosuppressive treatments in its fundamental approach, which consists of at least two courses of lymphocyte depletion followed by cellular repopulation. The reconstitution of lymphocytes is thought to be of particular importance not only for the beneficial clinical effects, but also for the long-term side effects [3]. Alemtuzumab is introducing a new therapeutic concept of an induction-like treatment strategy, but without the need of a maintenance treatment in the follow up in most of the treated patients. Such concepts are till now not well established in our clinical practice. Furthermore, other highly efficacious treatment options such as Natalizumab and Fingolimod are available. No clinical trials have directly compared Alemtuzumab with these medications making the clinical decision not straight forward.

Although the role of Alemtuzumab in RRMS was investigated in three active-controlled clinical studies [4–6], using it in clinical practice can be quite challenging as several questions are still to be answered: how to define patients who will most likely profit from Alemtuzumab? Where does Alemtuzumab stand in MS treatment scenario? And then if Alemtuzumab is to be given, how should we switch patients from other specific MS treatments to Alemtuzumab? What other MS medications could be given following Alemtuzumab? How could the infusion management be optimized? Which side effects can be expected and how should they be handled? What is the most applicable monitoring strategy in clinical practice?

The aim of this review is to summarize our experience with Alemtuzumab in clinical practice of the last two years following a structured approach starting with treatment selection followed by preparation and infusion management up to the longterm monitoring.

The innovative treatment concept of alemtuzumab

Alemtuzumab is a monoclonal antibody that selectively binds to CD52, which is a surface glycoprotein molecule

* Correspondence: Tjalf.Ziemssen@uniklinikum-dresden.de
MS Center Dresden, Center of Clinical Neuroscience, Department of Neurology, University Hospital Carl Gustav Carus, Dresden University of Technology, Fetscherstr. 74, 01307 Dresden, Germany

of unknown function [7]. It is expressed on the surface of T- and B-cells and other cell populations but not on the hematological precursors [8]. Alemtuzumab infusion results in rapid depletion of the CD52 positive cells [9], leading to lymphopenia, which lasts for several years [10]. While B-cells recover relatively quickly within a range of 3–8 months, the repopulation of T cells occurs more slowly, as it needs up to 3 years and in another study up to 60 months for CD4+ and 30 months for CD8+ T cells in average [11, 12]. The experimental data using humanized CD52 mice have shown, that the depletion of lymphocytes upon anti-CD52 treatment was predominant in peripheral circulation, while the number of those cells was clearly less affected in spleen, thymus, bone marrow and lymph nodes [13, 14]. This may represent an explanation for the unexpected low rate of infections in patients receiving Alemtuzumab. As mentioned before, the depletion of CD52-positive cell is followed by a recovery phase that can vary between treated patients. However, it was shown that different repopulation kinetics among patients was not able to predict the risk of MS reactivation [14–16].

This process is considered as part of the reprogramming of the dysregulated immune system. Some authors suggest that the observed prolonged effect of Alemtuzumab lies in the slow reconstitution of T lymphocytes after the initial depletion, and not in the depletion itself [3].

The radical approach of Alemtuzumab which leads to its prolonged therapeutical effect is actually also associated with the well-described side effects. In addition to the infusion-associated reactions (IAR), which will be described in more details later, the increased incidence of antibody-mediated autoimmune diseases upon Alemtuzumab therapy is remarkable [17]. Taking into consideration the previously described mechanism of immune cells depletion and the potential side effects, the need arises to find appropriate criteria that are useful for patient selection.

No biomarker to detect predisposition for secondary autoimmunity has been found yet. IL-21 was previously described as a promising candidate but these results could not be reproduced in another following study, which was attributed to the use of different kits [18, 19].

Different treatment strategies

Alemtuzumab therapy consists of two courses with 12 months in between. In spite of this non-frequent intermittent administration of the medication, this approach guarantees a long-term stabilization of the disease activity and to achieve the therapeutic effect, keeping in mind that Alemtuzumab infusions should take place under close monitoring. Until now, all available highly-efficacious therapies as Natalizumab and Fingolimod follow a continuous treatment strategy. After stopping these drugs, disease activity is returning or even overshooting as it has

been described for Natalizumab [20, 21] and also even in fewer cases for fingolimod [22–25]. On the other side, treatment switches are easier to perform if a more or less reversible treatment as Fingolimod or Natalizumab is applied. The disadvantage is that the use of other treatment approaches after Alemtuzumab is more complicated due to the effects of irreversible depletion and repopulation, on the other side patient is practically off treatment after the second Alemtuzumab infusion. The rapid onset of Alemtuzumab treatment effects can be explained by depletion of both cells of the acquired and innate immune system, including the impairment in activation as well as cytokine release [9].

Comparing side effects, Alemtuzumab has specific windows where side effects are increased specifically (IARs during infusion, infections directly after infusion, secondary autommunity with a maximum in the third year) [26, 27] which is different to risk of adverse events of eg. Natalizumab presenting an increased PML risk after a certain treatment duration [28]. In the field of MS treatment, we have for the first time different treatment strategies with different efficacy and risk profiles during the treatment duration which should be considered before treatment is selected (Fig. 1). Alemtuzumab presents with characteristics of induction treatment although strategy is not correctly defined by the term induction treatment as in the most cases no maintenance treatment is necessary at least for the 5 year window after treatment start [29].

Patient selection: who is the right patient for Alemtuzumab?

According to the European Medicines Agency (EMA), Alemtuzumab is approved for the treatment of patients with active RRMS [30], whereas disease activity is defined by clinical and/or imaging criteria. According to the criteria for assessment of MS activity proposed by Lublin and colleagues [31], a patient with RRMS would be considered as having an active course if a clinical relapse took place or the brain MRI showed new Gadolinium-enhancing and/or the increase in size or number of T2 lesions. MRI monitoring should be done in regular annual intervals [32]. In the clinical trials, the disease duration was limited to 5 years in treatment naïve and to 10 years in pretreated patients [4, 6] probably because Alemtuzumab was not able to cause improvement in SPMS patients in a small pivotal study [11]. So in our opinion, the benefit of the patients regarding Alemtuzumab treatment is optimal if significant inflammatory signs are present clinically and by MRI. So Alemtuzumab is not indicated for patients who do not show any disease activity, and it is also not considered as a standard alternative for patients who are stable on current therapy.

It should be emphasized that for MS patients with high disease activity, highly efficacious therapy options

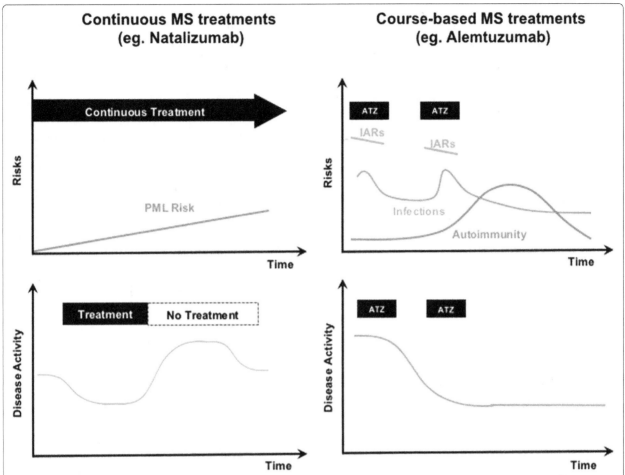

Fig. 1 Comparison of different highly efficacious RRMS therapy strategies Alemtuzumab (right), and Natalizumab (left). The upper diagrams show the adverse effects, which happen usually within specific time windows, the lower diagrams the clinical efficacy

such as Alemtuzumab should be used early within a "window of opportunity" [33]. That implies that the optimal timing would be in the presence of significant clinical and MRI inflammatory activity without significant disability [34]. Therapeutical efficacy of Alemtuzumab is most prominent in early stages of disease by reducing inflammatory activity to counteract the development and accumulation of disability [11, 35]. Patients presenting with an EDSS value up to 3–4 still potentially have predominant inflammatory processes, while irreversible damage is increasingly assumed to be associated with higher EDSS values [36]. Accordingly, Alemtuzumab is most appropriately to be used before an EDSS score of 4 is reached. This should not be interpreted that patients with higher EDSS scores can not benefit from treatment with Alemtuzumab, as the indication should be considered based on clinical and/or radiological disease activity Actually in some patients Alemtuzumab is used as "last option" treatment as many treatments before have failed. The efficacy of Alemtuzumab as last option treatment

strategy has to be investigated by defined cohort or real world studies [37, 38].

In addition to the disease activity as a determining factor in the therapeutic decision, other factors, such as patient personality and cognitive skills, should be taken into consideration. Because of necessary long-term monitoring patient's discipline is demanded, as Alemtuzumab treatment is potentially associated with severe adverse effects which have to be identified early [39].

Keeping in mind that different forms of MS are mediated by different pathological processes, possibly implicating different therapeutical approaches, the diagnosis and classification of MS should be definitely confirmed. Neuromyelitis optica (NMO) which was long been considered as a special form of MS, is associated with different etiology. Alemtuzumab is not considered as a first line treatment option in this disease, as several case reports showed a worsening of NMO under Alemtuzumab treatment [40–42].

As no previous studies have yet compared the efficacy of Alemtuzumab directly with other highly active therapies, such as Natalizumab or Fingolimod, the clinical decision to choose one of the above mentioned medications is largely based on other factors. That would include on top of the list the potential side effects of each drug versus the expected benefit. Additionally the relative and absolute contraindications should be carefully assessed to choose the most suitable drug. For example, patients with positive anti-JCV status represent high-risk group for PML development on longterm Natalizumab treatment [43]. For female patients in child-bearing age, Alemtuzumab can be the choice, but the it should be planned 4 months after the last infusion [44].

There are relative and absolute contraindications for Alemtuzumab treatment, which should be taken into consideration (Table 1).

Patient preparation: pretreatment

The strategy how to initiate the treatment with Alemtuzumab depends on pretreatment status of the patient (Fig. 2). In treatment-naïve MS patients, an immediate start of Alemtuzumab is possible. Moreover, Alemtuzumab treatment accompanied with high dose steroids can itself even be used as an acute relapse treatment. Direct switching from Interferon-beta or Glatiramer Acetate to Alemtuzumab is also possible without any specific washout period if no relevant laboratory abnormalities (for example lymphocytopenia) are present. In case of Teriflunomide and Dimethylfumarate, it is advised to wait at least one month before Alemtuzumab administration, as it is

Table 1 Absolute and relative contraindications of Alemtuzumab

Absolute contraindication

Hypersensitivity to the active substance, or to any of the excipients.

Severe active infections. Additionally, this drug should not be used in the presence of active chronic or recurrent bacterial or viral infections, such as TB, HCV. HBV or HIV.

Pregnancy or lactation.

Relative contraindication

Blood coagulation disorders such as dysfibrinoginemia, factor IX deficiency, hemophilia, von Willebrandt disease, or anti-coagulation therapy.

Significant infection liability, such as aspiration susceptibility or frequent urinary tract infection.

Malignant diseases in the patient history, which is not curatively treated.

Thrombocytopenia.

Negative Varicella-zoster IgG status

Severe liver or kidney insufficiency

Children under 18 years of age

required that the levels of lymphocytes are within normal range (>1.5 GPt/l). It is also recommended to accelerate Teriflunomide elimination by Cholestyramine application and determine its blood concentration before the Alemtuzumab start. Patients stopping Fingolimod should have recovered to physiological absolute lymphocyte counts as well which is an important pharmacodynamics parameter considering the mechanism of action of Fingolimod [45]. In patients switching from Fingolimod, we are not as strict with a recovered absolute lymphocyte count (>1.0 GPt/l) as with Dimethylfumarate (>1.5 GPt/l) as Fingolimod is only affecting lymphocyte redistribution between lymphoid tissues and blood.

Prior therapy with Natalizumab represents a special situation as the switching protocol depends on the actual PML risk which is closely linked to the JCV status and treatment duration [28]. The challenge is to find a way between returning disease activity after Natalizumab and PML risk. Because of the irreversible and acutely immunosppressive mechanism of action of Alemtuzumab, a carryover PML after natalizumab treatment which has been described occurring even up to 6 months after Natalizumab cessation has to be excluded before treatment start [46, 47]. So if there is only a low PML risk which means treatment duration with Natalizumab less than 2 years and/or negative anti-JCV antibodies, a washout period between two and three months is considered sufficient until pharmacodynamic effects of Natalizumab have disappeared. MRI and possibly CSF analysis should be performed as part of the work up as described later. For patients with higher PML risk (JCV antibody positive and treatment duration > 2 years) we recommend a stepwise approach. 3 months after last infusion first MRI should be performed to exclude PML and monitor return of disease activity. If no MRI activity is present, follow up MRI will be performed 4 weeks later which will be repeated until 6 months. If there is MRI activity (or clinical activity) present, CSF analysis with JCV DNA and cell count should be performed before Alemtuzumab is started. This procedure has been applied many times in our clinical practice and can avoid return of clinical activity and makes PML much more unlikely. This means that a strict 6 months washout period cannot be applied in all PML high risk patients on Natalizumab. It is crucial to implement an individual approach for the switch of natalizumab to Alemtuzumab. As irreversible, cell depleting therapy, a carry over of a Natalizumab-associated PML has to be avoided in potential Alemtuzumab patients. In our hands, identifying patients with MRI activity was mostly sufficient to avoid clinical rebound activity as Alemtuzumab demonstrates a rapid onset of action. After immunosuppressive therapies, such as Azathioprine, Cyclosporine A, Mitoxantrone or Cyclophosphamide, which are rarely used nowadays, wash-out period of 3–6 months is necessary in

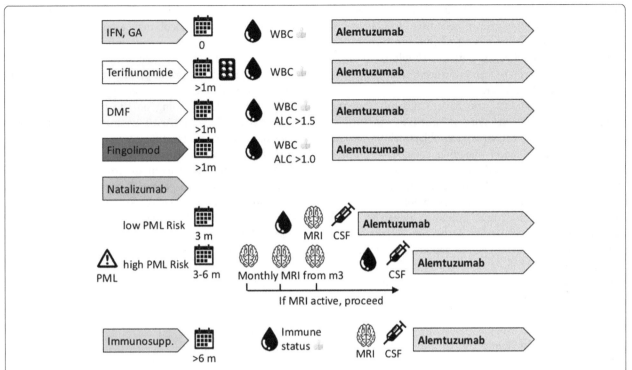

Fig. 2 Recommended protocols for switching to Alemtuzumab, regarding different pretreatments. Special attention should be paid for patients who were previously treated with natalizumab, two different protocols are suggested depending on the individual PML risk

addition to physiological white blood cell counts. Nevertheless patients after immunosuppressive pretreatment are not the ideal patients although case reports have reported beneficial effects [37].

In general, it should be kept in mind that these recommendations are general. In everyday clinical practice we are confronted with special individual patient cases that may require deviation from the general recommendations. These adjustments are justified depending on the individual disease activity and progression, and it is advisable to document the reason for the different approach appropriately [48].

Patient preparation: preparatory steps

Taking into consideration the well-known side-effects and contraindications of Alemtuzumab, a detailed patient history and physical examination should be performed to exclude possible contraindications. Effective treatment should be given in case of acute infections. It is required to wait until the infection is cured before going on with the Alemtuzumab infusion. On the other hand, chronic Infections such HBV, HCV, TBC and syphilis (except HIV) do not represent absolute contraindications, but their presence demands additional carefulness. An active infection should be excluded. In case of a positive quantiferon test, active TBC has to be excluded by chest X-ray and prophylactic treatment with Isoniacid for at least half a year has to be started before Alemtuzumab treatment can begin 6–8 weeks later

[49]. Neoplasms, which are considered as relative contraindication, should be cured before initiating Alemtuzumab treatment. Recommended lab tests before starting treatment with Alemtuzumab are described in Table 2. This workup should be done before every Alemtuzumab infusion later on.

MRI of the complete neuroaxis (not older than three months) should be performed as documentation for baseline status before Alemtuzumab start. All the above-mentioned tests should be accomplished and managed before the first treatment course; and these safety investigations should be repeated prior to the commencement of

Table 2 Recommended lab testing before Alemtuzumab treatment/retreatment

Differential blood count, and optionally an immune status depending on the pretreatment and on the number of lymphocytes

Liver panel including SGOT, SGPT, GGT, bilirubin

Kidney panel including Creatinine, GFR

Thyroid panel including TSH, T3, T4

Infection status including Syphilis, VZV, HIV, hepatitis serology, TB test (eg. Quantiferon test)

Coagulation panel including INR, PTT

Urine panel including quantitative urinalysis by sediment microscopic analysis

HPV screening and pregnancy test in women

Infection screening panel including CRP, BSG

the second treatment course. There are no specific requirements regarding lymphocyte or leukocyte cell counts which have to be reached before second Alemtuzumab course.

Women with childbearing potential should be informed to use an effective contraception during treatment phase and four months thereafter.

Especially for patients who have a history of neither chicken pox infection nor of previous vaccination against Varicella-Zoster virus, it is obligatory to measure its antibodies level before initiating Alemtuzumab treatment. We recommend VZV testing in all patients before Alemtuzumab application. For those who are VZV antibody negative the vaccination should be given, followed by measuring the VZV antibody titer four to six weeks after VZV vaccination. As vaccinations may be complication by the depleting-repleting mechanism of action vaccination status should be checked and necessary vaccinations should be performed before first Alemtuzumab application.

Before first Alemtuzumab treatment, patients should be informed about potential side effects and the need for regular monitoring which is mandatory for a beneficial risk-benefit ratio of Alemtuzumab.

Alemtuzumab infusion management

Treatment with Alemtuzumab consists of at least two courses of infusion therapy with twelve months in between. During the first course ("the induction course") the monoclonal antibody is intravenously infused over five consecutive days with the recommended dose of 12 mg/day. Out of practical reasons it is useful to start the treatment course on Monday to avoid infusions during weekends. One year later, Alemtuzumab is infused in a second course of treatment ("the maintenance course") over three consecutive days. Between the two treatment courses no immunomodulatory treatment should be applied. Shortening the interval between these two courses is not recommended as there is no experience. To reduce the infusion-associated reactions (IAR), a specific schedule of infusion should be applied (Table 3).

The day before Alemtuzumab infusion, H1 and H2 blockade should be initiated which could be applied beyond the infusion week if necessary [30, 50]. An antipyretic, given 30–60 min before infusion, may help to reduce the infusion reaction.

In addition, a short infusion of methylprednisolone (1 g) is recommended for the first three days of treatment. Cytokine release and lymphocyte activation could account for such infusion-associated reactions [51, 52]. Induction of serum cytokines could be due to cross-linking of NK cells in addition to cell lysis [52]. Pivotal studies not using standardized infusion procedure and methylprednisolone pre-treatment demonstrated higher levels of serum cytokines and significant more IARs after initial alemtuzumab infusions [51]. Pre-and concomitant

methylprednisolone treatment incorporated into the standard infusion protocol may attenuate cytokine release syndrome and help reduce infusion-associated reactions to enhance patient tolerance [50]. This protocol is based on the procedure in pivotal studies. However, in deviation from this study experience, the steroid infusion may be adjusted depending on the individual situation and the patient's response. This mean extension over 5 days or potential pretreatment one day before Alemtuzumab infusion which is actually investigated in a clinical trial. If the Alemtuzumab course could not be completed over the consecutive 5 days, if the course has to be interrupted because of eg. acute infection with fever, the remaining Alemtuzumab infusions should be performed as soon as possible in the next weeks. In this case, methylprednisolone should be applied before all remaining Alemtuzumab infusions.

Alemtuzumab infusion should be started after methylprednisolone infusion. Mixing these preparations is not allowed, as this can lead to precipitation of the drug. Alemtuzumab itself is diluted immediately before the infusion in 100 ml of 0.9 % sodium chloride solution or 5 % glucose solution (chemically stable at 2–8 °C for up to 8 h). Other infusions could be applied using the same intravenous port as Alemtuzumab, a paravenous infusion is not critical as Alemtuzumab is a monoclonal antibody and not a chemotherapy. The infusion-associated reactions (IAR) occur in up to 90 % of patients treated with Alemtuzumab [50]. Skin reactions are observed predominantly. With mild symptoms, symptomatic treatment with anti-histamergic treatments or anti-pyretics/anti-inflammatory treatments and slower infusion rate are usually sufficient. In case of severe reactions such as fever, urticaria, atrial fibrillation, nausea, chest discomfort or hypotension, the infusion should be stopped immediately. Because of these potential acute infusion-associated reactions, anaphylaxis therapy should be kept ready although the reaction to Alemtuzumab is generally not anaphylactic, so that the infusion can be further continued. The observation for two hours after the end of the infusion is necessary. In our hand, monitoring of the patient's temperature seems to be an effective method for early detection of an infusion-associated reaction in everyday practice [30]. It is therefore recommended to monitor and document the body temperature every half hour. Heart rate and blood pressure should also be measured every one hour. In addition to this reaction, reappearance of old neurological deficits, which occurred in the context of past relapses, can also occur, which it is caused by the release of cytokines due to cell depletion in a process similar to Uhthoff effect (Cytokine Uhthoff syndrome) [51]. The highest drug level is reached after the last infusion [53]. However, even if this falls in the next few days, its effect with regard to lymphocyte depletion goes on, so that it is still possible to experience reactions related to cells depletion [9].

Table 3 Recommended infusion protocol

Pre-Infusion	Concomitant medication: The evening before the 1st Alemtuzumab infusion for all infusion stages, orally:
	– H1 blockade eg. Cetirizine 1-0-1 (non-sedating H1 antihistamine)
	– H2 blockade eg Ranitidine 300 mg 1-0-1 (H2 receptor antagonist)
	– Herpes prophylaxis eg. Aciclovir 200 mg 1-0-1 (for HSV/VZV prophylaxis; for at least 4 weeks)
Infusion	1st year: infusion 5 days (Mon.-Fri.)
	2nd year infusion 3 days (3 consecutive days)
	Cardiovascular (BP, heart rate) + Body temperature (1×/30 min) Monitoring
	– 1st day of infusion course: Perform pregnancy test in female patients with childbearing potential
	– Insertion of peripheral permanent port (can also be used for other medications)
	1. 60 min. before Alemtuzumab infusion:
	a) Methylprednisolone 1 g i.v. as short infusion at the first 3 infusion days
	b) Paracetamol 1 g. i.v. as short infusion at all infusion days
	2. Alemtuzumab 12 mg i.v. via infusion pump (12 mg per day on each of 5 (or 3) days), is prepared as ready-to-use solution supply (volume 112 mL). Storage time of the infusion 8 h after preparation.
	- Target infusion period about 4 h (in case of side effects-especially at the start of the infusion-reduction of the infusion speed)
	3. NaCl infusion 100 mL over 30 min (infusion pump), to flush residual medication out of the infusion line (tube)
	Also to note:
	– Monitoring until 2 h after infusion
	– Drinking adequate liquids (at least 2 l/d)
	– Availability of trained physician and medical personnel during the entire period of the infusion
Potential acute adverse events	1. Anaphylaxia/anaphylactic shock (quite rare)
	2. Infusion-associated reactions (IAR):
	– Erythema, urticaria, pruritis, (fever, headache, fatigue)
	– Intensified neurological symptoms (Uhthoff Phenomenon!)
	→ STOP infusion and inform physician immediately!
	→ Fenistil 1 A (4 mg) i.v.
	→ In case of insufficient effect → 250 mg prednisolone i.v.
	Depending on severity of the IAR, continue infusion, but more slowly.
Routine follow-up care	1. Aciclovir 200 mg 1-0-1 for 4 weeks from the first day of the infusion
	2. Antihistamine (e.g. cetirizine 1-0-1) for an additional week
	3. Paracetamol standby (if headache or fever appear)
	First check-up appointment MS centre 4 weeks after infusion.
Procedural measures/follow up checks	– Adequate infection protection including adjusting diet (no cheese from raw milk, raw fish/raw meat)
	– During the infusion course, avoid stomach-irritating foods such as fruit acids, carbonates, sharp or strong-smelling foods, no sodium glutamate-"bland diet"
	– If applicable, safe contraception methods for at least 4 months after the infusion course
	– Due to the known potential side effects, the regimen of follow-up check-ups organised and implemented by the MS centre must be strictly observed
	– Patients are instructed to observe a low threshold for making an acute appointment in case of infections. In this respect, the reduced immune competence and reduced lymphocyte count must be considered, especially in the first months after infusion, and a complete focus screening must be conducted.
	– The patient should be informed of the symptoms of possible side effects (eg. ATP, glomerulonephritis), and should inform the treating physician of them. An early appointment with the physician should also be made in case of infection.

Post-infusion monitoring

Alemtuzumab treatment is associated with an increased risk for the development of autoimmune diseases, for this reason a regular monitoring is indicated to allow for an early recognition and thereby early treatment of these diseases [10, 17, 19, 54–57]. Most of the autoimmune phenomena have a beneficial prognosis if they are identified early and anti-inflammatory treatment is started early. So monthly check-ups should take place up to 48 months after the last infusion, including a complete differential blood count to detect the development of Alemtuzumab-induced thrombocytopenic purpura (ATP) [58, 59]. In addition, monthly monitoring of serum creatinine levels and urine tests with microscopy for an early detection of possible glomerulonephritis are necessary [59]. Thyroid function test using the TSH value should also be performed every three months. In pregnant patients with special interest in thyroid monitoring monthly TSH testing is recommended [55, 57, 60].

The monitoring does not need to be performed by the treating neurologist. Good experiences are reported in terms of the cooperation with general practitioners, who can perform or arrange for the check-ups. However, it is essential that the treating neurologist ensures that the control tests are carried out according to previous specifications and the obtained results are evaluated. Treating neurologist has to organize and supervise monitoring after Alemtuzumab treatment. Patients should be clearly informed not to wait for problems to happen, but immediately and regularly communicate with their physician. Modern communication tools as email reminders, smartphone could be nicely implemented in the patient management [61].

Collecting real world data in an alemtuzumab registry

Although the clinical experience with the agent has substantially increased since market introduction, there are only few reports yet on the long-term use of the drug in the routine of physicians and MS centers [10, 16, 44]. That is why real world data about Alemtuzumab data should be collected as the German non-interventional long-Term study foR obsErvAtion of Treatment with Alemtuzumab (TREAT-MS) which is documenting physician and patient experience in daily clinical practice for six years [62]. Data for this non-interventional study will be collected on a widely unselected patient population eligible for Alemtuzumab treatment. It is expected that compared to the clinical studies, patients with more concomitant diseases and/or more concomitant medications will be documented. Together with the high patient numbers and long follow-up period, a substantial number of patient years will be documented and the option for relevant subgroup analyses provided [48].

For this observational study, a protocol was developed based on the risk management plan for alemtuzumab. By participation in the study, physicians are reminded about the investigations and precautions. The documentation system MSDS3D has been shown to be efficient to guide physicians through the study procedures and to collect the relevant information in clinical practice and for the use in previous non-interventional studies such as PANGAEA [63]. It interactively collects data, but also assists neurologists in the execution of complex processes required for comprehensive management of MS patients (Fig. 3a, b) [64–66].

Infections

As infections can be facilitated by cellular depletion of the adaptive and innate immune system together and infusion-associated reaction symptoms like fever, headache, and fatigue may mimic infectious signs, routine blood analysis is usually a suitable tool to identify infectious conditions. But laboratory monitoring during infusion therapy is not needed, and it can even be affected by cell depletion-related artifacts [9]. During the the first infusion week, rapid cellular depletion and impairment of activation of different adaptive and innate immune cell subtypes take place accompanied by marked serum cytokine increases. Nevertheless, these acute Alemtuzumab-mediated effects are assumed to lead to several effects observable by standard blood testing, such as the non-infectious increase in leukocyte count, CRP, and PCT, which are of particular importance in identification and monitoring of infectious conditions. Furthermore, transient elevation of liver enzymes, thrombocytopenia, and TSH modulation are demonstrated. So we recommend clinicians to be aware of clinical symptoms and vital data to initiate supportive analysis rather than standard laboratory testing within the first alemtuzumab treatment week [9].

In general, patients should also be advised to avoid the consumption of raw foods such as raw milk products because of possible contamination with listeria [30]. The ability of Alemtuzumab to deplete dendritic cells as well may explain cases of Listeria meningitis linked to the initial Alemtuzumab infusions [9, 67, 68]. Listeria meningitis infection may be facilitated by immune cell depletion in the adaptive as well as the innate immune system, possibly by an outburst of a pre-existing, clinically silent and CD8+ T cell controlled infection due to cellular depletion and activation blockade. These findings highlight the relevance of certain infections, which could be promoted by the depletion and blockade of innate immune subsets, that clinicians should be aware of within the first days after initial Alemtuzumab infusion.

Patients who have acute or chronic infections should not start with Alemtuzumab therapy. As mentioned above the presence of acute infections under Alemtuzumab therapy

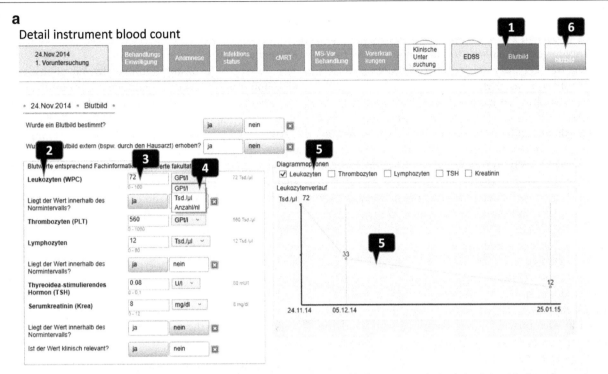

1 – blood count instrument in red state because of clinical significant values 2 – blood count parameter 2 – blood count parameter value 4 – selection of value unit 5 – history of selectable blood count parameter 6 – automatically added checkup blood count due to significant values in previous blood count

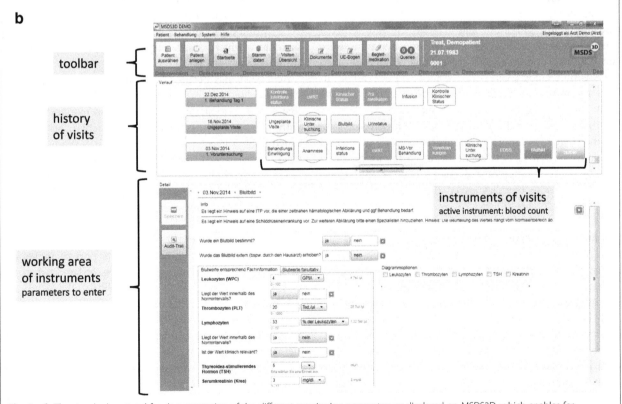

Fig. 3 a/b The standard protocol for documentation of the different monitoring parameters as displayed on MSDS3D, which enables for monitoring laboratory, clinical, and radiological progression, as well as planning the next step in approaching patients who showed abnormalities

demands immediate diagnostic and therapeutic procedures. Taking into consideration that human papilloma virus infections (including cervical dysplasia) were described, it is obligatory for female patients to perform an annual HPV-screening with cervical cytology, especially when no former HPV vaccination was given.

Due to the observed increased rate of herpes infections, prophylaxis with acyclovir is recommended [69]. In the phase 3 clinical studies, this prophylactic regimen was introduced not from the beginning on [4, 6, 59]. But the patients receiving 200 mg of acyclovir twice daily or an equivalent for this purpose demonstrated less herpetic infections. Prophylaxis should begin on the first day of each treatment phase and should be maintained throughout the course of treatment for at least for 1 month. It should be noted that acyclovir can cause several immunological phenomena including rash itself, which has to be differentiated from IARs and could be improved by the transition to a newer treatments, such as Valacyclovir, as an alternative.

In the approval trials infections were moderately increased in Alemtuzumab group compared with interferon group, represented mainly by mild to moderate infections in the upper respiratory tract, gastroenteritis and urinary tract infections [70]. This is a completely different profile compared to hematological patients treated by higher doses of Alemtuzumab demonstrating specific opportunistic infections of immunosuppression [71]. In MS patients, infections were not prolonged and receded under traditional medical therapy. Serious or opportunistic infections were not noticed to be increased. Pre-existing chronic diseases, such as tuberculosis, can be reactivated. No data are available regarding reactivation of controlled chronic HBV/HCV infections. In a recent observation period of 7 years no change in the malignancy rate has been detected [44]. As the thyroid is carefully investigated because of thyroid autoimmunity by eg. ultrasound, a rise in the incidence of thyroid papillary carcinoma diagnosis may be the consequence suggesting overdiagnosis [72].

Autoimmune adverse events

In a recent study for long-term safety evaluation an incidence of 48 % for secondary autoimmune diseases was reported [44]. This is attributed to dysregulated B cells, resulting in secondary autoimmunity [17]. Because of this high incidence of secondary autoimmune diseases, determining biomarkers that can predict which patients are more susceptible to develop secondary autoimmunity is of high importance. Even though a high value of interleukin 21 at baseline could successfully predict the occurrence of autoimmune diseases in Alemtuzumab treated patients, it is inadvisable to rely on these values when taking the treatment decision, because of problems related to the confirmation of results by the currently available kits [18, 19]. An

overview about the lab testing as part of the risk monitoring plan is demonstrated in Fig. 4.

Thyroid disease

The development of autoimmune thyroid diseases is of high importance as it can be detected in more than 35 % of patients treated with Alemtuzumab in the 4 years after first Alemtuzumab infusion [60]. Both hypo- and hyperthyroidism may occur, and the development of Graves' disease was highly prevalent [55].

The peak of incidence is reported to be in the third year after the first dose of Alemtuzumab. Most events are of mild to moderate severity and can respond to conventional therapies. However, surgical intervention may be needed in less than 1 % of patients. The occurrence of thyroids side effects requires careful assessment of the clinical status of the patient and the necessity of medical and/or surgical therapies before continuing Alemtuzumab treatment. According to data derived from clinical studies, the baseline value of anti-TPO antibodies before starting alemtuzumab could not predict the development of thyroid side effects. Almost 80 % of patients who manifested with thyroidal problems after alemtuzumab therapy, showed negative anti-TPO antibody status at the beginning of the study [60].

Alemtuzumab-induced thrombocytopenia

In addition, Alemtuzumab-induced autoimmune-mediated thrombocytopenia was reported in more than 1 % of patients, which represents a form of idiopathic thrombocytopenia (ITP) [26, 58, 73].

Acute ITP has occured in ab to 2 % of the treated patients in clinical MS-studies within 14–36 months after the first exposure to alemtuzumab. ATP can manifest clinically with higher tendency to bruises, petechias, spontaneous mucosal bleedings (epistaxis, hemoptysis), severe or irregular menstrual bleeding or symptoms of anemia due to blood loss including serious hemodynamic complications. Complete blood count including platelet value should be performed monthly over at least 48 months after the last alemtuzumab infusion. The platelet control should be performed weekly in case that platelet count drops to less than 30 % of its initial value or below the normal range, and hematological consultation should be ordered when the platelet number is less than 100.000 GPt/l.

Normally the acute treatment of thrombocytopenia is usually low to high dose corticosteroids, it does not tend to develop a chronic condition. Reports about continuing alemtuzumab therapy after the development of ATP are limited and giving a new alemtuzumab infusion should be assessed on an individual basis [2].

Nephropathies

Nephropathies and individual cases of Goodpasture's syndrome with renal and pulmonary infection were reported

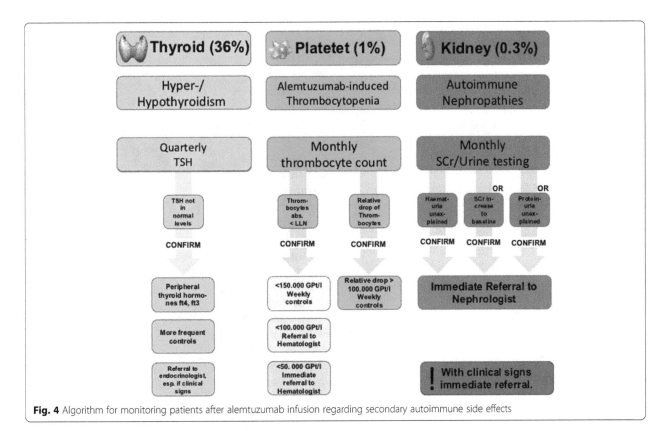

Fig. 4 Algorithm for monitoring patients after alemtuzumab infusion regarding secondary autoimmune side effects

in 0.3 % of the patients [44, 74]. Nephropathies including anti-glomerular basement membrane (anti-GBM) disease, occured in 0.3 % of the patients in clinical MS-studies up to 39 months after the last administration of Alemtuzumab. These cases were early recognized by clinical and laboratory control, so that they could follow favorable course after effective treatment. The development of anti-glomerular basement membrane (anti-GBM) disease without suitable monitoring had led to renal failure, which in case of delayed treatment led to dialysis and/or kidney transplantation. Such side effects can be detected by laboratory monitoring through the presence of hematuria, proteinuria and/or creatinine elevation. Consequently, an urgent specialized nephrological consultation will be necessary.

Vaccinations

The efficacy of vaccines during and closely after Alemtuzumab application can be limited. That is why it is recommended to check the success of the vaccinations by determining their respective titers. The use of attenuated living vaccination should be avoided. Patients should fulfill the vaccination requirements at least six weeks before starting the Alemtuzumab therapy. It should be emphasized that for patients treated with Alemtuzumab the flu-vaccine should be delayed at least six months after the last infusion; however this vaccination can be repeated in case the first vaccination was not efficient.

One pilot study showed that for patients treated with Alemtuzumab the humoral immunological response after different vaccinations was not different from that detected in respective controls [6, 75], implying that the immune competence is restored after lymphocytes depletion induced by Alemtuzumab therapy. This is in line with the data derived from clinical studies which demonstrated low incidence of opportunistic infections following Alemtuzumab infusions. However this study was small and only 5 patients were vaccinated within the first 6 months after Alemtuzumab [16, 76, 77].

Moreover different studies suggested that the long lasting lymphopenia is neither associated with higher incidence of infections nor with higher activity of MS compared with accelerated lymphocyte reconstitution [12, 15, 78].

Pregnancy

No safety data are available till now regarding the potential influence of Alemtuzumab on male fertility. The concerns regarding potential effect on fertility remains not well investigated, as the target antigen CD52 is also found in the tissues of the reproductive system.

Alemtuzumab is contraindicated during pregnancy and lactation, as animal studies have shown reproductive toxicity because Alemtuzumab, as well as human immunoglobulins, can cross the placenta. The same applies during lactation as they can be transferred by breast milk, and the risk to the infant is unknown. Additionally, the increased incidence of autoimmune diseases such as thyroid disease, particularly by the use of Alemtuzumab in women of childbearing age represents potential concern [79].

The development of autoimmune diseases had been observed during the study period within a maximum in the third year after first infusion followed by a decrease in risk [44]. So it makes sense to plan for pregnancy either after this period has passed or before the third year which means 4 months after the second infusion, and then profit from the prolonged high efficiency without the need for additional medication.

Treatment following the 2 Alemtuzumab courses
The majority of MS patients treated with Alemtuzumab do not need additional Alemtuzumab infusions or different MS treatments in the first 5 years after Alemtuzumab treatment. In a recent analysis for ECTRIMS 2015, 68 % of CARE-MS1 and 60 % of CARE-MS2 have not received additional Alemtuzumab infusions. 22.1 % resp. 8.0 % of CARE-MS1 and 28.8 % resp. 9.9 % of CARE-MS2 patients have received one resp. two Alemtuzumab retreatments. In both clinical trials, the threshold for Alemtuzumab retreatment was quite low with one relapse activity or two new T2 lesions resp. one new Gd + lesion in the follow up MRI. If the treatment strategy of Alemtuzumab has been selected after careful consideration, this selected strategy should be generally maintained which means that retreatments should be applied at least once or twice if needed. Every retreatment should be accompanied with careful consideration about retreatment, disease activity, response to Alemtuzumab and additional treatment options. If the patient seems to be an Alemtuzumab-non-responder, alternative treatment strategies should be considered as eg. Fingolimod or B-cell depleting therapies.

In the clinical trials, 2.3 % resp. 7.6 % of the CARE-MS 1 resp. 2 patients have been treated with other MS treatments in the first 5 years after Alemtuzumab start. The majority of these 96 out of 1496 patients used baseline medication (interferon and GA), 10 % each were treated with Fingolimod and Natalizumab. Switching after Alemtuzumab to Interferon-beta or Glatiramer Acetate can be done quite quickly after the last Alemtuzumab infusion after excluding relevant lymphopenia especially for interferon treatment. There is not a lot of experience with the new oral medications Teriflunomide and Dimethylfumarate. Especially with Dimethylfurmarate, the previous immunosuppression with Alemtuzumab has to be considered. By switching to Natalizumab it should be kept in mind that Alemtuzumab leads to significant long-lasting changes in the adaptive immunity cells. As Alemtuzumab works as an immunosuppressive, changing to Natalizumab is associated with higher risk for PML development especially in patients with positive JCV

antibodies. The better treatment option of highly active MS treatments which has already been used in our center is Fingolimod. Because of the individually very different prolonged effect of Alemtuzumab on the adaptive immunity, it is not possible to give a general waiting period after the last Alemtuzumab infusion. A complete immune status can be helpful including differential blood count, CD4+ T cells, CD8+ T cells, B cells, NK cells.

Conclusions
Alemtuzumab is a highly efficacious disease-modifying therapy which offers a new treatment principle for the treatment of relapsing-remitting MS. It shows clear benefits on relapses, disability outcomes, and freedom from clinical disease and magnetic resonance imaging activity. Infusion-associated reactions are common with Alemtuzumab, but rarely serious. Infection incidence was elevated with Alemtuzumab in clinical studies; most infections were mild or moderate in severity. Autoimmune adverse events occurred in approximately a third of patients, manifesting mainly as thyroid disorders, and less frequently as immune thrombocytopenia or nephropathy. A comprehensive monitoring program lasting at least 4 years after the last alemtuzumab dose allows early detection and effective management of autoimmune adverse events. Further experience with alemtuzumab in the clinic will provide needed long-term data.

Authors' contributions
LH and TZ designed and drafted the manuscript. JE and KT added important contact. All authors read and approved the final manuscript.

Competing interests
Tjalf Ziemssen has received reimbursements for participation in scientific advisory boards from Bayer Healthcare, Biogen Idec, Novartis Pharma AG, Merck Serono, Teva, Genzyme, and Synthon. He has also received speaker honorarium from Bayer Healthcare, Biogen Idec, Genzyme, Merck Sharp & Dohme, GlaxoSmithKline, Novartis Pharma AG, Teva, Sanofi Aventis, and Almirall. He has also received research support from Bayer Healthcare, Biogen Idec, Genzyme, Novartis Pharma AG, Teva, and Sanofi Aventis. Katja Thomas received honorarium from Novartis and Bayer. Lina Hassoun and Judith Eisele have no disclosures.

References
1. Coles A, Deans J, Compston A. Campath-1H treatment of multiple sclerosis: lessons from the bedside for the bench. Clin Neurol Neurosurg. 2004;106:270–4.
2. Kousin-Ezewu O, Coles A. Alemtuzumab in multiple sclerosis: latest evidence and clinical prospects. Ther Adv Chronic Dis. 2013;4:97–103.
3. Cox AL, Thompson SAJ, Jones JL, Robertson VH, Hale G, Waldmann H, et al. Lymphocyte homeostasis following therapeutic lymphocyte depletion in multiple sclerosis. Eur J Immunol. 2005;35:3332–42.
4. Cohen JA, Coles AJ, Arnold DL, Confavreux C, Fox EJ, Hartung H-P, et al. Alemtuzumab versus interferon beta 1a as first-line treatment for patients with relapsing-remitting multiple sclerosis: a randomised controlled phase 3 trial. 2012.
5. CAMMS223 Trial Investigators, Coles AJ, Compston DAS, Selmaj KW, Lake SL, Moran S, et al. Alemtuzumab vs. interferon beta-1a in early multiple sclerosis. N Engl J Med. 2008;359:1786–801.
6. Coles AJ, Twyman CL, Arnold DL, Cohen JA, Confavreux C, Fox EJ, et al. Alemtuzumab for patients with relapsing multiple sclerosis after disease-modifying therapy: a randomised controlled phase 3 trial. 2012.

7. Watanabe T, Masuyama J-I, Sohma Y, Inazawa H, Horie K, Kojima K, et al. CD52 is a novel costimulatory molecule for induction of CD4+ regulatory T cells. Clin Immunol. 2006;120:247–59.

8. Xia MQ, Tone M, Packman L, Hale G, Waldmann H. Characterization of the CAMPATH-1 (CDw52) antigen: biochemical analysis and cDNA cloning reveal an unusually small peptide backbone. Eur J Immunol. 1991;21:1677–84.

9. Thomas K, Eisele JC, Rodriguez-Leal FA, Hainke U, Ziemssen T. Acute effects of alemtuzumab infusion in active relapsing remitting multiple sclerosis patients. Neurology: Neuroimmunology & Neuroinflammation. 2016;3, e228.

10. Willis MD, Harding KE, Pickersgill TP, Wardle M, Pearson OR, Scolding NJ, et al. Alemtuzumab for multiple sclerosis: Long term follow-up in a multi-centre cohort. Mult Scler. 2015.

11. Coles AJ, Cox A, Le Page E, Jones J, Trip SA, Deans J, et al. The window of therapeutic opportunity in multiple sclerosis: evidence from monoclonal antibody therapy. J Neurol. 2006;253:98–108.

12. Cossburn MD, Harding K, Ingram G, El-Shanawany T, Heaps A, Pickersgill TP, et al. Clinical relevance of differential lymphocyte recovery after alemtuzumab therapy for multiple sclerosis. Neurology. 2012;80:55–61.

13. Freedman MS, Kaplan JM, Markovic-Plese S. Insights into the Mechanisms of the Therapeutic Efficacy of Alemtuzumab in Multiple Sclerosis. J Clin Cell Immunol. 2013;4.

14. Hu Y, Turner MJ, Shields J, Gale MS, Hutto E, Roberts BL, et al. Investigation of the mechanism of action of alemtuzumab in a human CD52 transgenic mouse model. Immunology. 2009;128:260–70.

15. Kousin-Ezewu O, Parker RA, Tuohy O, Compston A, Coles A, Jones J. Accelerated lymphocyte recovery after alemtuzumab does not predict multiple sclerosis activity. Neurology. 2014;82:2158–64.

16. Hill-Cawthorne GA, Button T, Tuohy O, Jones JL, May K, Somerfield J, et al. Long term lymphocyte reconstitution after alemtuzumab treatment of multiple sclerosis. J Neurol Neurosurg Psychiatr. 2012;83:298–304.

17. Cossburn M, Pace AA, Jones J, Ali R, Ingram G, Baker K, et al. Autoimmune disease after alemtuzumab treatment for multiple sclerosis in a multicenter cohort. Neurology. 2011;77:573–9.

18. Jones JL, Phuah C-L, Cox AL, Thompson SA, Ban M, Shawcross J, et al. IL-21 drives secondary autoimmunity in patients with multiple sclerosis, following therapeutic lymphocyte depletion with alemtuzumab (Campath-1H). J Clin Invest. 2009;119:2052–61.

19. Harding KE, Cossburn M, Robertson N, Compston A, Coles AJ, Jones JL. Predicting autoimmunity after alemtuzumab treatment of multiple sclerosis. J Neurol Neurosurg Psychiatr. 2014;85:795–8.

20. Sørensen PS, Koch-Henriksen N, Petersen T, Ravnborg M, Oturai A, Sellebjerg F. Recurrence or rebound of clinical relapses after discontinuation of natalizumab therapy in highly active MS patients. J Neurol. 2014;261:1–8.

21. Vellinga MM, Castelijns JA, Barkhof F, Uitdehaag BMJ, Polman CH. Postwithdrawal rebound increase in T2 lesional activity in natalizumab-treated MS patients. Neurology. 2008;70:1150–1.

22. La Mantia L, Prone V, Marazzi MR, Erminio C, Protti A. Multiple sclerosis rebound after fingolimod discontinuation for lymphopenia. Neurol Sci. 2014;35:1485–6.

23. Havla JB, Pellkofer HL, Meinl I, Gerdes LA, Hohlfeld R, Kümpfel T. Rebound of disease activity after withdrawal of fingolimod (FTY720) treatment. Arch Neurol. 2012;69:262–4.

24. Piscolla E, Hakiki B, Pasto L, Razzolini L, Portaccio E, Amato MP. Rebound after Fingolimod suspension in a pediatric-onset multiple sclerosis patient. J Neurol. 2013;260:1675–7.

25. Sempere AP, Berenguer-Ruiz L, Feliu-Rey E. Rebound of disease activity during pregnancy after withdrawal of fingolimod. Eur J Neurol. 2013;20:e109–10.

26. Havrdova E, Horakova D, Kovarova I. Alemtuzumab in the treatment of multiple sclerosis: key clinical trial results and considerations for use. Ther Adv Neurol Disord. 2015;8:31–45.

27. Weber MS, Menge T, Lehmann-Horn K, Kronsbein HC, Zettl U, Sellner J, et al. Current treatment strategies for multiple sclerosis-efficacy versus neurological adverse effects. Curr Pharm Des. 2012;18:209–19.

28. Plavina T, Subramanyam M, Bloomgren G, Richman S, Pace A, Lee S, et al. Anti-JCV antibody levels in serum or plasma further define risk of natalizumab-associated PML. Ann Neurol. 2014;76:802–12.

29. Fenu G, Lorefice L, Frau F, Coghe GC, Marrosu MG, Cocco E. Induction and escalation therapies in multiple sclerosis. Antiinflamm Antiallergy Agents Med Chem. 2015;14:26–34.

30. Bayas A, Baum K, Bitsch A, Haas J, Hellwig K, Lang M, et al. One Year Alemtuzumab – What have we Learned in Clinical Practice? Exchange of

31. Experience between Experts on Treatment of Multiple Sclerosis. Akt Neurol. 2015; 42(09):535-41.

31. Lublin FD, Reingold SC, Cohen JA, Cutter GR, Sørensen PS, Thompson AJ, et al. Defining the clinical course of multiple sclerosis: the 2013 revisions. Neurology. 2014;83:278–86.

32. Bermel RA, Naismith RT. Using MRI to make informed clinical decisions in multiple sclerosis care. Curr Opin Neurol. 2015;28:244–9.

33. Ziemssen T, De Stefano N, Pia Sormani M, Van Wijmeersch B, Wiendl H, Kieseier BC. Optimizing therapy early in multiple sclerosis: An evidence-based view. Multiple Sclerosis and Related Disorders. 2015;4:460–9.

34. Ziemssen T, Derfuss T, Stefano N, Giovannoni G, Palavra F, Tomic D, et al. Optimizing treatment success in multiple sclerosis. J Neurol. Springer Berlin Heidelberg; 2015;1–15.

35. Coles AJ, Wing M, Smith S, Coraddu F, Greer S, Taylor C, et al. Pulsed monoclonal antibody treatment and autoimmune thyroid disease in multiple sclerosis. Lancet. 1999;354:1691–5.

36. Leray E, Yaouanq J, Le Page E, Coustans M, Laplaud D, Oger J, et al. Evidence for a two-stage disability progression in multiple sclerosis. Brain. 2010;133:1900–13.

37. Le Page E, Deburghgraeve V, Lester M-A, Cardiet I, Leray E, Edan G. Alemtuzumab as rescue therapy in a cohort of 16 aggressive multiple sclerosis patients previously treated by Mitoxantrone: an observational study. J Neurol. 2015;262:1024–34.

38. Rothenbacher D, Capkun G, Uenal H, Tumani H, Geissbühler Y, Tilson H. New opportunities of real-world data from clinical routine settings in life-cycle management of drugs: example of an integrative approach in multiple sclerosis. Curr Med Res Opin. 2015;31:953–65.

39. Garnock-Jones KP. Alemtuzumab: a review of its use in patients with relapsing multiple sclerosis. Drugs. 2014;74:489–504.

40. Gelfand JM, Cotter J, Klingman J, Huang EJ, Cree BAC. Massive CNS monocytic infiltration at autopsy in an alemtuzumab-treated patient with NMO. Neurology: Neuroimmunology & Neuroinflammation. 2014;1:e34–4.

41. Azzopardi L, Cox AL, McCarthy CL, Jones JL, Coles AJ. Alemtuzumab use in neuromyelitis optica spectrum disorders: a brief case series. J Neurol. 2015;263:1–5.

42. Fujihara K, Nakashima I. Secondary progression and innate immunity in NMO: A possible link to alemtuzumab therapy? Neurology: Neuroimmunology & Neuroinflammation. 2014;1:e38–8.

43. Nali LHDS, Moraes L, Fink MCD, Callegaro D, Romano CM, Oliveira ACP D. Natalizumab treatment for multiple sclerosis: updates and considerations for safer treatment in JCV positive patients. Arq Neuropsiquiatr. 2014;0:0.

44. Tuohy O, Costelloe L, Bjornson I, Harding K, Robertson N, May K, et al. Alemtuzumab treatment of multiple sclerosis: long-term safety and efficacy. J Neurol Neurosurg Psychiatr. 2014;0:1–8.

45. Thomas K, Ziemssen T. Management of fingolimod in clinical practice. Clin Neurol Neurosurg. 2013;115(1):S60–4.

46. Berger JR, Centonze D, Comi G, Confavreux C, Cutter G, Giovannoni G, et al. Considerations on discontinuing natalizumab for the treatment of multiple sclerosis. Ann Neurol. 2010;68:409–11.

47. Hauser SL, Johnston SC. Balancing risk and reward: the question of natalizumab. Ann Neurol. 2009;66:A7–8.

48. Ziemssen T, Hillert J, Butzkueven H. The importance of collecting structured clinical information on multiple sclerosis. BMC Med. 2016;14:81.

49. Diel R, Hauer B, Loddenkemper R, Manger B, Krüger K. Recommendations for tuberculosis screening before initiation of TNF-alpha-inhibitor treatment in rheumatic diseases. Pneumologie. 2009;63:329–34.

50. Caon C, Namey M, Meyer C, Mayer L, Oyuela P, Margolin DH, et al. Prevention and Management of Infusion-Associated Reactions in the Comparison of Alemtuzumab and Rebif ®Efficacy in Multiple Sclerosis (CARE-MS) Program. Int J MS Care. 2015;17:191–8.

51. Moreau T, Coles A, Wing M, Isaacs J, Hale G, Waldmann H, et al. Transient increase in symptoms associated with cytokine release in patients with multiple sclerosis. Brain. 1996;119(Pt 1):225–37.

52. Wing MG, Moreau T, Greenwood J, Smith RM, Hale G, Isaacs J, et al. Mechanism of first-dose cytokine-release syndrome by CAMPATH 1-H: involvement of CD16 (FcgammaRIII) and CD11a/CD18 (LFA-1) on NK cells. J Clin Invest American Society for Clinical Investigation. 1996;98:2819–26.

53. Rebello P, Hale G. Pharmacokinetics of CAMPATH-1H: assay development and validation. J Immunol Methods. 2002;260:285–302.

54. Klotz L, Berthele A, Bruck W, Chan A, Flachenecker P, Gold R, et al. Monitoring of blood parameters under course-modified MS therapy: Substance-specific relevance and current recommendations for action. Nervenarzt: Springer Berlin Heidelberg; 2016. p. 1–14.

55. Tsourdi E, Gruber M, Rauner M, Blankenburg J, Ziemssen T, Hofbauer LC. Graves' disease after treatment with Alemtuzumab for multiple sclerosis. Hormones (Athens). 2015;14(1):148–53.

56. Williams KM, Dietzen D, Hassoun AA, Fennoy I, Bhatia M. Autoimmune thyroid disease following alemtuzumab therapy and hematopoietic cell transplantation in pediatric patients with sickle cell disease. Pediatr Blood Cancer. 2014;61(12):2307–9.

57. Aranha AA, Amer S, Reda ES, Broadley SA, Davoren PM. Autoimmune Thyroid Disease in the Use of Alemtuzumab for Multiple Sclerosis: A Review. Endocr Pract. 2013;11:1–25.

58. Cuker A, Coles AJ, Sullivan H, Fox E, Goldberg M, Oyuela P, et al. A distinctive form of immune thrombocytopenia in a phase 2 study of alemtuzumab for the treatment of relapsing-remitting multiple sclerosis. Blood. 2011;118:6299–305.

59. Jones JL, Coles AJ. Mode of action and clinical studies with alemtuzumab. Exp Neurol. 2014;262:37–43.

60. Daniels GH, Vladic A, Brinar V, Zavalishin I, Valente W, Oyuela P, et al. Alemtuzumab-Related Thyroid Dysfunction in a Phase 2 Trial of Patients With Relapsing-Remitting Multiple Sclerosis. J Clin Endocrinol Metab. 2014;99:80–9.

61. Haase R, Schultheiss T, Kempcke R, Thomas K, Ziemssen T. Use and acceptance of electronic communication by patients with multiple sclerosis: a multicenter questionnaire study. J Med Internet Res. 2012;14, e135.

62. Ziemssen T, Engelmann U, Jahn S, Leptich A, Kern R, Hassoun L, et al. Rationale, Design, and Methods of a Non-interventional Study to Establish Safety, Effectiveness, Quality of Life, Cognition, Health-Related and Work Capacity Data on Alemtuzumab in Multiple Sclerosis Patients in Germany (TREAT-MS). BMC Neurol. 2016. in press.

63. Ziemssen T, Kern R, Cornelissen C. The PANGAEA study design–a prospective, multicenter, non-interventional, long-term study on fingolimod for the treatment of multiple sclerosis in daily practice. BMC Neurol BMC Neurology. 2015;18:1–8.

64. Ziemssen T, Kempcke R, Eulitz M, Großmann L, Suhrbier A, Thomas K, et al. Multiple sclerosis documentation system (MSDS): moving from documentation to management of MS patients. J Neural Transm. 2013;120 Suppl 1:61–6.

65. Rieckmann P, Boyko A, Centonze D, Elovaara I, Giovannoni G, Havrdova E, et al. Achieving patient engagement in multiple sclerosis_ A perspective from the multiple sclerosis in the 21st Century Steering Group. Multiple Sclerosis and Related Disorders. 2015;4:202–18.

66. Schultheiß T, Kempcke R, Kratzsch F, Eulitz M, Pette M, Reichmann H, et al. Multiple sclerosis management system 3D: Moving from documentation towards management of patients. Nervenarzt: Springer Berlin Heidelberg; 2011.

67. Rau D, Lang M, Harth A, Naumann M, Weber F, Tumani H, et al. Listeria Meningitis Complicating Alemtuzumab Treatment in Multiple Sclerosis–Report of Two Cases. IJMS. 2015;16:14669–76.

68. Thomas K, Dietze K, Wehner R, Metz I, Tumani H, Schultheiss T, et al. Accumulation and therapeutic modulation of 6-sulfo LacNAc (+) dendritic cells in multiple sclerosis. Neurology: Neuroimmunology & Neuroinflammation. 2014;1:e33–3.

69. Morrison VA. Immunosuppression associated with novel chemotherapy agents and monoclonal antibodies. Clin Infect Dis. 2014;59(5):S360–4.

70. Coles AJ. Alemtuzumab therapy for multiple sclerosis. Neurotherapeutics. 2013;10:29–33.

71. Safdar N, Smith J, Knasinski V, Sherkow C, Herrforth C, Knechtle S, et al. Infections after the use of alemtuzumab in solid organ transplant recipients: a comparative study. Diagn Microbiol Infect Dis. 2010;66:7–15.

72. Ibitoye R, Wilkins A. Thyroid papillary carcinoma after alemtuzumab therapy for MS. J Neurol. 2014;261(9):1828–9.

73. Brown W, Coles A. Alemtuzumab: evidence for its potential in relapsing– remitting multiple sclerosis. Drug Des Devel Ther. 2013;7:131.

74. Coles AJ, Fox E, Vladic A, Gazda SK, Brinar V, Selmaj KW, et al. Alemtuzumab more effective than interferon-1a at 5-year follow-up of CAMMS223 Clinical Trial. Neurology. 2012;78:1069–78.

75. McCarthy CL, Tuohy O, Compston DAS, Kumararatne DS, Coles AJ, Jones JL. Immune competence after alemtuzumab treatment of multiple sclerosis. Neurology. 2013;81:872–6.

76. Zhang X, Tao Y, Chopra M, Ahn M, Marcus KL, Choudhary N, et al. Differential Reconstitution of T Cell Subsets following Immunodepleting Treatment with Alemtuzumab (Anti-CD52 Monoclonal Antibody) in Patients with Relapsing-Remitting Multiple Sclerosis. J Immunol. 2013; 191:5867–74.

77. Robertson NP, Scolding NJ. Immune reconstitution and treatment response in multiple sclerosis following alemtuzumab. Neurology. 2014;82:2150–1.

78. Tchao NK, Turka LA. Lymphodepletion and homeostatic proliferation: implications for transplantation. Am J Transplant. 2012;12:1079–90.

79. Vukusic S, Marignier R. Multiple sclerosis and pregnancy in the 'treatment era'. Nat Rev Neurol. 2015;11:280–9.

4

Epidemiology of MS in Russia, a historical review

A. Boyko[*], N. Smirnova, S. Petrov and E. Gusev

Abstract

Background: This review summarizes several epidemiological studies of multiple sclerosis (MS) in Russia.

Methods: The Authors selected the most well-organized population-based studies of MS prevalence and incidence in the huge territory of Russia. These studies were mostly published in Russian language and were unknown to international readers.

Results: In the majority of Russian territories MS prevalence ranged from 30 to 70 cases per 100,000 population inhabitants. At most places where the epidemiology of MS had been assessed more than once, an increase in prevalence has been reported over time. Incidence showed fluctuations with an increase in Eastern parts of the country. This increased prevalence despite a relatively stable incidence in the European part of the country may reflect the increased survival of the MS population.

Conclusions: Russia as a whole can be considered at medium risk for MS. Significant increase of prevalence rates have been recently reported, especially in Siberia and in the Far East regions of the country.

Keywords: Multiple sclerosis, Epidemiology, Prevalence rates, Russia

Background

One of the most striking epidemiological characteristics of MS is the distribution of the disease across the world. The traditional view, based on numerous early studies and reviews, is that MS is particularly prevalent in low temperate zones, less common in subtropical zones, and uncommon in tropic zones. Both in the Northern and Southern hemisphere the characteristic pattern have been increasing prevalence towards the poles, although deviations from this pattern can be seen both in Europe and North America as well as in Australia and New Zealand. This distribution suggests an interplay between at least three overlapping factors, a) the genetic makeup of a population; b) geographically determined environmental factors; and c) socio-economic conditions, including access to medical facilities. Data from the former USSR and late from Russia have never been reported so far in the English literature. In 1960-1970's, the prevalence of MS on the huge territory of the former Soviet Union was reported as at "probably high risk of MS". Ten years later, the famous world distribution MS map by John Kurtzke had no definite information on the majority of regions of the Soviet Union [20]. A first review was performed in 1994 and was mainly based on hospital registers. Although a number of factors may have affected the validity of these first observations, including inconsistencies of diagnostic facilities among different territories [2, 3], bad cases ascertainment, differences in ethnic features, high migration rate and different epidemiological methods. In any case, overall MS prevalence was reported in the low to medium frequency range [23, 26].

Since then, the availability of medical service has had a profound impact on the diagnostic accuracy and probability ascertainment, and these factors have improved in most parts of the world and have been more uniform throughout the last three to four decades. After the 1990s, the quality of medical care and the availability of diagnostic methods, including MRI, has become uniform in all Russian territories. A special national program on MS epidemiology was launched in 2002 and new studies, performed according to generally accepted methodologies, provided new information which could be compared with previous studies [5, 6]. The structure and design of these studies were established by a special

* Correspondence: boykoan13@gmail.com
Department of Neurology, Neurosurgery and Medical Genetics of the Prigorov's Russian National Research Medical University and MS Center at Neuroclinica at the Usupov's Hospital, Moscow, Russia

Recommendation of the Russian Ministry of Health Care [11]. Recently the majority of these studies were reviewed [12]. The goal of this publication is to present data on MS prevalence and incidence in Russia, which were published previously only in Russian language.

Materials and methods

Russia is the largest country in the World. Its territory is 17.1 million of km^2 and it accounts approximately for 1/8 of the land mass of the Earth. One third of this country in located in Europe, while 2/3 belongs to Asia. Climate in Russia is quite heterogeneous. For example, in Sochi – Olympic capital of 2014 – average winter temperature is +5 °C, i.e. a temperate zone; Novosibirsk, the biggest city of Siberia with a population of 1.5 million, shows an average winter temperature of – 15 °C; at the same time in Oimyakon area of Yakutia, known as the "cold pole", the average winter temperature is – 61 °C: obviously, people cannot live or work in such low temperature. Approximately 20 % of the Russian population resides in the 13 biggest cities: Moscow, St Petersburg, Novosibirsk, Nizhniy Novgorod, Yekaterinburg, Samara, Omsk, Kazan, Chelyabinsk, Rostov-on-Don, Ufa, Volgograd, Perm. The largest cities of Russia are located in the European part of the country – Moscow (11.54 million) and Saint-Petersburg (4.8 million), while more than 10 million are living in the republics of the Northern Caucasus. With 145 million people Russia is the seventh most populated nation in the world. While some 79 % of the residents are Russians, more than 160 ethnic groups live in this huge territory (each of them carrying its own genetic predisposition to MS), including Tatars (20 %), Ukrainians (10 %), Bashkirs (6 %), Chuvash (6 %), Chechen (5 %), Armenians (4 %), and Mordva (3 %). In Russia there are 1147 women per 1000 men [7]. This overrepresentation of women becomes more evident from 33 years of age on. Russia is young country, with a mean population age of 38.8 years in 2010, 36.1 in men and 41.1 in women. The oldest inhabitants are in the Central European area (in the city of Tula mean 42.2 years old, 38.5 for men and 45.2 for women), the youngest in Northern Caucases (in the Ingushetia republic, mean age is 29.6 years old; 28.8 for men and 30.4 for women). Able-bodied population (men 16-59 age and women 16-54 age) is 89,0 million (61 %), while the remaining is either younger – 26,3 million (18 %) – or elder – 29,8 million (21 %). For Russia, as for most European countries, progressive ageing of inhabitants is increasingly common. According to the national census of 1989, mean age of the population is 34,7 years; 31,9 for man, 37,2 for woman [7]. Since then, mean age of residents has increased by 3 years and reached 37,7 years; 35,2 for man,

40,0 for woman. Literacy in Russia is 99 %. There are about 3 million students and 567 institutes of higher education including 48 universities.

The National program on MS epidemiology in Russia was started in 2002. The first step was to establish a network of MS Centers covering the entire country, using as a model the successful Moscow MS Center (established in 1998). The program mostly contemplates two actions: descriptive epidemiology – i.e. analysis of prevalence and incidence using unified methodology of population-based studies and analytical epidemiology – case-control studies in different populations analyzing environmental risk factors for MS, case-control pairs matched by age, gender, ethnicity and place of birth. All studies are conducted using a unique methodology that includes the validated questionnaire proposed by the Oslo International Think-tank on MS Epidemiology published in Neurology in 1997 [4].

At present more than 90 studies analyzing MS prevalence and incidence in periods between 1980 and 2013 have been published within this program: they may be compared with some of the best quality studies, done in the 1970-1980 decade. Is several regions (Moscow, Novosibirsk, Blagoveshensk) longitudinal observations for 30 and more years have been done. For this review we have selected data from 68 population-based studies of the best quality from different regions of Russia. These studies used unified design of data collection, evaluation of MS clinical course and methods of statistical analysis.

Results

The majority of studies used clinical Poser diagnostic criteria while more recent studies, performed after 2005 (7 from 68 to 10.3 %), used the 2001 McDonald criteria. Generally, MS prevalence varied from 10 to 70 cases per 100,000 population with higher MS frequencies at the West, East and Central parts of the country (Fig. 1). A lower prevalence was recorded in Northern areas and in the Far East of Russia, where a low population density and higher representation of populations of Asian origin including Northern tribes, still less affected by MS, occurs.

Data from some of the studies done in different time periods are presented in the Table and show that there is a general tendency of increasing of MS prevalence almost everywhere in Russia. Explanations for this worldwide occurring phenomenon include: 1) better cases ascertainment because of early diagnosis with a percentage increase of mild cases; 2) free access to DMT, active symptomatic and antibacterial therapy extending the life of MS patients; and 3) no loss of information about these patients because of the general use of MS-registers and electronic data-bases. This improved

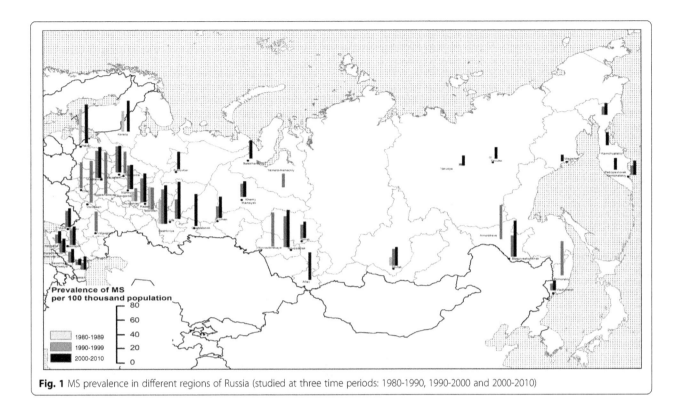

Fig. 1 MS prevalence in different regions of Russia (studied at three time periods: 1980-1990, 1990-2000 and 2000-2010)

management has certainly increased life expectancy and reduced the percent of severely affected MS patients.

The most striking increase of MS prevalence and incidence was noted in Eastern Siberia and in the Far East, where MS frequency increased among third generation of migrants from the European part of Russia. The risk of MS appears to be very homogeneous and varies from 20 to 60 cases per 100,000 population [6] with the majority of populations predominantly Russian, Ukrainian or from other European Caucasoid origin (e.g. Slavonics). Table 1 includes prevalence data from the East to the West of the Russian Federation; Table 2 includes incidence data.

Eastern and Central part of Russia

The most recent rates of MS prevalence vary from 35 cases per 100,000 in Kostroma up to 67 in Voronezh. Recent MS incidence rates were 2.8 in Yaroslavl and 2.6 in Moscow region, 2.1 in Voronezh, 2.0 in Kostroma and 1.9 in Orel and Nizhniy Novgorod cities [13, 15, 18]. An increase in MS incidence in the Yaroslavl region was seen from 1975 (0.5 per 100,000 population) up to mean 3.0 between 1996 and 2001 (highest rate: 3.1 in 1998) but then decreased to 2.5 between 2001 and 2006 [15]. In the Moscow region, MS incidence was 2.1 between 1995 and 2000 and rose to 2.6 between 2001 and 2006 [6].

Volga river region

The ethnicity of the population of this area is very different from the Moscow region, with many non-Slavic ethnic groups (Turks) – Tatars, Bashkirs, Chuvashes, as well as the Finno-Ugric group – Mari and Udmurts. MS epidemiological studies in this area showed lower incidence and prevalence rates compared to the Central region of the country with some variation. For example, in Bashkiria the lowest MS prevalence rate reported was 21 per 100,000 population but up to 79 per 100,000 in Northern parts of the republic (the highest in recent studies). Surprisingly, MS prevalence in Ufa, the capital of this republic, was the highest among the Tatars (36.4 per 100,000), intermediate in Russians (near 23 per 100,000), and lowest in Bashkirs (9 per 100,000) [1]. By comparison, at the Moscow region MS is significantly less frequent in Tatars then in Russians. Mean MS incidence in these republics were 2.6 per 100,000, the highest in the city of Kazan (2.9 per 100,000) [14, 19].

Southern parts of Russia and the Northern Caucasus

In these areas rates are again lower than in the Central part of Russia, varying from 20 to 35 per 100,000 [30], while in some cities the mean MS incidence was very high: in the past few years it increased up to 9.8 in 2000-2005 period in the city of Volgograd [8]. In the neighboring Rostov, region the prevalence of MS also varies from district to district with the lowest – 19.5 per 100,000 – in the rural eastern part, and the highest – 53.6 per 100,000 – in the northwestern part with industrial enterprises and cities [10]. MS is relatively rare in

Table 1 MS prevalence in Russia at different time periods

Cities/regions	1980-1989	1990-1999	2000-2010
Eastern and Central parts of Russia (near 50 mlns of population, 90 % Slavonik)			
Karelia	30		45
Pskov	55		62
Moscow		44	55
Orel		42	
Yaroslavl		42	43
Kostroma		35	
Voronezh		67	
Nizhniy Novgorod		38	39
Ryazan		61	
Volga-river regions (near 30 mlns of population, 40 % Slavonik, 50 % Turks, 10 % others)			
Republic of Tatarstan		32	33
Kazan (capital of Tatarstan)		38	46
Republic of Bashkiria	35	50	56
Northern parts of Bashkiria		79	
Ufa (capital of Bashkiria)		31	59
Republic of Chuvashia	14	19	
Southern parts of Russia and the Northern Caucuses (near 30 mlns of population, 40 % Slavonik, 60 % others – ethnic groups of the Northern Caucuses)			
Stavropol		24	30
Rostov-na-Dony		26	30
Volgograd		32	
Republic of Karachaero-Cherkessia		17	20
Republic of Dagestan		10	19
Republic of Adigea		13	18
Republic of Northern Osetia		16	20
Republic of Chechnya		5	9
Ural region and the Western Siberia (near 10 mlns of population, 70 % Slavonik, 30 % others)			
Tyumen		19	34
Chanti-Mansiysk region		21	25
Yamalo-Nentskyi region		20	
Salechadr			29
Tomsk		22	27
Siktivkar			28
Cheliabinsks			51
Novosibirsk		50	60
The Eastern Siberia and the Far East (near 5 mlns of population, 80 % Slavonik, 20 % others)			
Irkutsk	14	27	30
Blagoveshensks		34	58
Amur region		50	
Yakutsk	4		19

Table 1 MS prevalence in Russia at different time periods *(Continued)*

Altay region		40
The Primorsk region	10	17
Vladivostok	11	16
The Northern part of Sakhalin		19
The Southern part of Sakhalin		17
The Northern part of Kamchatka	12	17
The Southern part of Kamchatka	15	23
Magadan		11

the republics of the Northern Caucuses with MS prevalence less than 20 at majority of sites (Table 1).

Ural region and the Western Siberia

Several population-based studies were recently completed in the Tyumen region and in the city of Novosibirsk. The Tyumen region is divided in three parts: the Northern Yamal region, scarcely populated, where 6.8 % of the population descends from the Northern tribes (Nentsi, Mansy, Khanti and others) and shows a medium level MS prevalence – 27.8 per 100,000 [27, 28]. Conversely, the Khanti-Mansi region, consistently more populated and with only

Table 2 Some recent MS incidence rates in Russia (according to latest published data)

Cities	MS incidence
Eastern and Central parts of Russia	
Moscow	2.6
Orel	1.9
Yaroslavl	2.8
Voronezh	2.1
Nizhniy Novgorod	1.9
Volga-river regions	
Kazan	2.9
Ufa	2.0
Southern parts of Russia and the Northern Caucuses	
Stavropol	1.8
Rostov-na-Dony	1.5
Volgograd	9.8
Ural region and the Western Siberia	
Tyumen	1.8
Tomsk	2.1
Novosibirsk	3.5
The Eastern Siberia and the Far East	
Irkutsk	1.6
Blagoveshensks	2.1
Yakutsk	1.2

1.5 % of the population coming from the Northern tribes – has an MS prevalence of only 14.3 per 100,000. The highest prevalence, close to 40.5 per 100,000, was found in the Southern part of the region with mostly populated by Russians and hosting many chemical factories. A very important result of this study was the first recorded cases of definite MS in the Northern tribes – overall the prevalence in this area was 2.8 per 100,000 population (highest in Komi-Ziriane ethnic group – up to 16 per 100,000) [29].

A retrospective study covering 25 years in Novosibirsk demonstrated a significant increase in MS incidence in this territory between 1980 and 2000 that rose from 1.6 up to 5.4 cases per 100,000 [21]. Current incidence in this area has stabilized between 2.5 and 3.5 cases per 100,000 population. MS prevalence here in one the highest in the entire Siberia region – near 60 cases per 100,000 population [22].

The Eastern Siberia and the Far East

A population-based study was performed in Yakutia. Previous studies in this area were completed in the 1980's, apparently based mainly on hospital cases. MS prevalence (2.1 per 100,000) and incidence (0,2 per 100,000) were reported to be extremely low. The first MRI scanner in this region started to work in 1993. The first clinically definite MS case according to Poser criteria in native Yakuts was reported only in 1995, with the first autopsy confirmed MS case obtained in 1998. In the following years native Yakuts witnessed a surge of the disease in their community. More than half young cases were women with numerous lesions at spinal cord at early stages of the disease ("Asian" type of MS). Between 2000 and 2005 the rates in Russians were higher than in Yakuts, but in this ethnic group the prevalence rate was 13.4 per 100,000 in the city and 4.2 per 100,000 in rural regions, while the incidence was 1.8 and 0.4, respectively. Mean MS prevalence in 2002-2007 was 19 cases per 100,000 [24]. MS incidence at the Amur region varied from 2.8 in 1980-1985 to 0.3 in 2000-2005 [16, 17]. Overall, MS prevalence (1985-2010) varied in this area from 30 to 50 cases per 100,000 [25]. Recent studies of MS prevalence and incidence at the Far East region show relatively low frequencies with MS prevalence from 11 to 23 cases per 100,000 population [9].

Conclusions

This short review shows that the majority of territories of Russia fall into the medium MS risk zone with a prevalence ranging mostly from 30 to 70 cases per 100,000 population. At most places where the prevalence of MS has been studied on more than once, a definite increase has occurred, similarly to the rest of the Western world [26]. Incidence rates displayed a fluctuating trend, with a clear-cut increase in Eastern parts of the country. This increased prevalence, despite a relatively stable incidence in

the European part of the country, may be partially due to an increased survival of the patients as a result of a combination of positive changes. An overall improved medical care, more complete ascertainment procedures and differential emigration of unaffected people [MS was more frequent in Caucasoids Slavoniks then in non-Caucasoid ethnic groups (Turks, Yarutes, etc.)] were all considered as possible contributing factors.

Although an influence of environmental factors must be taken into consideration in determining the sketchy epidemiology if MS in Russia, our data do not allow strong conclusions. The influence of temperature could not be properly assessed because of instability and great variations at the majority of the regions. The increase of MS prevalence in the third generation of the migrants to the Far East suggest a role for ecological and other unknown urban factors. Improvement in diagnosis and/or case ascertainment could certainly lead to a technology-driven increased incidence and prevalence rates, especially in the1980-1990 period. Therefore, the data on increase in incidence of MS across this time period should be interpreted with caution. The correction for delay in ascertainment may be inaccurate to some degree. On the other hand, it is now evident that many territories and ethnic groups from Russia, thought to be free of MS, actually display low and medium levels of MS prevalence.

In conclusion, for this review we have selected population-based, peer-reviewed studies of MS prevalence and incidence in Russia, performed according to modern technology. We are not providing age-standardized, ethnic-specific or sex-specific data, which were not recorded in the majority of the studies. A further analysis and classification of the data presented in Russian-speaking literature along with consistently designed, perspective epidemiological studies are clearly needed to clarify the complex scenario of MS in the Russian confederation.

Authors' contributions
AB reviewed and analyzed literature data, selection the most appropriate, prepared the manuscript. NS participated in data collection and helped to draft the manuscript. SP participated in data collection and the figure preparation. EG participated in the design of the study and manuscript preparation. All authors read and approved the final manuscript.

Competing interests
The authors declare that they have no competing interests.

References
1. Bakhtiiarova KZ, Magzhanov RV. Multiple sclerosis in ethnic groups of Bashkortostan Republic. Zh Nevrol Psikhiatr Im S S Korsakova. 2006;3:17–21. (in Russian).

2.   Boyko AN. Multiple sclerosis prevalence in Russia and other countries of the former USSR. In: Firnhaber W, Lauer K, editors. Multiple sclerosis in Europe: an epidemiological update. Alsbach: LTV Press; 1994. p. 219–30.

3.   Boyko AN. Epidemiology of multiple sclerosis in Russia and other countries of the former Soviet Union: investigations of environmental and genetic factors. Acta Neurol Scand. 1995;91(Suppl161):71–6.

4.   Boyko A. Guidelines for questionnaires to be used in case-control studies of MS. In: The epidemiologic study of exogenous factors in the ethiology of multiple sclerosis. Riise T, Wolfson C (eds.) Neurology. 1997, 49, 2 (Suppl.2) :S75–S80.

5.   Boyko A, Zavalishin IA, Spirin NN, et al. Epidemiology of MS in Russia: first data of United Study of Multiple sclerosis epidemiology in Russia. Mult Scler. 2004;10(Supl):157.

6.   Boyko AN. Epidemiology of MS in Russia. Mult Scler. 2009;15:S15.

7.   Demographic statistics in Russia, Rosstat, 2010. 157p (in Russian).

8.   Dokuchaeva NN, Boyko AN. Clinical and epidemiological study of multiple sclerosis in Volgograd city. Zh Nevrol Psikhiatr Im S S Korsakova. 2006;3:4–10. (in Russian).

9.   Gavrilenko AA, Evdokimova ZS, Vasilkovskaya GA, Boyko AN. Epidemiology of multiple sclerosis in Primorsky Krai and the Far East regions. Zh Nevrol Psikhiatr Im S S Korsakova. 2012;2:5–8. (in Russian).

10. Goncharova ZA, Balyazin VA. Risk factors of multiple sclerosis development in the population of the Rostov region. Zh Nevrol Psikhiatr Im S S Korsakova. 2009;7:10–5. (in Russian).

11. Gusev EI, Boyko AN, Zavalishin IA et al. Epidemiological studies of multiple sclerosis. Methodological recommendations of the Ministry of Health Care of Russian Federation. №2003/82, Moscow; 2003.

12. Gusev EI, Zavalishin IA, Boyko AN. Multiple sclerosis. Moscow: Guide for neurologists; 2011. (in Russian).

13. Horoshilova NL. Prevalence and risk factors of a multiple sclerosis in the Orel city. Kursk: Thesis on candidate of medical sciences; 2005. (in Russian).

14. Ishmanova SA. Environmental and internal factors defining features of clinic and current of a multiple sclerosis. Kazan: Thesis on candidate of medical sciences; 2003. (in Russian).

15. Kachura DA. Clinical research of a multiple sclerosis on model of a city population of the Yaroslavl area. Ivanovo: Thesis on candidate of medical sciences; 2003. (in Russian).

16. Karnauch VH. Dynamics and clinical presentation of multiple sclerosis in Amur region for the period of 1960 to 2005. Zh Nevrol Psikhiatr Im S S Korsakova. 2009;7:75–8. in Russian.

17. Karnauch VN. Multiple sclerosis in Amur region – 35-year prospective study (epidemiology, clinical course and prognosis). Irkutsk: Thesis on doctor of medical sciences; 2011. (in Russian).

18. Kim ER. The clinical characteristic and epidemiology a multiple sclerosis in the Nizhniy Novgorod area. Nizhniy Novgorod: Thesis on candidate of medical sciences; 2004. (in Russian).

19. Kondratyeva OS. Prevalence and socially-ecomonic features of multiple sclerosis in the Republic of Tatarstan. Kazan: Thesis on candidate of medical sciences; 2003. (in Russian).

20. Kurtzke JF. Epidemiology of multiple sclerosis. In: Koetsier JC, editor. Handbook of clinical neurology, vol.3 (47). Amsterdam: Elsevier; 1985. p. 259–87.

21. Malkova NA. Epidemiology and clinical course of multiple sclerosis (20 years prospective research in Western Siberia). Novosibirsk: Thesis on doctor of medical sciences; 2005. (in Russian).

22. Malkova NA, Shperling LP, Riabukhina OV, Merkulova EA. Multiple sclerosis in Eastern Siberia: a 20-year prospective study in Novosibirsk city. Zh Nevrol Psikhiatr Im S S Korsakova. 2006;3:11–6. (in Russian).

23. Marrie RA. Environmental risk factors in multiple sclerosis aetiology. Lancet Neurol. 2004;3:709–18.

24. Minurova AR. Clinical and epidemiological study of multiple sclerosis in Yakutia. Moscow: Thesis on candidate of medical sciences; 2008 (in Russian).

25. Molchanova EE. Risk factors and epidemiology of a multiple sclerosis on model of a city population of the Amur area. Vladivostok: Thesis on candidate of medical sciences; 2002. (in Russian).

26. Pugliatti M, Rosati G. Epidemiology of multiple sclerosis. In: Multiple sclerosis: a comprehensive text. CS Raine, HF McFarland, R Hohlfeld (eds). Elsevier; 2008. p. 126–34.

27. Sivertseva SA. Epidemiological and immunogenetic features of a multiple sclerosis in the Tyumen region. Moscow: Thesis on doctor of medical sciences; 2009. (in Russian).

28. Sivertseva SA, Zhuravlyov MN, Muravyov SA, Boyko AN. Epidemiology of a multiple sclerosis in the Tyumen area. Zh Nevrol Psikhiatr Im S S Korsakova. 2006;3:22–5. (in Russian).

29. Sivertseva SA, Kandala NS, Zhuravlev MN, et al. Multiple sclerosis in the native population of Yamal. Zh Nevrol Psikhiatr Im S S Korsakova. 2010;1:97–9.

30. Trinitatskij JV. Clinical and MRI data in diagnosis and treatment of a multiple sclerosis. Moscow: Thesis on doctor of medical sciences; 2003. (in Russian).

5

The still under-investigated role of cognitive deficits in PML diagnosis

Cristina Scarpazza[1,2], Nicola De Rossi[1], Lucia Moiola[3], Simonetta Gerevini[4], Mirco Cosottini[5], Ruggero Capra[1], Flavia Mattioli[2*], on behalf of the Italian PML Group

Abstract

Background: Despite cognitive deficits frequently represent the first clinical manifestations of Progressive Multifocal Leukoencephalopathy (PML) in Natalizumab-treated MS patients, the importance of cognitive deficits in PML diagnosis is still under-investigated. The aim of the current study is to investigate the cognitive deficits at PML diagnosis in a group of Italian patients with PML.

Methods: Thirty-four PML patients were included in the study. The demographic and clinical data, the lesion load and localization, and the longitudinal clinical course was compared between patients with ($n = 13$) and without ($n = 15$) cognitive deficit upon PML suspicion (the remaining six patients were asymptomatic). Clinical presentation of cognitive symptoms was described in detail.

Result: After symptoms detection, the time to diagnosis resulted to be shorter for patients presenting with cognitive than for patients with non cognitive onset ($p = 0.03$). Within patients with cognitive onset, six patients were presenting with language and/or reading difficulties (46.15%); five patients with memory difficulties (38.4%); three patients with apraxia (23.1%); two patients with disorientation (15.3%); two patients with neglect (15.3%); one patients with object agnosia (7.7%), one patient with perseveration (7.7%) and one patient with dementia (7.7%). Frontal lesions were less frequent ($p = 0.03$), whereas temporal lesions were slightly more frequent ($p = 0.06$) in patients with cognitive deficits. The longitudinal PML course seemed to be more severe in cognitive than in non cognitive patients ($F = 2.73$, $p = 0.03$), but differences disappeared ($F = 1.24$, $p = 0.29$) when balancing for the incidence of immune reconstitution syndrome and for other treatments for PML (steroids, plasma exchange (PLEX) and other therapies (Mefloquine, Mirtazapine, Maraviroc).

Conclusion: Cognitive deficits at PML onset manifest with symptoms which are absolutely rare in MS. Their appearance in MS patients should strongly suggest PML. Clinicians should be sensitive to the importance of formal neuropsychological evaluation, with particular focus on executive function, which are not easily detected without a formal assessment.

Keywords: Progressive multifocal leukoencephalopathy, Natalizumab, Cognition, Neuropsychological impairment, Italian database

* Correspondence: flaviacaterina.mattioli@gmail.com
[2]Neuropsychology Unit, Spedali Civili di Brescia, Via Nikolajewka 13, 25123 Brescia, Italy
Full list of author information is available at the end of the article

Background

Progressive multifocal leukoencephalopathy (PML) is an uncommon brain disease emerging in the setting of immune deficiency [1], caused by the reactivation of the John Cunningham virus (JCV) in the brain. Despite widely studied in HIV patients [1], in the last decade PML has also been observed in Multiple Sclerosis (MS) patients treated with Natalizumab (NTZ) [2]. Critically, the infection is present in the brain before the occurrence of the first clinical symptoms [3, 4], thus a delay in PML recognition and Natalizumab cessation can often occur. Furthermore, due to the relative lack of specificity in PML related neurological symptoms, the occurrence of new focal deficits can be misinterpreted as a MS relapse. As rapid immune reconstitution by removal of Natalizumab appears to determine prognosis, early diagnosis is mandatory [5].

Focal neurological syndromes as well as neuropsychological deficits are described as presenting symptoms in PML [3, 6, 7], but the prevalence of specific cognitive disorders as distinctive signs of PML in differential diagnosis with other MS related cognitive impairments has not been yet clarified. Dong-Si et al. [8] described 372 PML patients, who experienced during the course of PML cognitive/behavioral or speech symptoms in 75.5% of the cases. However, these data refer to a later stage of the PML course. In Clifford et al. [6] series, 57.1% of the patients showed cognitive, behavioral or speech symptoms at PML onset, but no specifications about the nature of cognitive deficits were provided by the authors. Finally, Hoepner et al. [7] showed that, although only half of the patients with PML complained of cognitive deficits, all of them demonstrated neuropsychological impairment at formal evaluation, suggesting a higher prevalence of cognitive impairment than what was subjectively reported. However, the authors did not consider aphasia as a cognitive deficit, and described only 8 PML patients, thus limiting the generalizability of the results. Hence, the importance of cognitive deficits in PML diagnosis is still underinvestigated.

The current paper describes the neuropsychological symptoms at onset and the longitudinal clinical course of a group of Italian MS patients treated with Natalizumab, who experienced PML, with the aim to better identify the possible peculiar aspects of PML related cognitive symptoms. The current study includes 34 Natalizumab treated MS patients who developed PML between 2009 and 2015 and were retrospectively collected from 25 Italian MS sites. Firstly, the whole sample has been analyzed. Secondly, we focused on patients presenting with cognitive deficits and compared their demographic and clinical features with those ones of patients presenting with other symptoms at PML diagnosis. Moreover, for patients with cognitive symptoms at onset, we considered the type of neuropsychological deficits reported the possible anatomo-clinical correlation between lesion location and the neuropsychological deficit.

Methods
Patients inclusion

An Italian, independent spontaneous collaborative repository initiative made a registry for the collection of patients with MS treated with NTZ who developed possible or definite PML according to the American Academy of Neurology criteria [8], as described in detail elsewhere [9]. In the current paper, the data from 25 Italian MS Centers, which took part to the initiative were included, resulting in 34 PML patients who received diagnosis of definite PML between 2009 and June 2015. To our knowledge, one NTZ-PML italian patient with was not included in the registry since he/she denied his consent for data sharing.

In each Center patients were regularly followed-up, and their data were retrospectively collected from members of the Italian PML group, were included in a centralized database and were stored by the MS centre of Montichiari (Brescia). The retrospective analysis of patients' data was approved by the ethical committee of the Spedali Civili of Brescia and was conducted in accordance with specific national laws and the ethical standards laid down in the 1964 Declaration of Helsinki and its later amendments.

Data collection

A detailed description of the data collected is present elsewhere [9]. Here, we only describe the data relevant for the current paper, extracted from patient charts.

Demographic data included: gender; age at NTZ start; age at PML diagnosis.

Clinical data included: disease duration (years); previous immune suppression; total number of NTZ infusions; annual relapse rate (ARR) in the year before NTZ start and during NTZ treatment; symptomatic or asymptomatic PML (i.e. detection of PML lesions at brain MRI scan in presence or absence of new signs or symptoms respectively); number of JCV-DNA copies detected with quantitative polymerase chain reaction performed on cerebrospinal fluid sample at PML suspect; clinical symptom (if any) manifested at PML suspect; diagnosis delay, defined as days elapsed between the day when the treating neurologist become aware of the symptomatology and the day in which cerebrospinal fluid was sampled for JCV search; whether or not a neuropsychological (NPS) formal assessment has been performed; longitudinal Expanded Disability Status scores (EDSS [10]) collected at NTZ start (hereafter referred as baseline), at PML diagnosis (M0), at 2 months (M2), 6 months (M6) and 12 months (M12) from PML diagnosis; whether or not patients were treated with steroids, plasma exchange (PLEX) and other therapies (Mefloquine, Mirtazapine, Maraviroc).

Magnetic resonance images (MRI) data included: lesion patterns classified as unilobar (confined to one lobe), multilobar (involving two or more contiguous lobes), widespread (involving two or more non-contiguous lobes and/ or present in both hemispheres) [11] and infratentorial [9]; lesion localization; presence or absence of the radiological features of immune reconstitution inflammatory syndrome (IRIS) as defined in Prosperini et al. [9].

Statistical analysis
First, we present the data of the whole sample ($n = 34$). Secondly, we compared patients with and without cognitive onset.

Categorical variables are expressed as count (percentage) and continuous variables as mean (SD) or median (range), as appropriated. Between-group differences were tested using the Chi-squared or the U Mann-Whitney test/ two independent sample t-tests for categorical and continuous variables, respectively.

The EDSS scores distribution at all time intervals were not different from a normal distribution (Kolmogorov-Smirnov tests, all ps > .20). A repeated measures (RM) ANOVA with Group (two levels: Cognitive; no Cognitive) as between subjects variable and Time (5 levels: NTZ beginning; Baseline; M2; M6; M12) as within subjects variable was used in order to compare the longitudinal clinical course of patient with or without cognitive deficits. Plasma exchange, therapy with steroids and other therapies (i.e. Mirtazapine, Mefloquine, Maraviroc) were included in the model as covariates, in order to remove their effects from the results. Newmann-Keuls post hoc test was used when necessary.

Results
Whole group analysis ($n = 34$)
Socio-demographic and clinical data
The 34 patients consisted in ten males and 24 females, with a mean age of 41.7 ± 9.3 years. The mean EDSS at PML diagnosis is 4.9 ± 2.0. The mean number of infusions of NTZ before PML onset was 36.94 ± 17.0 (range 11–78). Annualized Relapse Rate resulted significantly lower in the NTZ treatment interval than in the pre NTZ period (0.13 vs. 1.76, respectively, $t = 9.76$, df = 66, $p < 0.001$), confirming NTZ efficacy in reducing the progression of the MS disease in terms of relapses. The mean time elapsed between the symptoms onset and the PML diagnosis was 50.2 ± 31.4 days. The mean number of viral copies in the whole sample was 1750 ± 4682 copies/mL, ranging from 10 to 5174 copies/mL with an outlier patient with 26300 viral copies/mL. IRIS emerged in 24 out of 34 patients (70.5%). The survival rate was 91%: at one-year follow up 31 out of 34 patients were still alive. One patient died

within the first 6 months from PML onset due to the complication of acute acalculous cholecystitis, while two patients died within 1 year from PML onset due to IRIS complications. All of them were symptomatic at PML onset. Twenty-three out of 34 (67.6%) of PML patients developed IRIS.

Lesion load and localization at PML onset
the MRI scan was available for 31 out of 34 patients. For the three remaining patients, the MRI scan was acquired but images were not available and information were obtained from the neuroradiologist' s report. Thirteen (38.2%) patients had a unilobar lesion at PML onset; 9 (26.4%) had multilobar lesions; 6 (17.6%) had widespread lesions and 6 (17.6%) had infratentorial lesion (cerebellum or brainstem). Within the encephalic lesions (i.e. excluding the brainstem lesions, $n = 28$), occipital lesions were present in six patients (21.4%), temporal lesions in 12 patients (42.8%), parietal lesions in 11 patients (39.2%), frontal lesions in 17 patients (60.7%) and diencephalic lesions in three patients (10.7%). Thus, frontal lesions were preminent within this cohort of patients.

Clinical presentation of PML
Six patients (17.6%) were asymptomatic, while 28 (82.3%) manifested ≥1 symptom. Within this group, ten patients (35.7%) presented with pure cognitive symptoms; three patients (10.7%) with cognitive and motor symptoms; six patients (21.42%) with pure motor symptoms; three patients (10.7%) with symptoms indicative of brainstem involvement; two patients (7.14%) with both motor and brainstem symptoms; two patients (7.14%) with epilepsy; one patient (3.5%) with visual loss and one patient (3.5%) with hallucination.

Longitudinal clinical course
The RM ANOVA on longitudinal EDSS scores revealed a main effect of the variable Time (F[4132] = 25.25, $p < 0.001$). Post hoc tests highlight an EDSS worsening between NTZ beginning (mean:3.89) and PML onset (4.98, $p < 0.001$), which is likely to reflect PML insurgence. EDSS at NTZ beginning is also better than EDSS at the following observations (all ps < 0.001). EDSS at PML diagnosis (4.98) better than EDSS at M2 (5.94, $p < 0.001$), M6 (6.39, $p < 0.001$) and M12 (6.04, $p < 0.001$), while no difference between M2, M6 and M12 emerged (all ps > 0.21).

Patients with cognitive symptoms at PML onset ($n = 13$)
Socio-demographic and clinical data
Table 1 presents the comparison between the demographic and clinical features of PML patients who had a cognitive symptom at onset ($n = 13$) and the remaining patients with a symptomatic onset without cognitive symptoms ($n = 15$). The two groups do not differ in any

Table 1 Demographic and clinical features of patients with and without cognitive deficit at PML diagnosis

	Cognitive onset	No cognitive onset	
	$n = 13$	$n = 15$	Significance
Gender (♂)[a]	7 (53.8%)	14 (93.3%)	0.016*
Age at MS diagnosis[b]	25.6 (11.5)	23.3 (10.3)	0.414
Age at PML diagnosis[b]	39.0 (14.1)	37.5 (13.8)	0.584
MS duration (years)[b]	12.9 (7.3)	12.0 (9.6)	0.740
Number of infusions [b]	33.0 (19.5)	34.5 (20.0)	0.856
Prior Immunesoppression[a]	5 (34.7%)	4 (29.4%)	0.505
Viral Load[c]	324 [12–26300]	64 [11–4403]	0.271
IRIS insurgence (yes)[a]	11 (84.6%)	8 (53.3%)	0.077
Steroids administration (yes)[a]	12 (92.3%)	14 (93.3%)	0.912
Other therapies (yes)[a]	8 (61.5%)	10 (66.6%)	0.825
PLEX (yes)[a]	11 (84.6%)	8 (53.3%)	0.077

Number denotes row number ([a]), mean (standard deviation) ([b]) and median [range] ([c]). Statistical significance was evaluated using Chi Square ([a]), two independent samples t test ([b]) and Mann Whitney test ([c]). *asterisk denotes statistical significance

of clinical and demographic features considered but gender. IRIS, though not significantly, appears to be more frequent in patients with cognitive onset ($p = 0.077$). Plasma Exchange (PLEX) results to be slightly more frequently administered in patients with cognitive onset ($p = 0.077$). Two patients within the cognitive onset and one patients within the non cognitive onset group died.

Of note, the time elapsed between the symptoms onset and the PML diagnosis significantly differs between patients with cognitive onset and patients with non cognitive onset, being significantly shorter for patients with cognitive onset (27.5 ± 27.2 days) than for patients with non cognitive onset (56.6 ± 39.7, two independent t test = 2.24, df = 26, $p = 0.03$).

Lesion load and localization at PML onset

MRI scan was available for 12 out of 13 patients. For the remaining patient, MRI was acquired but images were not available and information were obtained from the neuroradiologist' s report. Four (30.6%) patients had a unilobar lesion at PML onset; 5 (38.4%) had multilobar lesions; 3 (23.0%) had widespread lesions and 1 (7.6%) had infratentorial lesion (cerebellum). Within the supratentorial lesions, occipital lesions were present in four patients (33.3%), temporal lesions in nine patients (75%), parietal lesions in six patients (50%), frontal lesions in three patients (25.0%) and diencephalic lesions in one patient (8.3%). Interestingly, frontal lesions were hypo-represented in patients with cognitive onset compared with the whole cohort (25.0% vs 60.7%, chi square = 4.28, p = 0.03), whereas temporal lesions were hyper-represented

within patients with cognitive onset (42.8% vs 75%, chi square = 3.48, $p = 0.06$). Lesions are shown in Fig. 1.

Clinical presentation of cognitive PML

Table 2 shows the PML lesion site at MRI, the type of neuropsychological deficits manifested and/or complained by the patients, the possible anatomo clinical correlation between the lesion site and the cognitive deficit. Six patients (46.15%) presented language and/or reading difficulties (from mild anomia to severe aphasia); five patients (38.4%) memory difficulties; three (23.1%) patients apraxia; two patients (15.3%) disorientation; two patients (15.3%) neglect; one patients (7.7%) object agnosia, one patient (7.7%) perseveration and one patient (7.7%) dementia. An at least partial anatomo-clinical correlation was present in 12/13 patients. Moreover, in the table was also specified how the symptoms were detected. Formal neuropsychological (NPS) assessment has been conducted in 10 out of 13 patients (76.9%). In five out of ten of these cases we were provided with the NPS tests performed (reported in Table 2), whereas in the remaining five cases, only a clinical description of the cognitive deficits manifested by patients was available. In particular, NPS assessment was performed in seven cases (53.84%) because of patient's complaint, in one case (7.7%) upon observation of neuropsychological symptoms during the neurological examination, whereas in two patients (15.3%) the deficits were found during their routing monitoring.. In the remaining three cases, NPS deficit was diagnosed basing on patient complaint only (one case), evidence of the deficit during neurological examination only (one case) and both patient's complain and evidence during neurological examination (one case).

Longitudinal clinical course

The longitudinal clinical course in terms of disability of patients with and without cognitive symptoms at onset is shown in Fig. 2. The RM ANOVA on longitudinal EDSS scores revealed a significant Group x Time interaction (F[4104] = 2.73, $p = 0.03$). Post hoc tests highlight different clinical course in the two groups. Indeed, in patients without cognitive impairment at PML onset, the EDSS at NTZ beginning (mean 4.36) is slightly better than the EDSS at PML diagnosis (5.4, $p = 0.06$), and is better than the EDSS at M2 (5.83, $p = 0.009$), M6 (6.36, $p < 0.001$) and M12 (5.93, $p = 0.008$). However, EDSS at PML diagnosis do not differ from EDSS at all the following observations (all ps > 0.15) and no differences in EDSS between M2, M6 and M12 emerged (ps > 0.34). On the contrary, in patients with cognitive impairment at PML diagnosis, EDSS at NTZ beginning (mean 3.92) is better than EDSS at PML diagnosis (5.3, $p = 0.009$), M2 (6.9, $p < 0.001$), M6 (7.3, $p < 0.001$)

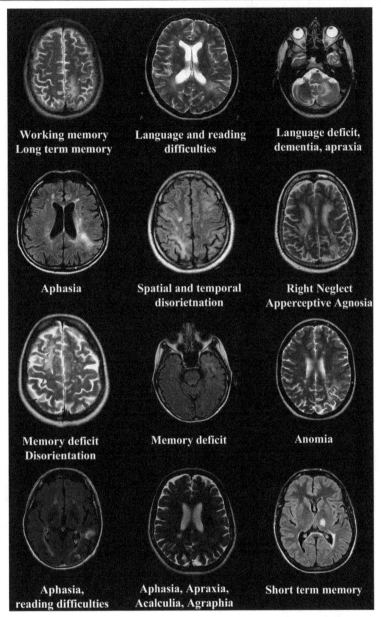

Fig. 1 For each patient with cognitive onset is represented the lesion localization and the presenting symptom. The MRI images are available for 12 out of 13 patients. The data of the last patient, reported in Table 2, was derived from the neuroradiologist's report

and M12 (7.11, $p < 0.001$). Statistical worsening also emerged between EDSS at PML diagnosis at EDSS at M2 ($p = 0.008$), M6 ($p < 0.001$) and M12 ($p = 0.002$). No differences in EDSS between M2, M6 and M12 emerged (ps > 0.55).

The RM ANOVA was repeated using gender, IRIS insurgence and PLEX as covariates, in order to remove their effects on the results. Including these covariates into the ANOVA, the ANOVA is no more significant ($F[4,92] = 1.24$, $p = 0.29$), i.e. no differences in EDSS between patients with and patients without cognitive onset was found.

Discussion

Despite the high prevalence of cognitive deficit at PML diagnosis, their importance on the clinical point of view and their diagnostic relevance has often been neglected. In the present observational study, we aimed at describing the main features of patients presenting with cognitive symptoms, in order to underline the possible identification of specific symptoms as red flag for PML, and to compare their clinical course with that oneof patients presenting with different symptoms at PML diagnosis. The current paper provides several interesting findings, namely, the prevalence and type of cognitive

Table 2 Anatomo-clinical correlation and diagnosis details

	Lesion site	Cognitive deficit	Anatomo clinical correlation	How symptoms were detected	Neuropsychological tests
1	L_Parietal	Verbal memory	X	Patient's complain + formal NPS assessment	N/A
2	L_Tempo Parietal	Language and reading deficits	X	Evident at neurological examination	-
3	L_Cerebellum	Language deficit, dementia, apraxia	-	Patient's complain + formal NPS assessment	Mini mental state examination; Language test, apraxia test, drawing test
4	L_Temporal	Aphasia	X	Evident at neurological examination + formal NPS assessment	N/A
5	Bilateral Fronto temporo and Parietal	Spatial and temporal disorientation + perseveration + apraxia + left neglect	X	Patient's complain + formal NPS assessment	Mini mental state examination for disorientation; Apraxia test; drawing test; Verbal fluency; Line bisection
6	L_Parieto occipital	Right neglect Objects' Agnosia	X	Patient's complain + formal NPS assessment	Line bisection; Apraxia test; Agnosia test
7	R_ Fronto temporal	Memory deficit Disorientation	X	Patient's complain	-
8	L_Insula, ippocampus and parahippocampus (temporal lobe)	Memory deficit	X	Patient's complain + formal NPS assessment	N/A
9	L_Parieto-temporal occipital	Anomia + semantic paraphasias	X	Patient's complain + formal NPS assessment	Verbal fluency
10	L_Temporo occipital	Aphasia, reading difficulties	X	Patient's complain + Evident at neurological examination	-
11	L_Temporo parietal	Aphasia, acalculia, apraxia, agraphia	X	Patient's complain + formal NPS assessment	Aachener Aphasia test; Apraxia test; drawing test; acalculia test
12	L_ Thalamus	Memory	X	formal NPS assessment	N/A
13[a]	R_Fronto-temporo occipital	Memory and attention	X	formal NPS assessment	N/A

For each patient is reported: the PML lesion site, the type of cognitive deficits manifested and /or complained by the patients, the possible anatomo clinical correlation between the lesion site and the neuropsychological difficulties and how the symptoms have been diagnosed. [a]the MRI is missing (neuroradiological report provided). *L* left, *R* right, *NPS* neuropsychological, *N/A* not available

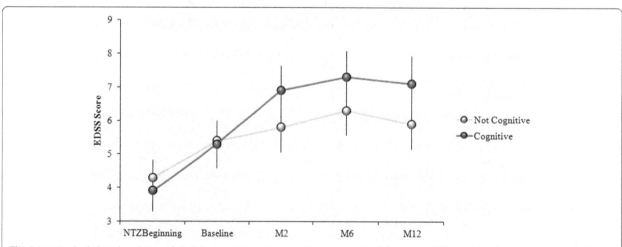

Fig. 2 Longitudinal clinical evolution of disability in patients with and without cognitive deficits upon PML suspicion. Bars denotes standard error of the mean

deficit in our population, the time-to-diagnosis of PML; the PML lesion localization and the anatomo-clinical correlation.

13 out of 34 (38.2%) MS patients with Natalizumab associated PML were presenting with cognitive deficit as a suggestive symptom of PML onset. This percentage is lower than the one reported by Clifford et al. [6], who showed a percentage of 57.1% of cognitive onset, although without any specification of the nature of cognitive deficits. On the other hand, in our sample, though limited, the symptoms were carefully described at individual level and reported mainly as disorders in memory, attention, neglect, reading, calculation, naming or orientation. Unfortunately, neuropsychological tests were available for a minority of patients and the performed test widely differed across patients, thus preventing a better analysis and interpretation of neuropsychological tests scores.

Another interesting finding is that the aforementioned cognitive deficits are not peculiar of MS patients' cognitive impairment. Indeed, typical cognitive impairment in MS is described as a general cognitive slowdown and mainly involves information processing speed, attention, working memory and executive functions [12, 13], which are likely to worsen with the disease evolution [14], typically sparing language and orientation. Furthermore, neglect, acalculia, apraxia agraphia are notably not peculiar of MS patients. Since these symptoms are absolutely rare in MS, their appearance in MS patients treated with NTZ should be considered as a red flag and should give rise to a suspicion of PML, thus prompting a rapid MR scan. Indeed, evidences are now available regarding the positive effects of NTZ on cognitive deterioration of MS patients over long follow ups, as well as on cognitive improvement of MS patients treated with NTZ over time [15–21]. Furthermore, a rebound of cognitive impairment has also been described following natalizumab discontinuation [22]. For these reasons, any new cognitive symptom emerging during treatment with Natalizumab should alert the treating neurologist to consider a potential sign of PML.

Another interesting finding is that amongst the 28 symptomatic PML cases, we observed a shorter time to diagnosis in patients presenting with cognitive symptoms than in those ones presenting with other symptoms. We may speculate that cognitive and behavioral changes, differently from new or worsening motor symptoms, alerted clinicians toward a possible PML diagnosis. Similarly to newly appearing MRI lesions in NTZ treated patients, any new cognitive symptom or symptoms occurring beyond the first year of treatment should be considered with suspicion [23]. However, fluctuations of motor function, which are frequent in patients with MS and sometimes misinterpreted as MS relapses, could

have delayed PML diagnosis [24]. Literature data report that another diagnosis is considered before PML in nearly two-thirds of PML patients, and that more than three-quarters of PML patients suffered from diagnostic delay, irrespective of their underlying immunosuppressive condition [25].

As we reported shorter time to diagnosis in patients with cognitive presentation compared to those without cognitive presentation, consequently smallest lesion size, less viral copies and presumably better prognosis would be expected in the cognitive onset sample of patients, which was not the case. The possible interpretation of this mismatch is that, in our opinion, cognitive deficits' identification really occurred late in its course, maybe due to the lack of a careful neuropsychological investigation and assessment in the majority of the patients. This may have caused a delay in the "red flag" recognition by the neurologists and, as a consequence, larger lesions, more viral copies and worse prognosis in patients with cognitive presentation. What is worth noting is the need of sensitizing both physicians and patients toward the appearance/worsening of cognitive deficit, that might be also subtle and difficult for the patients to understand and describe, and for the neurologist to detect, in particular if related to the frontal lobe.

Furthermore, lesion analysis in PML patients with cognitive onset revealed that the anatomo-clinical correlation was present in the large majority of cases, even when the lesion size was small; thus giving strength to the clinical diagnosis of such cognitive deficit. Similarly to Richert et al. [11], we also found in the whole PML group of patients a prevalence of frontal lesions at PML onset; on the other hand, considering PML patients with cognitive symptom at onset only, a prevalence in temporal lesions was found. It is possible that some cognitive signs of prefrontal involvement could have been under-diagnosed by clinicians: noteworthy frontal signs may be less clinically evident, particularly in the right hemisphere. It might also be possible that, for this reason, in our patients with PML without cognitive symptoms at onset, and even in the asymptomatic one, some peculiar neuropsychological deficits would have been present and not clinically detected.

Finally, a careful neuropsychological examination in MS patients assuming NTZ should be regularly performed, including not only tests measuring attention, information processing speed and memory, but also executive functions, language, visual exploration and scales assessing a possible behavioral abnormalities. This could reveal early cognitive deficits suggestive of PML and allow the neurologist to quickly obtain MR scans, CSF sampling for JCV searching and withdrawing natalizumab if a strong suspicion of PML is present. It is worth noting that formal neuropsychological evaluation with appropriate tests would not only allow an accurate measure of cognitive deficits, but also its repetition over follow up would be able to monitor the evolution of these deficits over time.

Conclusions

Cognitive deficits at PML onset present with symptoms that are absolutely rare in MS, such as apraxia, aphasia, neglect, disorientation. Their appearance should strongly suggest PML. Clinicians should be sensitized about the importance of formal neuropsychological evaluation, with particular focus on executive function, which are not easily detected without a formal assessment. Patients should be sensitized as well to tell the doctor every, even small, change in their clinical status.

Abbreviations

ARR: Annualized relapse rate; EDSS: Expanded disability status score; IRIS: Immune reconstitution inflammatory syndrome; JCV: John Cunningham virus; M12: Observation at twelve months from PML diagnosis; M2: Observation at two months from PML diagnosis; M6: Observation at six months from PML diagnosis; MRI: Magnetic resonance images; MS: Multiple sclerosis; NPS: Neuropsychological; NTZ: Natalizumab; PLEX: Plasma exchange; PML: Progressive multifocal leukoencephalopathy; RM ANOVA: Repeated measures analysis of variance

Acknowledgements

We would like to acknowledge all the members of the Italian PML group, who shared the data of patients. In alphabetic order: Maria Pia Amato; Carlo Alberto Artusi; Fabio Bandini; Valeria Barcella; Antonio Bertolotto; Vincenzo Bresciamorra; Marco Capobianco; Guido Cavaletti; Paola Cavalla; Diego Centonze; Marinella Clerico; Cinzia Cordioli; Giangaetano D'Aleo; Marilena de Riz; Luciano Deotto; Luca Durelli; Mario Falcini; Ernesta Ferrari; Maria Luisa Fusco; Claudio Gasperini; Angelo Ghezzi; Luigi Grimaldi; Mario Guidotti; Alice Laroni; Alessandra Lugaresi; Paola Naldi; Chiara Pane; Patrizia Perrone; Matteo Pizzorno; Carlo Pozzilli; Luca Prosperini; Monica Rezzonico; Marco Rovaris; Giuseppe Salemi; Marco Salvetti; Giuseppe Santuccio; Elio Scarpini; Edoardo Sessa; Claudio Solaro; Giulia Tabiadon; Carla Tortorella; Maria Trojano; Paola Valentino.

Funding

This studies was not funded.

Authors' contributions

CS: conception and design of the study, analysis and interpretation of the data; drafting a significant portion of the manuscript/figures; NDR: acquisition of the data, analysis and interpretation of the clinical data; SG: analysis and interpretation of the MRI data; LM: acquisition of the data, analysis and interpretation of the clinical data; MC: analysis and interpretation of the MRI data; RC: conception and design of the study, drafting a significant portion of the manuscript/figures. FM: conception and design of the study, drafting a significant portion of the manuscript/figures. All the authors has been involved in revising the manuscript critically for important intellectual content. All the authors read and approved the final manuscript.

Competing interests

Dr. Scarpazza declares that she have no competing interests. Dr. De Rossi received speaker honoraria from Biogen and Teva and travel grants from Biogen, Teva and Merk Serono. Dr. Moiola received honoraria for speaking or for advisory board from Sanofi-Genzyme, Biogen, Novartis and Teva. Dr. Gerevini received speaker honoraria from Biogen. Dr. Cosottini received speaker honoraria from Biogen. Dr. Capra received consulting fees from Novartis, Biogen and lecture fees and/or travel grants from Novartis,

Biogen, Genzyme and Sanofi-Aventis. Dr. Mattioli received travel grants from Merck Serono and advisory board honoraria from Novartis.

Author details

[1]Multiple Sclerosis Centre, Spedali Civili di Brescia, Via Ciotti 154, 25018, Montichiari, Brescia, Italy. [2]Neuropsychology Unit, Spedali Civili di Brescia, Via Nikolajewka 13, 25123 Brescia, Italy. [3]Department of Neurology, San Raffaele Scientific Institute, Vita-Salute San Raffaele University, Via Olgettina 60, 20132 Milan, Italy. [4]Department of Neuroradiology, Institute of Experimental Neurology, Division of Neuroscience, San Raffaele Scientific Institute, Vita-Salute San Raffaele University, Via Olgettina 60, 20132 Milan, Italy. [5]Department of Translational Research and of New Surgical and Medical Technologies, University of Pisa, Via Paradisa 2, Pisa (IT) 56124, Italy.

References

1. Pavlovic D, Patera AC, Nyberg F, Gerber M, Liu M, Consortium PML. Progressive multifocal leukoencephalopathy: current treatment options and future perspectives. Ther Adv Neurol Disord. 2015;8(6):255–73.
2. Dong-Si T, Gheuens S, Gangadharan A, Wenten M, Philip J, McIninch J, et al. Predictors of survival and functional outcomes in natalizumab-associated progressive multifocal leukoencephalopathy. J Neurovirol. 2015;21(6):637–44.
3. Dong-Si T, Richman S, Wattjes MP, Wenten M, Gheuens S, Philip J, et al. Outcome and survival of asymptomatic PML in natalizumab-treated MS patients. Ann Clin Transl Neurol. 2014;1(10):755–64.
4. Clifford DB. Neurological immune reconstitution inflammatory response: riding the tide of immune recovery. Curr Opin Neurol. 2015;28(3):295–301.
5. Vermersch P, Kappos L, Gold R, Foley JF, Olsson T, Cadavid D, et al. Clinical outcomes of natalizumab-associated progressive multifocal leukoencephalopathy. Neurology. 2011;76(20):1697–704.
6. Clifford DB, De Luca A, DeLuca A, Simpson DM, Arendt G, Giovannoni G, et al. Natalizumab-associated progressive multifocal leukoencephalopathy in patients with multiple sclerosis: lessons from 28 cases. Lancet Neurol. 2010;9(4):438–46.
7. Hoepner R, Klotz P, Faissner S, Schneider R, Kinner M, Prehn C, et al. Neuropsychological impairment in natalizumab-associated progressive multifocal leukoencephalopathy: implications for early diagnosis. J Neurol Neurosurg Psychiatry. 2016;87(2):224–6
8. Berger JR, Aksamit AJ, Clifford DB, Davis L, Koralnik IJ, Sejvar JJ, et al. PML diagnostic criteria: consensus statement from the AAN neuroinfectious disease section. Neurology. 2013;80(15):1430–8.
9. Prosperini L, De Rossi N, Scarpazza C, Moiola L, Cosottini M, Gerevini S et al. Natalizumab-related progressive multifocal leukoencephalopathy in multiple sclerosis: findings from an Italian independent registry. Plos One. 2016; 11(12):e0168376.
10. Kurtzke JF. Rating neurologic impairment in multiple sclerosis: an expanded disability status scale (EDSS). Neurology. 1983;33(11):1444–52.
11. Richert N, Bloomgren G, Cadavid D, et al. Imaging findings for PML in natalizumab-treated MS patients. Mult Scler. 2012;18((Suppl 4):27. Oral 99.
12. Chiaravalloti ND, DeLuca J. Cognitive impairment in multiple sclerosis. Lancet Neurol. 2008;7(12):1139–51.
13. Borghi M, Cavallo M, Carletto S, Ostacoli L, Zuffranieri M, Picci RL, et al. Presence and significant determinants of cognitive impairment in a large sample of patients with multiple sclerosis. PLoS One. 2013;8(7):e69820.
14. Borghi M, Carletto S, Ostacoli L, Scavelli F, Pia L, Pagani M, et al. Decline of neuropsychological abilities in a large sample of patients with multiple sclerosis: a two-year longitudinal study. Front Hum Neurosci. 2016;10:282.
15. Mattioli F, Stampatori C, Bellomi F, Capra R. Natalizumab efficacy on cognitive impairment in MS. Neurol Sci. 2011;31 Suppl 3:321–3.
16. Mattioli F, Stampatori C, Capra R. The effect of natalizumab on cognitive function in patients with relapsing-remitting multiple sclerosis: preliminary results of a 1-year follow-up study. Neurol Sci. 2011;32(1):83–8.
17. Iaffaldano P, Viterbo RG, Paolicelli D, Lucchese G, Portaccio E, Goretti B, et al. Impact of natalizumab on cognitive performances and fatigue in relapsing multiple sclerosis: a prospective, open-label, two years observational study. PLoS One. 2012;7(4):e35843.

18. Wilken J, Kane RL, Sullivan CL, Gudesblatt M, Lucas S, Fallis R, et al. Changes in fatigue and cognition in patients with relapsing forms of multiple sclerosis treated with natalizumab: the ENER-G study. Int J MS Care. 2013;15(3):120–8.

19. Portaccio E, Stromillo ML, Goretti B, Hakiki B, Giorgio A, Rossi F, et al. Natalizumab may reduce cognitive changes and brain atrophy rate in relapsing-remitting multiple sclerosis–a prospective, non-randomized pilot study. Eur J Neurol. 2013;20(6):986–90.

20. Kunkel A, Fischer M, Faiss J, Dähne D, Köhler W, Faiss JH. Impact of natalizumab treatment on fatigue, mood, and aspects of cognition in relapsing-remitting multiple sclerosis. Front Neurol. 2015;6:97.

21. Mattioli F, Stampatori C, Bellomi F, Scarpazza C, Capra R. Natalizumab significantly improves cognitive impairment over three years in MS: pattern of disability progression and preliminary MRI findings. PLoS One. 2015;10(7):e0131803.

22. Iaffaldano P, Viterbo RG, Trojano M. Natalizumab discontinuation is associated with a rebound of cognitive impairment in multiple sclerosis patients. J Neurol. 2016;263(8):1620–5.

23. Hunt D, Giovannoni G. Natalizumab-associated progressive multifocal leucoencephalopathy: a practical approach to risk profiling and monitoring. Pract Neurol. 2012;12(1):25–35.

24. Ytterberg C, Johansson S, Andersson M, Widén Holmqvist L, von Koch L. Variations in functioning and disability in multiple sclerosis. A two-year prospective study. J Neurol. 2008;255(7):967–73.

25. Miskin DP, Ngo LH, Koralnik IJ. Diagnostic delay in progressive multifocal leukoencephalopathy. Ann Clin Transl Neurol. 2016;3(5):386–91.

6

Stroop event-related potentials as a bioelectrical correlate of frontal lobe dysfunction in multiple sclerosis

N. Amato, M. Cursi, M. Rodegher, L. Moiola, B. Colombo, M. Falautano, F. Possa, G. Comi, V. Martinelli and L. Leocani[*]

Abstract

Background: Dysfunction of higher cognitive abilities occurs in 40–60 % of people with multiple sclerosis (MS), as detected with neuropsychological testing, with predominant involvement of executive functions and processing speed. Event-related potentials to the Stroop are a bioelectrical correlate of executive function. We tested whether event-related potentials to the executive Stroop test may reflect executive dysfunction in MS.

Methods: 29 MS patients (M/F:14/15; mean age 40 ± 8), and 16 healthy control subjects were included in the study (M/F:7/9; mean age 36 ± 10). Patients underwent a neuropsychological battery and, according to the performance obtained, they were divided in two groups: 13 frontal patients (F-MS; M/F:6/7; mean age: 40 ± 8) and 16 non frontal patients (NF-MS; M/F:8/8; mean age: 41 ± 7). Simple and complex reaction times to the Stroop task were measured using a computerized system. Event-Related Potentials (ERPs) to the same stimuli were obtained from 29 channel EEG, during mental discrimination between congruent and incongruent stimuli. Multivariate analysis was performed on reaction times (RTs) and ERPs latencies; topographic differences were searched with low resolution brain electromagnetic tomography (LORETA).

Results: Significant group effects were found on the percentage of correct responses: F-MS subjects committed more errors than the other two groups. F-MS patients showed delayed P3 and N4 compared to NF-MS patients and delayed P2, N2, P3 and N4 compared to controls. NF-MS subjects showed significantly slower P2, N2 and P3 compared to control subjects. Moreover, frontal score correlated negatively with ERPs' latency and with complex RTs. At source analysis F-MS patients presented significantly reduced activation predominantly over frontal, cingulate and parietal regions.

Conclusions: Taken together, these findings suggest that bioelectrical activity to the Stroop test may well reflect the speed and extent of neural synchronization of frontal circuits. Further studies are needed to evaluate the usefulness of Stroop reaction times and ERPs for detecting frontal involvement early at a subclinical stage, allowing early cognitive therapy, and as a paraclinical marker for monitoring treatment outcomes.

Keywords: MS, Executive function, Stroop task, ERPs, Source analysis

* Correspondence: letizia.leocani@hsr.it
Neurological Department, Institute of Experimental Neurology (INSPE),
Scientific Institute Hospital San Raffaele, University Vita-Salute San Raffaele,
Via Olgettina, 60, 20132 Milan, Italy

Background

Cognitive dysfunction is a common finding in multiple sclerosis (MS), being reported in 40–60 % of all patients [18, 58, 62], typically consisting of deficits in attention, memory, executive functions and speed of information processing. This pattern of dysfunctions resembles that typical of subcortical dementia and is considered as mostly dependent on the disruption of connections between cortical associative areas, related to demyelination and/or axonal loss within the white matter immediately underlying the cortex [39].

Several neuroimaging studies investigated these deficits in MS patients trying to establish a relationship to lesion load as detected on MRI; some of these studies proposed that cognitive impairment is better explained by cortical structural abnormalities rather than subcortical white matter lesions [13, 14, 59], other recent studies instead, which compared the role of cortical lesions and white matter lesions in the development of cognitive impairments in MS, documented a higher role of white matter integrity changes than previously assumed [50].

During performance of cognitive tasks, a greater extent of brain activation has been reported in patients compared to healthy subjects, [6, 44, 64] indicating cortical reorganization possibly owing to compensatory mechanisms. Moreover, MS patients with mild cognitive impairment presented increased and additional activation during attention tasks compared to controls, while MS patients with severe cognitive impairments presented no additional activation [53]. These findings suggest that the compensation depends on the possibility to access additional brain structures and the exhaustion of these resources would determine severe cognitive impairment.

Electrophysiological studies have widely examined cognitive dysfunction in MS patients. Coherence analysis is a useful indicator of functional connections between different cortical areas [39], which are disrupted in multiple sclerosis. Cognitive impaired MS patients had a significant increase of theta power over the frontal regions [39] as well as an increase in beta and gamma bends [69] and a diffuse coherence decrease [19, 39].

Event Related Potentials (ERPs) are among the most suitable electrophysiological methods to examine processing speed, which appears to be the most common cognitive deficit in MS [8, 20]. Delayed latency and decreased amplitude of the main ERPs components, particularly of the P3 to oddball paradigm, representing the discrimination of stimuli differing in some physical dimension and whose latency reflects processing speed [36], have been reported in MS [38, 42]. Delayed P3 is associated with higher EDSS scores [22, 67], disease duration [25], low performance on attention and memory tasks and total MRI lesion burden [30, 49, 63]. Previous neuroimaging and neuropsychological studies pointed out the need for early detection of cognitive impairment in MS [1, 46], possibly at the subclinical level. ERPs could be particularly helpful in the early recognition of cognitive dysfunction and have been already successfully used to this end [43]. However, the oddball task, used to evoke P3, is not specifically challenging executive function, which is generally a key feature of cognitive involvement observed in MS [5, 16, 17, 21, 47, 57]. Among the cognitive tests which are suitable for ERPs analysis, the Stroop test [65] can be a good candidate and has been already applied in the study of executive functions in MS patients, in healthy subjects and in other neuropsychiatric disorders [4, 16, 32, 37, 71]. Cognitive control and flexibility are the most impaired in MS among executive functions [16], and the Stroop task is particularly suitable to detect deficits in these components of executive function [26]. We aimed at investigating the electrophysiological correlates of executive dysfunction in MS using ERPs to Stroop stimuli in persons with MS with and without executive dysfunction. As a performance correlate of the ERP task, reaction times to Stroop stimuli were measured.

Methods

Subjects

Twenty-nine patients (15 females; mean age 40 ± 8) with clinically definite multiple sclerosis according to McDonald criteria [45, 55, 56], and 16 healthy controls (9 females; mean age 36 ± 10) were included in the study. Patients with Expanded disability status scale [35] higher than 6.5 or with severe cognitive, motor or visual impairment interfering with task compliance, as well as with steroid or psychoactive drug treatment in the previous 3 months days were excluded from the study. The protocol was approved by the Institutional Ethics Committee at the Hospital San Raffaele and all subjects gave their written informed consent for participation.

Prior to the beginning of the study, patients underwent a neuropsychological battery including: Stroop test [65], Tower of Hanoi [29], Dual task [48], Wisconsin Card Sorting [7, 73], semantic and fonemic verbal fluency tests. According to their performance on these tests, a "frontal score" was assigned to each patient, who were subdivided in two groups: 13 frontal patients (F-MS; 7 females, mean age 40 ± 8 years) and 16 non frontal patients (NF-MS; 8 females, mean age: 41 ± 7).

Computerized Stroop Performance

Reaction times (RTs) in the Stroop task were measured using a computerized version implemented in commercial STIM software (Neuroscan, Herndon, VA, USA). Responses were recorded using a computer mouse with two response buttons. Four colour words (green, red, yellow, and blue) written in congruent (50 %) or incongruent

(50 %) colour were randomly presented (stimulus duration, 200 ms; intertrial interval, 3.5 s) in four different series of 32 stimuli each.

In the first condition (simple RT - SRT), the subjects had to press a button for every stimulus presentation, regardless of stimulus type. The second condition (go/no-go RT) consisted of two series, in which a response was required to either the incongruent (go/no-go I) or congruent (go/no-go C) stimuli. In the third condition (choice RT), the subjects had to press one button after the congruent stimuli (choice C) and the other button after the incongruent stimuli (choice I). For each series, the response latency was measured only for correct responses. Trials with latencies that exceeded 2.3 s were considered omissions and excluded from the calculation of average RTs and accuracy. The latter was calculated in the complex RTs (go/no-go and choice) as the percentage of correct responses.

Event-related potential recording

Twenty-nine EEG channels with binaural reference were recorded using scalp electrodes set on an elastic cap (Electrocap International, Eaton, OH, USA). The EEG signal was amplified (Synamps, Neuroscan, Herndon, VA, USA), filtered (DC–50 Hz), and digitized (sampling frequency, 250 Hz). The electrooculogram and electromyogram of the right and left extensor pollicis brevis were also recorded to detect eye movements and relaxation failure.

A series of 120 of the same Stroop stimuli (stimulus duration, 200 ms; intertrial interval, 6 s) used for the RT measurement were presented using the same computerized version implemented in commercial STIM software (Neuroscan, Herndon, VA, USA). The subjects were instructed to mentally discriminate between congruent and incongruent stimuli. This condition was chosen for ERP recording to avoid movement interference. Attention was monitored every 10–15 trials by randomly asking subjects to verbally define the congruency of the last stimulus presented. Recordings were performed in the morning (8:30–10:00 a.m.) to reduce variability due to circadian fluctuations.

Event-related potential analysis

Epochs from –500 to 1200 ms from stimulus onset were obtained. Linear detrending was performed over the entire epoch to correct for DC drifts. The baseline was then corrected between –500 and 0 ms. Epochs that contained artefacts or muscle relaxation failure upon visual inspection were excluded from the analysis. Initially, separate averages were obtained for congruent and incongruent stimuli. After a preliminary comparison between and within groups, which did not show significant differences between the parameters obtained in the

two conditions, data from the congruent and incongruent trials were collapsed into a single ERP for each subject to reduce signal noise.

The latency of the main ERP components (i.e., N1 [O1 or O2 electrode], P2, N2, P3 and N4 [Fz electrode]) was measured for each subject. The amplitude and topographic analysis was performed at time intervals of the same components (time intervals = group mean latency value of each component ± 30 ms) using low-resolution brain electromagnetic tomography (LORETA; [51, 52]; see *Statistical analysis* section below).

Statistical analysis

The significance of group effects with regard to the number of correct responses (in the choice condition, go/no-go C condition, and go/no-go I condition), RT latency in the choice C condition, choice I condition, go/no-go C condition, go/no-go I condition, and simple RT condition, and latency of the main ERP components (N1, P2, N2, P3 and N4) was tested using three separate multivariate analyses of variance (MANOVAs). *Post hoc* tests were performed using Bonferroni correction. Correlations between frontal score and RTs and between frontal score and ERP latencies were also performed using Spearman's coefficient. All of the statistical tests were performed using SPSS 17 software (Technologies, Chicago, IL, USA). Group differences in the amplitude and topography of ERP waveforms were investigated using LORETA with a statistical nonparametric voxelwise comparison between the F-MS, NF-MS and control groups. The level of significance was set at $p < 0.05$.

Results

Stroop RTs

Significant group effects were found on the percentage of correct responses (Fig. 1) at MANOVA ($p = 0.001$): in

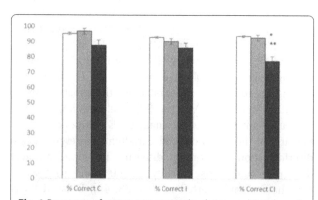

Fig. 1 Percentage of correct responses in the choice condition, the go/no-go condition and the simple reaction time condition, in controls (white), NF-MS (grey) and F-MS (black). F-MS vs CNT: ∗ $p = 0.001$; F-MS vs NF-MS ∗∗ $p = 0.001$. Line bars over each column indicate standard error

the choice condition F-MS patients committed significantly more errors than controls ($p = 0.001$) and NF-MS patients ($p = 0.001$).

There were no significant group effects on RTs at MANOVA.

ERPs latency
Significant group effect was found (Fig. 2) at MANOVA (F = 21.699; $p = 0.000$); F-MS patients showed significantly delayed P2, N2, P3 and N4 latencies compared to controls (P2: $p = 0.000$; N2: $p = 0.001$; P3: $p = 0.000$; N4: $p = 0.000$) and P3 and N4 latencies compared to NF-MS patients (P3: $p = 0.015$; N4: $p = 0.000$). NF-MS patients showed significantly delayed P2, N2 and P3 latencies compared to controls (P2: $p = 0.007$; N2: $p = 0.021$; P3: $p = 0.033$).

Correlations
There was a negative correlation between frontal score and N1 latency ($\rho = -0.426$, $p = 0.024$), P2 latency ($\rho = -0.643$, $p = 0.000$) and N4 latency ($\rho = -0.566$, $p = 0.002$). Moreover, frontal score correlated negatively with RTs speed in the go/no-go I condition ($\rho = -0.425$, $p = 0.022$) and in the choice C condition ($\rho = -0.381$, $p = 0.042$) (Fig. 3), and correlated positively with the percentage of correct responses in the go/no-go C condition ($\rho = 0.431$, $p = 0.019$) and in the choice condition ($\rho = 0.550$, $p = 0.002$) (Fig. 4).

ERPs amplitude and topography
LORETA statistical non-parametric voxel-wise analysis revealed significant group differences. In the N1 time window (time interval = group mean N1 latency value ± 20 ms), the F-MS group, compared to the other two groups, had a significantly reduced activation of the right supramarginal gyrus, the right inferior parietal lobule, the right middle and inferior temporal gyri and the superior and middle frontal gyri (Figs. 5 and 6). In the P2 time window (time interval = group mean P2 latency value ± 20 ms), there were not significant differences between groups. In the N2 time window (time interval = group mean N2 latency value ± 20 ms), F-MS patients showed a significantly decreased activity in the cingulate gyrus and in the parahippocampal gyrus compared to NF-MS patients (Fig. 7) but not significant differences compared to control subjects; significance was reached vs NF-MS and not vs controls, owing to a slight non significant increase in activation in NF-MS vs controls. In the P3 time window (time interval = group mean P3 latency value ± 20 ms), F-MS group presented a reduced activity reaching significance vs controls in the superior and medial frontal gyri, the cingulate gyrus, the precuneus and the precentral lobule (Fig. 8) and vs NF-MS in the anterior cingulate, the medial frontal gyrus and the cingulate gyrus (Fig. 9). In the N4 time window (time interval = group mean N4 latency value ± 20 ms), F-MS patients showed a significant decreased activity compared to healthy subjects in the cingulate gyrus, the paracentral lobule and the precuneus (Fig. 10).

Discussion
Compared to NF-MS patients and control subjects, our sample of F-MS patients showed delayed ERPs' latencies, reduced frontoparietal activity and less accuracy in the execution of the Stroop task. Moreover, frontal score correlated negatively with ERPs' latency and with complex RTs. These findings are discussed in details below.

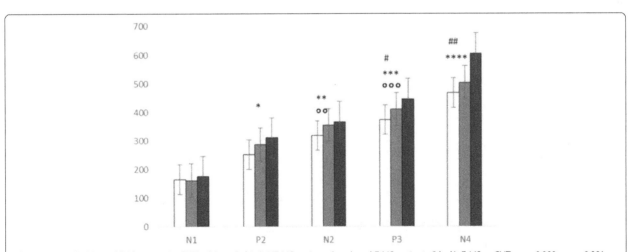

Fig. 2 N1, N2, P3, N4 and P6 latencies in CNT subjects (white), NF-MS patients (grey) and F-MS patients (black). F-MS vs CNT: * $p = 0.000$; ** $p = 0.001$; *** $p = 0.000$; **** $p = 0.000$. F-MS vs NF-MS: # $p = 0.015$; ## $p = 0.000$. NF-MS vs CNT: ○ $p = 0.007$; ○○ $p = 0.021$; ○○○ $p = 0.033$. Line bars over each column indicate standard error

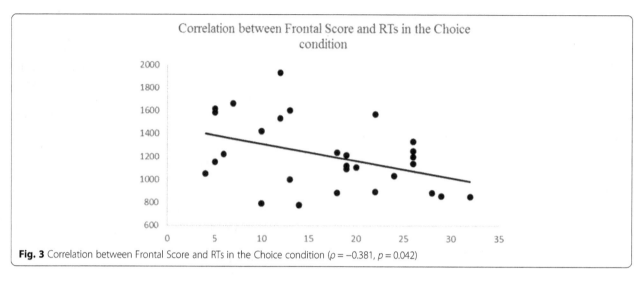

Fig. 3 Correlation between Frontal Score and RTs in the Choice condition ($\rho = -0.381$, $p = 0.042$)

RTs

The lower level of accuracy observed in frontal patients compared with the other two groups, but not in non frontal patients compared with controls, suggests an impairment, in the first group, of conflict monitoring function, necessary to process competing information and select the adequate response, reported to be mediated by frontal structures as the anterior cingulate cortex [10, 12]. Moreover, accuracy and speed in the complex tasks were correlated with frontal score obtained from neuropsychological assessment. Overall, these findings suggest that computerized RTs may provide useful measures for the assessment of executive functions in these patients. Although a learning effect may have certainly occurred during RTs measurements, the tasks were performed in a sequence with increasing difficulty. This choice was made to facilitate learning as much as possible for the subsequent ERPs recordings, to minimize an additional source of between-subject variability across RT tasks and to limit the number of RT exclusions due

to errors. However, this methodological choice could not allow us to avoid two possible confounding factors. One is learning itself: subjects with MS-related learning impairment could present slower learning and therefore higher impairment in the most complex tasks because these were performed later, favoring the subjects with faster learning. The second is cognitive fatigue, defined as performance decay with test repetition and reported to affect MS patients to a greater extent than healthy controls [34, 41]. However, performance at the computerized RTs was more impaired in frontal compared with non frontal MS patients and correlated with the frontal score, suggesting that this tools reflects, at least partially, the severity of frontal involvement. To further interpret our findings more studies are needed specifically addressing the issues of whether this impairment is a direct correlate of executive function or it is at least partly mediated by learning difficulties or cognitive fatigue. In any case, both learning difficulties and cognitive fatigue may well represent other correlate of frontal dysfunction,

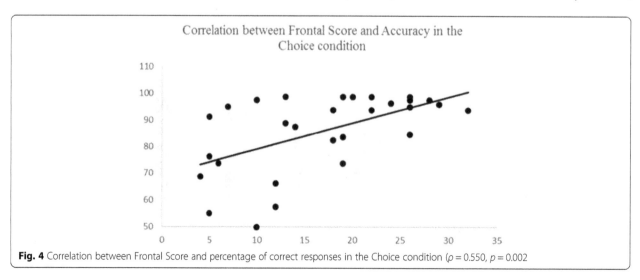

Fig. 4 Correlation between Frontal Score and percentage of correct responses in the Choice condition ($\rho = 0.550$, $p = 0.002$)

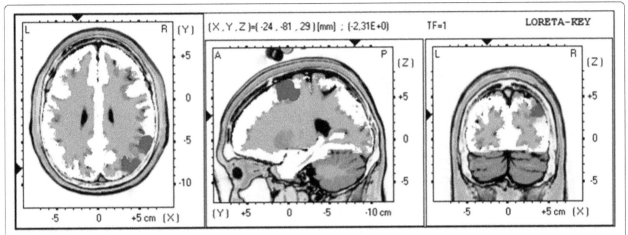

Fig. 5 LORETA non-parametric voxel-wise comparison map between F-MS and controls in the N1 time window. Blue: regions of significant decreased activity in F-MS

needing more work to disentangle the relative contribution of these factors to our findings.

ERPs latency

ERPs latencies were significantly increased in both patients groups compared with controls and in the F-MS group compared to NF-MS group. This finding is consistent with previous studies widely documenting cognitive ERPs latencies' delay in multiple sclerosis [3, 28, 72].

This delay was significant for all components measured but the earliest (N1). This result suggests that in our sample of patients visual discrimination processes, as reflected by the posterior N1 component, were not delayed and that the cognitive ERPs latencies' delay observed cannot be explained only in term of impaired information processing speed since in this case we would have observed a delay also at this earlier level of information processing.

These latter findings point out to the possibility that bioelectrical activity to the Stroop stimuli, particularly the later component, may well reflect the speed of neural synchronization of frontal lobe circuits, being especially involved in patients with frontal dysfunction.

ERPs amplitude and topography

LORETA topographic ERPs analysis showed reduced activity in the N1, N2, P3 and N4 time windows mostly over the frontal, cingulate and parietal regions evident in frontal MS patients compared with controls and with non frontal patients.

N1 is assumed to reflect selective attention to basic stimulus characteristics, initial selection for later pattern recognition, and intentional discrimination processing [70]. Its source is located in the inferior occipital lobe, occipito-temporal junction [31], and inferior temporal lobe [9]. Since the discrimination process, reflected by

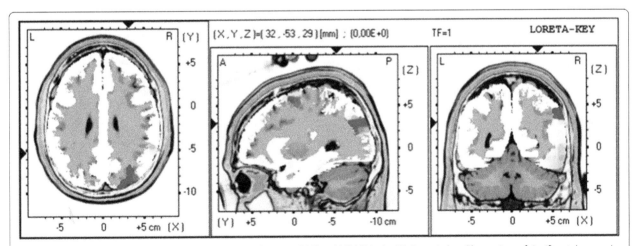

Fig. 6 LORETA non-parametric voxel-wise comparison map between F-MS and NF-MS in the N1 time window. Blue: regions of significant decreased activity in NF-MS

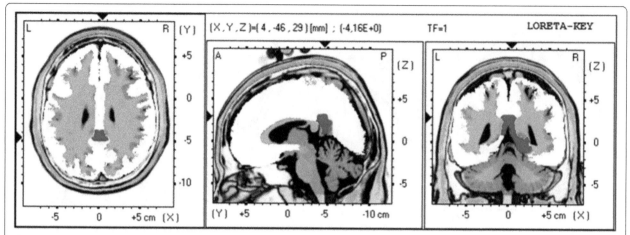

Fig. 7 LORETA non-parametric voxel-wise comparison map between F-MS and NF-MS in the N2 time window. Blue: regions of significant decreased activity in NF-MS

occipito-temporal N1, can be modulated by top-down executive control (the greater the difficulty of stimulus discrimination, the greater the need of top-down executive control modulation and therefore the greater the amplitude of the N1 component, cfr. [23]), the significant reduced activity observed here in the N1 time window in F-MS patients compared to both the other two groups, could be determined by executive control deficits in these patients: control and NF-MS groups would show a greater N1 amplitude, with respect to F-MS group, as a consequence of executive control modulation, which is instead lacking in frontal patients.

The N2 component in go/no-go-like tasks has been attributed to response inhibition mechanisms [27, 33]. However, the N2 component has also been reported to occur in relation to covert responses in the present study and in previous studies [2, 54]. This would indicate that it is not completely attributable to the inhibition of

responses and that it may at least partially account for conflict monitoring. N2 is especially pronounced over the fronto-central electrodes and has been proposed to reflect ACC sensitivity to conflict [68].

The P3 component is elicited in tasks related to stimulus differentiation and appears when a memory representation of the recent stimulus context is updated upon the detection of deviance from it [66]. The frontal P300 component in go/no-go-like tasks has been associated with an inhibitory mechanism [24]. However, in the present study, the subjects only had to mentally discriminate between congruent and incongruent stimuli; therefore, conflict did not arise at the response level. Thus, the P3 component observed herein most likely reflects the detection of conflict that arose at the level of the semantic encode.

The N4 component to the Stroop task is supposed to reflect anterior cingulate activity [40], which has been

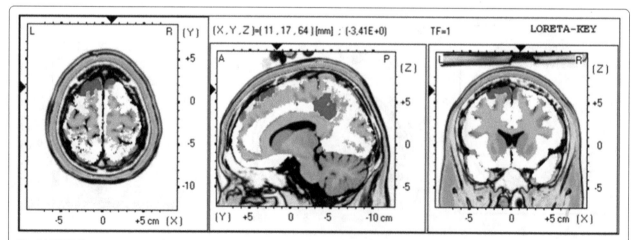

Fig. 8 LORETA Non-parametric voxel-wise comparison map between F-MS and controls in the P3 time window. Blue: regions of significant decreased activity in F-MS

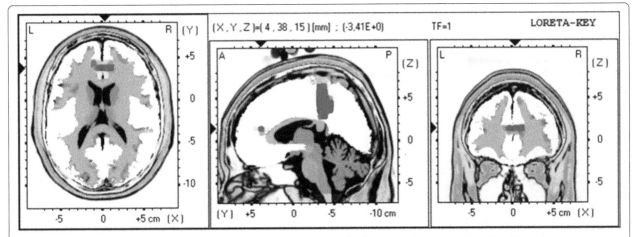

Fig. 9 Non-parametric voxel-wise comparison map between F-MS and NF-MS in the P3 time window. Blue: regions of significant decreased activity in F-MS

widely documented to account for conflict monitoring function and for triggering compensatory adjustment in cognitive control [11, 15, 27].

Taken together these findings reflect cognitive control impairment in frontal involved MS patients.

Previous functional neuroimaging studies to Stroop task [60, 61] showed a greater activation in MS subjects compared with healthy controls in several areas involved in the task execution, which resulted hypo-activated herein in cognitive impaired patients. These findings are only apparently inconsistent; in the studies by Rocca et al., in fact the increase in activation in MS patients, which, although not significant, was reported to occur also herein in NF-MS patients, seems to reflect compensatory mechanisms granting a normal performance, whereas our sample of patients with frontal involvement seems to be too compromised to compensate and just presented reduced activation accompanied by impaired

performance at complex tasks. Compensatory mechanisms depend on the possibility to access additional brain structures and the exhaustion of these resources seems to determine severe cognitive impairment, as documented elsewhere [53].

Conclusion

Our finding of decreased accuracy in frontal involved MS group suggests that this approach may provide useful objective measures for the assessment of executive functions in these patients. Topographic analysis of ERPs components to the Stroop stimuli showed predominant involvement of frontal, cingulate and parietal regions, probably reflecting the executive stage of stimulus processing. Also the latency of these components correlated with neuropsychological frontal score. Taken together, these findings suggest that bioelectrical activity to the Stroop test may well reflect the speed and extent of

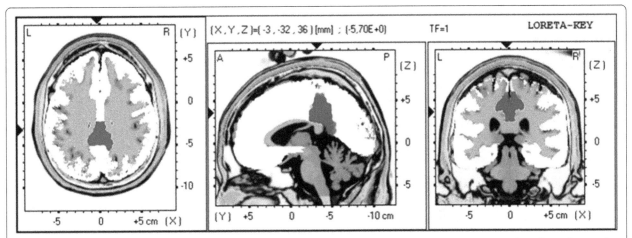

Fig. 10 Non-parametric voxel-wise comparison map between F-MS and controls in the N4 time window. Blue: regions of significant decreased activity in F-MS

neural synchronization of frontal circuits. Further studies are needed to evaluate the usefulness of Stroop reaction times and ERPs for detecting frontal involvement early at a subclinical stage, allowing early cognitive therapy, and as a paraclinical marker for monitoring treatment outcomes.

Competing interests

The authors declare that they have no competing interests.

Authors'contribution

NA data and statistical analysis and interpretation, manuscript draft and revision. MC supervision of source localization, manuscript revision. MR patients recruitment and clinical assessments, manuscript revision. LM patients recruitment and clinical assessments, manuscript revision. BC, patients recruitment and clinical assessments, manuscript revision. MF neuropsychological assessments, manuscript revision. FP neuropsychological assessments, manuscript revision. GC supervision to clinical and neuropsychological assessment, manuscript revision. VM supervision to clinical and neuropsychological assessment, manuscript revision. LL study design, supervision to data collection and analysis, manuscript revision. All authors read and approved the final manuscript.

Acknowledgements

The authors wish to thank A. Nossa, EEG technician, for EEG recordings.

References

1. Amato MP, Portaccio E, Goretti B, Zipoli V, Hakiki B, Giannini M, et al. Cognitive impairments in early stages of multiple sclerosis. Neurol Sci. 2010;31(S2):S211–4.
2. Amato N, Riva N, Cursi M, Martins-Silva A, Martinelli V, Comola M, et al. Different frontal involvement in ALS and PLS revealed by Stroop event-related potentials and reaction times. Front Aging Neurosci. 2013;5:82.
3. Aminoff JC, Goodin DS. Long-latency cerebral event-related potentials in multiple sclerosis. J Clin Neurophysiol. 2001;18(4):372–7.
4. Annovazzi P, Colombo B, Bernasconi L, Schiatti E, Comi G, Leocani L. Cortical function abnormalities in migraine: neurophysiological and neuropsychological evidence from reaction times and event-related potentials to the Stroop test. Neurol Sci. 2004;25 Suppl 3:S285–7.
5. Arnett PA, Rao SM, Bernardin L, Grafman J, Yetkin FZ, Lobeck L. Relationship between frontal lobe lesions and Wisconsin Card Sorting Test performance in patients with multiple sclerosis. Neurology. 1994;44(3 Pt 1):420–5.
6. Audoin B, Ibarrola D, Ranjeva JP, Confort-Gouny S, Malikova I, Ali-Chérif A, et al. Compensatory cortical activation observed by fMRI during a cognitive task at the earliest stage of MS. Hum Brain Mapp. 2003;20(2):51–8.
7. Berg EA. A simple objective technique for measuring flexibility in thinking. J Gen Psychol. 1948;39:15–22.
8. Bergendal G, Fredrikson S, Almkvist O. Selective decline in information processing in subgroups of multiple sclerosis: an 8-year longitudinal study. Eur Neurol. 2007;57(4):193–202.
9. Bokura H, Yamaguchi S, Kobayashi S. Electrophysiological correlates for response inhibition in a Go/NoGo task. Clin Neurophysiol. 2001;112:2224–32.
10. Botvinick MM, Braver TS, Barch DM, Carter CS, Cohen JD. Conflict monitoring and cognitive control. Psychol Rev. 2001;108(3):624–52.
11. Botvinick MM, Cohen JD, Carter CS. Conflict monitoring and anterior cingulate cortex: an update. Trends Cogn Sci. 2004;8(12):539–46.
12. Botvinick M, Nystrom LE, Fissell K, Carter CS, Cohen JD. Conflict monitoring versus selection-for-action in anterior cingulate cortex. Nature. 1999;402(6758):179–81.
13. Calabrese M, Agosta F, Rinaldi F, Mattisi I, Grossi P, Favaretto A, et al. Cortical lesions and atrophy associated with cognitive impairment in relapsing-remitting multiple sclerosis. Arch Neurol. 2009;66(9):1144–50.
14. Calabrese M, Rinaldi F, Grossi P, Gallo P. Cortical pathology and cognitive impairment in multiple sclerosis. Expert Rev Neurother. 2011;11(3):425–32.
15. Carter CS, van Veen V. Anterior cingulate cortex and conflict detection: an update of theory and data. Cogn Affect Behav Neurosci. 2007;7(4):367–79.
16. Cerezo García M, Martín Plasencia P, Aladro BY. Alteration profile of executive functions in multiple sclerosis. Acta Neurol Scand. 2015;131(5):313–20.
17. Chiaravalloti ND, DeLuca J. Cognitive impairment in multiple sclerosis. Lancet Neurol. 2008;7(12):1139–51.
18. Comi G, Filippi M, Martinelli V, Sirabian G, Visciani A, Campi A, et al. Brain magnetic resonance imaging correlates of cognitive impairment in multiple sclerosis. J Neurol Sci. 1993;115(Suppl):66–73.
19. Cover KS, Vrenken H, Geurts JJ, van Oosten BW, Jelles B, Polman CH, et al. Multiple sclerosis patients show a highly significant decrease in alpha band interhemispheric synchronization measured using MEG. Neuroimage. 2006;29(3):783–8.
20. DeLuca J, Chelune GJ, Tulsky DS, Lengenfelder J, Chiaravalloti ND. Is speed of processing or working memory the primary information processing deficit in multiple sclerosis? J Clin Exp Neuropsychol. 2004;26(4):550–62.
21. Drew M, Tippett LJ, Starkey NJ, Isler RB. Executive dysfunction and cognitive impairment in a large community-based sample with Multiple Sclerosis from New Zealand: a descriptive study. Arch Clin Neuropsychol. 2008;23(1):1–19.
22. Ellger T, Bethke F, Frese A, Luettmann RJ, Buchheister A, Ringelstein EB, et al. Event-related potentials in different subtypes of multiple sclerosis–a cross-sectional study. J Neurol Sci. 2002;205(1):35–40.
23. Fedota JR, McDonald CG, Roberts DM, Parasuraman R. Contextual task difficulty modulates stimulus discrimination: electrophysiological evidence for interaction between sensory and executive processes. Psychophysiology. 2012;49(10):1384–93.
24. Gajewski, Falkenstein. Effects of task complexity on ERP components in Go/Nogo tasks. Int J Psychophysiology. 2013;87(3):273–8.
25. Gil R, Zai L, Neau JP, Jonveaux T, Agbo C, Rosolacci T, et al. Event-related auditory evoked potentials and multiple sclerosis. Electroencephalogr Clin Neurophysiol. 1993;88(3):182–7.
26. Goldberg E, Bougakov D. Neuropsychologic assessment of frontal lobe dysfunction. Psychiatr Clin North Am. 2005;28(3):567–80.
27. Gonzalez-Rosa JJ, Inuggi A, Blasi V, Cursi M, Annovazzi P, Comi G, et al. Response competition and response inhibition during different Choice-discrimination tasks: Evidence from ERP measured inside MRI scanner. Int J Psychophysiol. 2013;89(1):37–47.
28. Gonzalez-Rosa JJ, Vazquez-Marrufo M, Vaquero E, Duque P, Borges M, Gomez-Gonzalez CM, et al. Cluster analysis of behavioural and event-related potentials during a contingent negative variation paradigm in remitting-relapsing and benign forms of multiple sclerosis. BMC Neurol. 2011;11:64.
29. Hofstadter DR. Metamagical Themas: Questing for the Essence of Mind and Pattern. New York: Basic Books; 1985.
30. Honig LS, Ramsay RE, Sheremata WA. Event-related potential P300 in multiple sclerosis. Relation to magnetic resonance imaging and cognitive impairment. Arch Neurol. 1992;49(1):44–50.
31. Hopf JM, Vogel E, Woodman G, Heinze HJ, Luck S. Localizing visual discrimination processes in time and space. J Neurophysiol. 2002;88:2088–95.
32. Hsieh YH, Chen KJ, Wang CC, Lai CL. Cognitive and motor components of response speed in the stroop test in Parkinson's disease patients. Kaohsiung J Med Sci. 2008;24(4):197–203.
33. Jodo E, Kayama Y. Relation of a negative ERP component to response inhibition in a Go/NoGo task. Electroencephalogr Clin Neurophysiol. 1992;82:477–82.
34. Krupp LB, Serafin DJ, Christodoulou C. Multiple sclerosis-associated fatigue. Expert Rev Neurother. 2010;10(9):1437–47.
35. Kurtzke JF. Rating neurologic impairment in multiple sclerosis: an expanded disability status scale (EDSS). Neurology. 1983;33(11):1444–52.
36. Kutas M, McCarthy G, Donchin E. Augmenting mental chronometry: the P300 as a measure of stimulus evaluation time. Science. 1977;197(4305):792–5.
37. Lapshin H, Audet B, Feinstein A. Detecting cognitive dysfunction in a busy multiple sclerosis clinical setting: a computer generated approach. Eur J Neurol. 2014;21:281–6.
38. Leocani L, Gonzalez-Rosa JJ, Comi G. Neurophysiological correlates of cognitive disturbances in multiple sclerosis. Neurol Sci. 2010;31 Suppl 2:S249–53.
39. Leocani L, Locatelli T, Martinelli V, Rovaris M, Falautano M, Filippi M, et al. Electroencephalographic coherence analysis in multiple sclerosis: correlation with clinical, neuropsychological, and MRI findings. J Neurol Neurosurg Psychiatry. 2000;69(2):192–8.
40. Liotti M, Woldorff MG, Perez R, et al. An ERP study of the temporal course of the Stroop color-word interference effect. Neuropsychologia. 2000;38:701–11.
41. MacAllister WS, Krupp LB. Multiple sclerosis-related fatigue. Phys Med Rehabil Clin N Am. 2005;16(2):483–502.
42. Magnano I, Aiello I, Piras MR. Cognitive impairment and neurophysiological correlates in MS. J Neurol Sci. 2006;245(1-2):117–22.

43. Magniè MN, Bensa C, Laloux L, Bertogliati C, Faure S, Lebrun C. Contribution of cognitive evoked potentials for detecting early cognitive disorders in multiple sclerosis. Rev Neurol. 2007;163(11):1065–74.

44. Mainero C, Pantano P, Caramia F, Pozzilli C. Brain reorganization during attention and memory tasks in multiple sclerosis: insights from functional MRI studies. J Neurol Sci. 2006;245(1-2):93–8.

45. McDonald WI, Compston A, Edan G, et al. Recommended diagnostic criteria for multiple sclerosis: guidelines from the International Panel on the diagnosis of multiple sclerosis. Ann Neurol. 2001;50(1):121–7.

46. Moccia M, Lanzillo R, Palladino R, Chang KC, Costabile T, Russo C, et al. Cognitive impairment at diagnosis predicts 10-year multiple sclerosis progression. Mult Scler. 2015;11:1–9.

47. Muhlert N, Sethi V, Schneider T, Daga P, Cipolotti L, Haroon HA, et al. Diffusion MRI-based cortical complexity alterations associated with executive function in multiple sclerosis. J Magn Reson Imaging. 2013;38(1):54–63.

48. Navon D, Gopher D. On the economy of the human-processing system. Psychol Rev. 1979;86:214–55.

49. Newton MR, Barrett G, Callanan MM, Towell AD. Cognitive event-related potentials in multiple sclerosis. Brain. 1989;112(Pt 6):1637–60.

50. Papadopoulou A, Müller-Lenke N, Naegelin Y, Kalt G, Bendfeldt K, Kuster P, et al. Contribution of cortical and white matter lesions to cognitive impairment in multiple sclerosis. Mult Scler. 2013;19(10):1290–6.

51. Pascual-Marqui RD, Esslen M, Kochi K, Lehmann D. Functional imaging with low-resolution brain electromagnetic tomography (LORETA): a review. Methods Find Exp Clin Pharmacol. 2002;24(Suppl C):91–5.

52. Pascual-Marqui RD, Michel CM, Lehmann D. Low resolution electromagnetic tomography: a new method for localizing electrical activity in the brain. Int J Psychophysiol. 1994;18(1):49–65.

53. Penner IK, Rausch M, Kappos L, Opwis K, Radü EW. Analysis of impairment related functional architecture in MS patients during performance of different attention tasks. J Neurol. 2003;250(4):461–72.

54. Pfefferbaum A, Ford JM, Weller BJ, Kopell BS. ERPs to response production and inhibition. Electroencephalogr Clin Neurophysiol. 1985;60:423–34.

55. Polman CH, Reingold SC, Banwell B, Clanet M, Cohen JA, Filippi M, et al. Diagnostic criteria for multiple sclerosis: 2010 revisions to the McDonald criteria. Ann Neurol. 2011;69(2):292–302.

56. Polman CH, Reingold SC, Edan G, Filippi M, Hartung HP, Kappos L, et al. Diagnostic criteria for multiple sclerosis: 2005 revisions to the "McDonald Criteria". Ann Neurol. 2005;58(6):840–6.

57. Rao SM, Hammeke TA, Speech TJ. Wisconsin Card Sorting Test performance in relapsing-remitting and chronic-progressive multiple sclerosis. J Consult Clin Psychol. 1987;55(2):263–5.

58. Rao SM, Leo GJ, Bemardin L, Unverzagt F. Cognitive dysfunction in multiple sclerosis. I. Frequency, patterns and prediction. Neurology. 1991;41(5):685–91.

59. Rinaldi F, Calabrese M, Grossi P, Puthenparampil M, Perini P, Gallo P. Cortical lesions and cognitive impairment in multiple sclerosis. Neurol Sci. 2010;31(2):S235–7.

60. Rocca MA, Bonnet MC, Meani A, Valsasina P, Colombo B, Comi G, et al. Differential cerebellar functional interactions during an interference task across multiple sclerosis phenotypes. Radiology. 2012;265(3):864–73.

61. Rocca MA, Valsasina P, Ceccarelli A, Absinta M, Ghezzi A, Riccitelli G, et al. Structural and functional MRI correlates of Stroop control in benign MS. Hum Brain Mapp. 2009;30(1):276–90.

62. Ron MA, Callanan MM, Warrington EK. Cognitive abnormalities in multiple sclerosis: a psychometric and MRI study. Psychol Med. 1991;21(1):59–68.

63. Sailer M, Heinze HJ, Tendolkar I, Decker U, Kreye O, v Rolbicki U, et al. Influence of cerebral lesion volume and lesion distribution on event-related brain potentials in multiple sclerosis. J Neurol. 2001;248(12):1049–55.

64. Staffen W, Mair A, Zauner H, Unterrainer J, Niederhofer H, Kutzelnigg A, et al. Cognitive function and fMRI in patients with multiple sclerosis: evidence for compensatory cortical activation during an attention task. Brain. 2002;125(6):1275–82.

65. Stroop JR. 2Studies of interference in serial verbal reactions. J Exp Psychol. 1935;18:643–62.

66. Sutton S, Tueting P, Zubin J, John ER. Evoked potential correlates of stimulus uncertainty. Science. 1965;150:1187–8.

67. Triantafyllou NI, Voumvourakis K, Zalonis I, Sfagos K, Mantouvalos V, Malliara S, et al. Cognition in relapsing-remitting multiple sclerosis: a multichannel event-related potential (P300) study. Acta Neurol Scand. 1992;85(1):10–3.

68. van Veen V, Carter CS. The anterior cingulate as a conflict monitor: fMRI and ERP studies. Physiol Behav. 2002;77:477–4820.

69. Vazquez-Marrufo M, Gonzalez-Rosa JJ, Vaquero E, Duque P, Borges M, Gomez C, et al. Quantitative electroencephalography reveals different physiological profiles between benign and remitting-relapsing multiple sclerosis patients. BMC Neurol. 2008;8:44.

70. Vogel EK, Luck SJ. The visual N1 component as an index of a discrimination process. Psychophysiology. 2000;37:190–203.

71. West R, Alain C. Effects of task context and fluctuations of attention on neural activity supporting performance of the Stroop Task. Brain Res. 2000;873:102–11.

72. Whelan R, Lonergan R, Kiiski H, Nolan H, Kinsella K, Hutchinson M, et al. Impaired information processing speed and attention allocation in multiple sclerosis patients versus controls: a high-density EEG study. J Neurol Sci. 2010;293(1-2):45–50.

73. Weigl E. On the psychology of so-called processes of abstraction. The Journal of Abnormal and Social Psychology. 1941;36(1):3–33.

7

Myelin-derived and putative molecular mimic peptides share structural properties in aqueous and membrane-like environments

Jussi Tuusa[1], Arne Raasakka[1,2], Salla Ruskamo[1] and Petri Kursula[1,2*] (iD)

Abstract

Background: Despite intense research, the causes of various neurological diseases remain enigmatic to date. A role for viral or bacterial infection and associated molecular mimicry has frequently been suggested in the etiology of neurological diseases, including demyelinating autoimmune disorders, such as multiple sclerosis. Pathogen mimics of myelin-derived autoimmune peptides have been described in the literature and shown to induce myelin autoimmune responses in animal models.

Methods: We carried out a structural study on myelin-derived peptides, and mimics thereof from various pathogens, in aqueous and membrane-like environments, using conventional and synchrotron radiation circular dichroism spectroscopy. A total of 13 peptides from the literature were studied, and 290 circular dichroism spectra were analysed. In addition, peptide structure predictions and vesicle aggregation assays were performed.

Results: The results indicate a high level of similarity in the biophysical and folding properties of the peptides from either myelin proteins or proteins from pathogenic viruses or bacteria; essentially all of the studied peptides folded in the presence of lipid vesicles or under other membrane-mimicking conditions, which is a sign of membrane interaction. Many of the peptides presented remarkable similarities in their conformation in different environments.

Conclusions: As most of the studied epitope segments in myelin proteins are associated with membrane-binding sites, our results support a view of molecular mimicry, involving lipid membrane interaction propensity and similar conformational properties, possibly playing a role in demyelinating disease. The results suggest mechanisms related to protein amphiphilicity and order-disorder transitions in the recognition of peptide epitopes in autoimmune demyelination.

Keywords: Myelin, Peptide, Folding, Lipid membrane, CD spectroscopy, Synchrotron, Molecular mimicry, Structure

Background

Myelin is a multilayered, tightly packed proteolipid membrane structure crucial for the rapid saltatory conduction of nerve impulses in vertebrates. It is formed when the plasma membrane of a myelinating glial cell wraps around an axon, with eventual compaction driving out excess cytoplasm and extracellular fluid. Demyelinating diseases are neurological conditions related to the loss of the myelin sheath around axons. Such diseases can be caused by inherited mutations, often concerning myelin-specific proteins, or autoimmune reactions against myelin components. For most demyelinating diseases, the corresponding molecular mechanisms remain unknown, directly impairing our understanding of these disorders and their potential treatment.

Multiple sclerosis (MS) is a central nervous system (CNS) demyelinating autoimmune disease with a complex, incompletely known etiology. The current understanding of the pathogenesis and immunological models of MS has been reviewed [1, 2]. MS is an autoimmune

* Correspondence: petri.kursula@uib.no
[1]Faculty of Biochemistry and Molecular Medicine & Biocenter Oulu, University of Oulu, Oulu, Finland
[2]Department of Biomedicine, University of Bergen, Bergen, Norway

disease with an initial autoreactive, T cell-mediated mechanism, while B cell-expressed autoantibodies likely play a role in disease progression. Several peptide epitopes from myelin proteins, including myelin basic protein (MBP) [3], proteolipid protein (PLP) [4, 5], myelin-oligodendrocyte glycoprotein (MOG) [6], and myelin-associated oligodendrocytic basic protein (MOBP) [7, 8] have been implicated as T cell epitopes in MS, and many such peptides have been used to induce experimental autoimmune encephalomyelitis (EAE), the most widely used animal model of MS [9]. In addition, the myelin proteins P0, P2, and PMP22 have similarly been implicated in the peripheral nervous system (PNS) autoimmune disease Guillain-Barré syndrome (GBS) and its corresponding animal model, experimental autoimmune neuritis (EAN) [10–12]. In GBS, a common disease-preceding infection is by *Campylobacter jejuni* [13, 14].

It is unclear, how autoreactive T cells are triggered, but environmental factors play a significant role in MS. Especially inflammations caused by viral or microbial infections have been implicated. For example, Epstein-Barr virus infection seems to correlate with MS morbidity [2]. A number of other viral pathogens have also been implicated in MS etiology [15–18]. The proposed immunological mechanisms behind infection-induced autoimmunity include molecular mimicry, bystander activation, and dual-specificity T cell receptor (TCR) expression. While in the latter two mechanisms, the response towards the infective agent either indirectly or co-operatively induces autoreactive T cell function, molecular mimicry predicts immunological identity or close similarity between the sequences and/or structures of self-epitopes and viral/bacterial proteins at the molecular level.

Several viral and bacterial peptides harbour structural epitopes that mimic the well-characterized immunodominant MBP85-99 peptide, albeit they share very limited sequence similarity, with only a few conserved amino acids required for major histocompatibility complex (MHC) or TCR binding [19]. However, it is not known whether the self-epitopes are present in the native physiological state, or whether they form after conformational changes or denaturation caused by insults against myelinating glial cells and subsequent antigen presentation. MBP isolated from nerve tissue has been for long known for its intrinsically disordered structure and conformational changes induced by lipids [20–27]; much of this work stems from isolation of native protein from tissue, which will inevitably produce heterogeneous samples. Full-length 18.5-kDa murine MBP and the MBP72-107 peptide underwent a disordered-to-ordered transition, when transferred from an aqueous to a membrane-like environment in a trifluoroethanol (TFE) titration experiment [28, 29]. We observed folding of recombinant 18.5-kDa MBP in various membrane-mimetic conditions, as well as in the presence of lipid vesicles [30]. Similarly, the MBP85-99 peptide acquired helical conformation in the presence of detergent micelles and lipid vesicles [31]. The main immunogenic epitope of MBP, represented by the MBP85-99 peptide, corresponds to the central membrane attachment site, and correlations between the strength of the membrane interaction and MS etiology have been suggested [32]. Taken into account recent theories on the formation of a protein phase consisting of MBP upon myelin membrane maturation [33], it is clear that membrane binding and related conformational changes in MBP are crucial for normal myelin formation and maintenance.

The above findings raise questions on whether molecular mimicry in the context of MS may focus on structural epitopes, which change during water-lipid environmental transitions. Importantly, conformation-specific anti-MOG antibodies are required for MS-type pathological changes in EAE [34]. Therefore, there exists significant interest to find out, whether the autoimmunogenic epitopes in myelin proteins undergo conformational changes, when shifted between aqueous and hydrophobic, membrane-like environments, and whether the pathogen epitopes, which share similar T cell recognition, behave similarly. Could similar behaviour of peptide epitopes from myelin proteins and putative pathogenic mimics in membrane-mimicking conditions be correlated to autoimmunogenic properties in the specific case of demyelinating autoimmune diseases?

Here, circular dichroism (CD) spectroscopy was used to follow conformational changes in several myelin self-epitope peptides from PLP, MOBP, MOG, and P2 and in four MBP85-99-mimicking viral/bacterial peptides in aqueous and membrane-like environments. All peptides were picked from relevant literature. We observed that the autoimmunogenic candidate peptides underwent folding, when shifted from an aqueous to a hydrophobic environment. The same change was evident for the MBP-mimicking peptides. All the results point towards shared biophysical and structural properties in the different peptide epitopes.

Methods

Peptides
Synthetic peptides were from GenScript, Piscataway, NJ, USA. Details of the peptides are given in Table 1. Peptides were dissolved in sterile water to get 10 mg/ml stock solutions. All peptides were acetylated at the N terminus and amidated at the C terminus.

Detergents and lipids
n-Dodecyl phosphocholine (DPC) was from Anatrace and sodium dodecyl sulfate (SDS) from Sigma. Dimyristoyl

Table 1 The peptides selected for the current study

Peptide	Sequence	Predicted structure	References
MOBP15-36	QKFSEHFSIHCCPPFTFLNSKR	beta/disordered	[7]
MOBP37-60	EIVDRKYSICKSGCFYQKKEEDWI	alpha/disordered	[8]
hMOG35-55	MEVGWYRPPFSRVVHLYRNGK	beta/disordered	[6]
mMOG35-55	MEVGWYRSPFSRVVHLYRNGK	beta/disordered	[6]
HSV-mimic	FRQLVHFVRDFAQLL	alpha	[19]
EB-mimic	TGGVYHFVKKHVHES	alpha	[19]
IA-mimic	YRNLVWFIKKNTRYP	beta/disordered	[19]
PA-mimic	DRLLMLFAKDVVSRN	alpha	[19]
P2gbs	ENFDDYMKALGV	alpha/disordered	[78]
PLP139-151	VSLGKWLGHPDKF	alpha/disordered	[4]
PLPextra2	FNTWTTCQSIAFPSKTSASIGSLCADARMYG	alpha/disordered	[5, 60]
PLPintra1	AEGFYTTGAVEQIFGDYKTTICGKGLSATVTGGQKGRG	mixed	[60, 100]
PLPintra2	SRGQHQAHSLERVCHCLGKWLGHPDKFVGI	alpha/disordered	[4, 60]

The predicted structure corresponds to that obtained from PEP-FOLD. References for the possible disease linkage of each peptide are also given

phosphatidylcholine (DMPC) and dimyristoyl phosphatidylglycerol (DMPG) were from Affymetrix. To prepare lipid vesicles, the lipids were dissolved in 1:1 methanol:chloroform. The lipid solutions were then mixed in a 1:1 molar ratio, and solvent was evaporated under a gentle air stream. The dried lipid mixtures were suspended to 10 or 20 mg/ml in water or 10 mM HEPES (pH 7.5). Hydration was completed and unilamellar vesicles prepared by sequential sonication (30 min Branson 3510 bath sonicator, followed by 60 s Branson 450 ultrasonifier with 10% power and a 1 s pulse–1 s chase protocol).

Circular dichroism spectroscopy

Environment-induced folding of peptides was analyzed by CD spectroscopy, using a Chirascan Plus spectropolarimeter (Applied Photophysics). Quartz cuvettes with a 1-mm light path were used to measure CD spectra from 260 to 190 nm. The samples were water-dissolved peptide samples of nominal concentrations of 50 to 100 µg/ml, with or without TFE, detergents, or lipids (added immediately before the measurement). A peptide form the *Plasmodium falciparum* formin was used as a negative control. Synchrotron radiation CD (SRCD) spectra were recorded at +30 °C on the DISCO beamline at the SOLEIL synchrotron (Paris, France) and on the AU-CD beamline at the ASTRID2 storage ring (ISA, Aarhus, Denmark), using 0.2- and 0.5-mm quartz cuvettes and 0.25 mg/ml peptide.

In the oriented CD (OCD) experiment, 200 µl of a peptide-lipid (1:30 molar ratio) mixture, containing 10 µg of peptide, or 200 µl of a DMPC:DMPG (1:1) lipid blank alone, were pipetted onto a quartz disk. The generation of multilamellar planar lipid bilayers was conducted by air-drying, followed by 10 h of re-hydration in a saturated K_2SO_4 atmosphere at +30 °C (relative

humidity 97%) [31]. OCD spectra were recorded with 45° rotation steps on the DISCO beamline at the SOLEIL synchrotron (Paris, France), and the resulting eight spectra, covering 360° of total rotation, were averaged. Due to the rather harsh sample preparation procedure and the tendency of the peptides to aggregate membranes, only the EB-mimic peptide gave a high enough signal for further analysis.

SRCD and OCD spectra were averaged and backgrounds subtracted with CDtool [35]. A total of 290 CD spectra were measured and analysed.

Structure prediction and CD deconvolution

De novo structure prediction of the peptides was done *in silico* using the PEP-FOLD server [36, 37]. Membrane association modes of protein and peptide models where predicted using PPM [38]. Secondary structure contents were inferred by deconvoluting the CD spectra with the DICHROWEB server using the CONTINLL algorithm with DICHROWEB reference databases 6 and 7 for SRCD and regular CD, respectively [39]. The Bestsel server [40] was also used. It should be noted that in the case of short peptides, deconvolution algorithms optimized for full proteins give semi-quantitative or qualitative results, and we think more information is available by simply observing and comparing the full spectra, instead of relying on numbers from deconvolution. Spectra of short peptides are strongly affected by amino acid composition, for example.

Turbidimetry

Peptide-induced vesicle agglutination was studied in 0.5 mM DMPC:DMPG lipid in water. Peptides or proteins were added at the start of the experiment, and the experiment was carried out essentially as described before [41]. The full-length human P2 protein was used as a positive control [41]. Another possible positive control could have been full-length MBP [42].

Turbidity changes as a function of peptide concentration were followed by absorbance measurement at 450 nm in 96-well format using a Tecan Infinite M1000 Pro plate reader (Tecan, Salzburg, Austria). The total volume was 150 μl, and 2 s orbital shaking with 1 mm amplitude and 150 ms settling time were used.

Results

Demyelinating autoimmune diseases, such as MS or GBS, are thought to present a molecular mimicry component related to relatively common viral or bacterial pathogens, many of which involve the nervous system in their infection. This research was sparked by our interest in studying putative common biophysical properties between myelin-derived autoimmune peptides and peptides from pathogens described in the literature and proposed to cause molecular mimicry in e.g. multiple sclerosis. Our hypothesis was that such peptides might share similar properties with respect to structure, conformational changes, and lipid membrane binding, and furthermore, that peptides affecting the CNS and PNS might have similar properties.

Myelin-derived or myelin-mimicking peptides of potential relevance to demyelinating disease

Nine peptides from four human or mouse compact myelin proteins with a putative autoimmunogenic character and four viral/bacterial peptides suggested [19] to mimic the well-known MS-associated MBP sequence (amino acids 85–99) were chosen for structural analysis; all peptides have been described in the literature earlier (see Table 1 and references therein). The corresponding MBP85-99 peptide was a subject of our earlier study [31]. An additional common denominator of the myelin protein peptides was known or suggested membrane contact. The N terminus of MOBP is predicted to have a membrane-associated FYVE domain [43]. The peripheral myelin protein P2 acts in the formation of myelin membrane stacks, with the two α helices involved in membrane contacts [41, 44]. MOG and PLP are transmembrane proteins, in which both the extracellular and cytoplasmic domains may interact with the next apposing lipid bilayer. In PLP, the autoimmunogenic peptides are in the close vicinity of the transmembrane domains, forming loops between them. Finally, pathogen-derived peptides were predicted to mimic the autoimmunogenic central membrane-anchoring segment of MBP, which has been shown to become embedded into the lipid bilayer [19, 31, 45–49].

Based on amino acid sequences, the peptides do not exclusively share obvious biophysical characteristics. However, most of the peptides are positively charged at neutral pH and contain hydrophobic amino acids, which may be important for membrane attachment (Additional file 1: Table S1). The charge distributions are evenly scattered along the sequence. However, most peptides showed amphipathic distribution of positively charged and hydrophobic residues on helical wheel models (Fig. 6b, Additional file 2: Figure S1), possibly reflecting propensity for interactions with phospholipid membrane surfaces. A predicted property for most, but not all, of the studied peptides is the presence of a membrane-induced amphipathic helix.

The peptide *de novo* structure was predicted *in silico* using the PEP-FOLD algorithm [36] (Additional file 3: Figure S2). The MOG-derived peptides, as well as the Influenza hemagglutinin peptide (IA mimic), were predicted to harbor β strands, whereas other MBP-mimicking peptides (HSV mimic, EB mimic, and PA mimic) as well as the P2-derived peptide P2gbs, contained an α helix as the dominant predicted secondary structure. The latter corresponds to α helix 1 in the crystal structure of human P2 [41, 44]. Peptides from PLP were predicted to consist of α-helical parts with a β strand (PLPintra1) or disordered sequences (Table 1), while MOBP15-36 and MOBP37-60 were predicted to have β strand and α helix, respectively, in addition to disordered regions (Table 1). While all peptides were experimentally observed to maintain an unfolded structure in aqueous solution, these predicted propensities of folding were, in fact, rather consistent with CD spectroscopic experiments under membrane-mimicking conditions (see results below).

During the formation of compact myelin, the peripheral membrane proteins of myelin, as well as the extra- and intracellular domains of integral myelin membrane proteins, experience change from an aqueous/single membrane physical environment to a dehydrated membrane multilayer. After mechanical damage, or an inflammation/infection-induced insult to myelin, an opposite environmental change is possible, whereby membrane-embedded epitopes may be exposed to aqueous conditions. CD spectroscopy is a powerful method to probe solvent effects on peptide structure. Previously, it has been shown that many myelin protein-derived peptides, indeed, undergo folding, when shifted from aqueous buffer into a more hydrophobic environment [31, 50]. We monitored the CD spectra of the 13 selected peptides (Table 1) by conventional and SRCD in the presence of different concentrations of TFE, DPC, and SDS, as well as with DMPC:DMPG (1:1) vesicles.

In general, all studied peptides were disordered in water and showed TFE-, SDS- (a negatively charged detergent, critical micellar concentration CMC = 8.2 mM; ~0.24%), and lipid vesicle-induced folding at variable levels, while DPC (a zwitterionic detergent, CMC = 1.1. mM; ~0.04%) did not induce folding of MOBP peptides (see below for details). Of note, a peptide from the formin of the malaria parasite did not fold upon membrane-mimicking conditions and was considered a negative control (Additional file 4: Figure S3). Consistently, CONTINLL predicted higher degrees of folding and higher α/β ratios than the Bestsel algorithm. However, these differences were minor in terms of quantity. Finally, as expected, the diagnostic value of the wavelength region 180–190 nm, which can be reliably measured only with SRCD, was significant. This could be observed by comparing the secondary structure content deconvolutions between conventional CD (190–260 nm) and SRCD (180–270 nm), as the programs inferred conventional CD spectra in favour of β strand content, which likely arose from random coil structure, as indicated by SRCD data. The results from secondary

structure deconvolution of all 290 CD spectra with both of the algorithms are given in Additional file 5: Table S2.

MBP85-99-mimicking peptides demonstrate a major disorder-to-helix transition induced by TFE, micelles, and lipid vesicles

The four MBP85-99-mimicking peptides (Fig. 1a), 'HSV-mimic' from tripartite terminase subunit 3 (UL15) of *Human herpes simplex virus 1*, 'EB-mimic' from *Epstein-Barr virus* DNA polymerase catalytic subunit (BALF5), 'IA-mimic' from *Influenza A* virus hemagglutinin, and 'PA-mimic' from *Pseudomonas aeruginosa* phosphomannomutase (algC), were selected based on earlier literature on their properties related to molecular mimicry in autoimmune response [19]. Structural information for the corresponding segment in MBP is available (Fig. 1b, c), and while it is helical when bound to membranes [31, 47], its conformation is extended when bound to MHC [51]. The residues most conserved between MBP and the mimic peptides lie slightly embedded in the membrane in

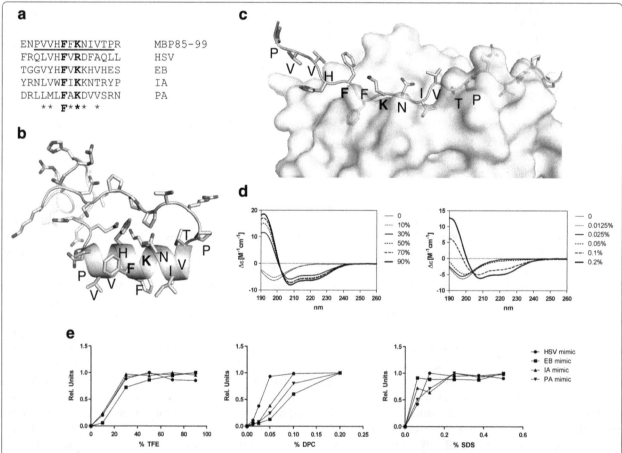

Fig. 1 Pathogen peptides mimicking MBP85-99 in membrane-like conditions. **a** Sequence alignment of MBP and the mimicking peptides. **b** NMR structure of the MBP72-107 peptide in micelles [46]. **c** Crystal structure of the MBP epitope bound to MHC [51]. **d** TFE (*left*) and DPC (*right*) titration of the EB mimic peptide. **e** Membrane-like conditions induced by TFE (*left*), DPC (*middle*), and SDS (*right*) for all four peptides. The y axis contains the relative signal at 195 nm

the helical conformation, and they point outward from the MHC complex; these are the positions that MHC presents to the T cell. Mutation of these positions in the MBP85-99 epitope lead to altered immunological response [52, 53].

In CD experiments, the mimic peptides were mainly disordered in water and acquired folded structure after moving into membrane-like environments (Fig. 1d, e and Additional file 5: Table S2). This behavior is highly similar to that of the MBP85-99 peptide [31]. From the SRCD spectra of peptide-lipid vesicle mixtures (Fig. 2), CONTINLL and Bestsel, respectively, calculated α-helical contents of 91 and 79% for EB-mimic, 57 and 58% for HSV-mimic, 63 and 62% for IA-mimic, and 43 and 38% for PA-mimic. Interestingly, while the predicted structure *de novo* (Table 1) was helical for EB-mimic, HSV-mimic, and PA-mimic, IA-mimic was predicted to have a β strand, which is also present for this segment in the hemagglutinin protein [54]. Similarly to MOG35-55 (see below), the IA-mimic peptide thus shows, at least as an isolated peptide, that it has a propensity for helical conformation under membrane-like conditions. Such common properties may explain the encephalitogenic properties of many myelin- and pathogen-derived peptides, despite the context of the corresponding sequence in the full protein.

The EB-mimic peptide membrane orientation is similar to MBP85-99

Previously, we [31] have shown by OCD that MBP85-99 is partially embedded into a lipid membrane leaflet in a tilted orientation. We repeated the experiment here for the EB mimic peptide, which had the highest helical content when mixed with vesicles (see above). Briefly, 10 μg of peptide was mixed with DMPC:DMPG (1:1) vesicles with a 1:30 P/L ratio, and OCD was measured from planar multilayered membranes. The 208-nm

minimum, typical for α-helical conformation, which was observed in isotropic solution CD spectra, was missing in OCD (Fig. 3), indicating either a conformational change or assembly of the peptide in a tilted orientation in the oriented membrane layers. This observation supports the hypothesis that the MBP85-99 self-epitope and the mimic peptides share similar conformational epitopes.

The MOG35-55 epitope has a propensity to adopt helical conformation

The MOG35-55 epitope (Fig. 4a) is a widely recognized inducer of encephalitogenic reactions, and it is routinely used to induce mouse EAE models [55, 56]. The mMOG35-55 epitope is highly immunogenic and induces EAE, while the corresponding peptide from human MOG is less active in causing EAE [57]. This is surprising, since only one residue distinguishes mMOG35-55 and hMOG35-55 from each other.

Both human and mouse MOG35-55 were largely disordered in water and acquired α-helical character in hydrophobic environments (Fig. 4). While these peptides differ only by a single amino acid (Pro/Ser42), the α/β ratio was in general higher for hMOG35-55 in membrane-mimicking conditions (Fig. 4, Additional file 5: Table S2). The SRCD spectra of the two peptides with lipid vesicles also suggest more β structure content for mMOG35-55 (Fig. 4b). In the crystal structure, the peptide sequence covers two β strands and a connecting loop [58] (Fig. 4a), which was also predicted for these peptides *de novo* in aqueous environment (Table 1). However, based on our results, this autoimmunogenic region in MOG has an intrinsic propensity to adopt α-helical conformation in the context of a peptide interacting with membranes. Subtle differences in folding between the mMOG35-55 and hMOG35-55 epitopes may be relevant

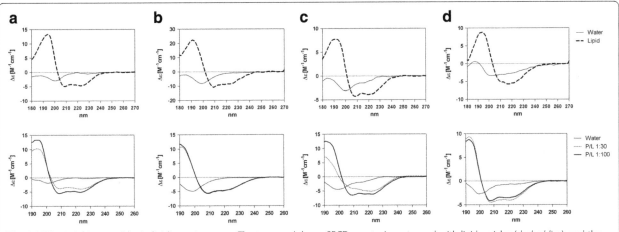

Fig. 2 MBP-mimicking peptides in lipidic environment. The *top panel* shows SRCD spectra in water and with lipid vesicles (*dashed line*), and the *bottom panel* conventional CD spectra at two different P/L ratios. **a** HSV-mimic. **b** EB-mimic. **c** IA-mimic. **d** PA-mimic

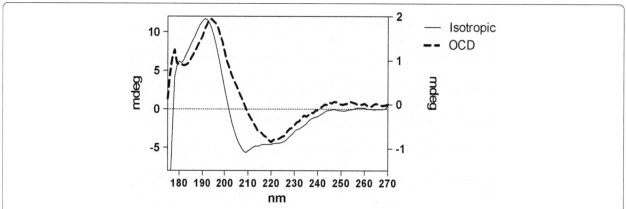

Fig. 3 Orientation of the EB-mimic peptide on a membrane. The figure shows comparison of isotropic and oriented SRCD spectra. The loss of the peak at 208 nm in OCD is a sign of tilting of the peptide with respect to the membrane surface plane

for inducing EAE with MOG peptides. Mutations in the mMOG35-55 peptide have also been linked to altered immune responses in mouse models [59]. Whether the recognition of the Pro/Ser residue itself or the variant-favored conformation determines the strength of autoimmunogenicity remains to be studied.

MOBP peptides fold into different structures in membranes

The N terminus of MOBP, shared by all known MOBP isoforms, is predicted to fold into a FYVE-like membrane interaction domain [43] (Fig. 5a, b). The epitope peptide segments correspond to areas predicted to

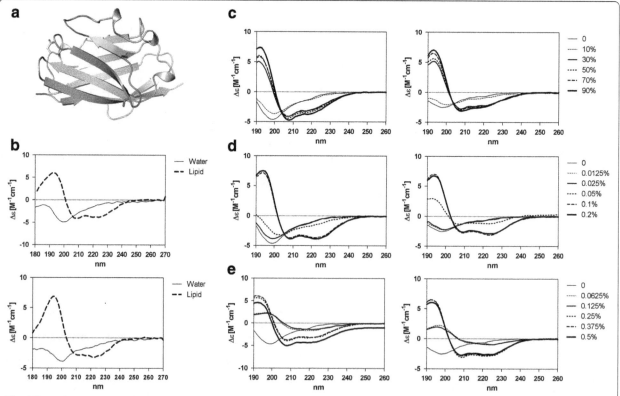

Fig. 4 The MOG35-55 peptides. **a** Location of the segment 35–55 in the MOG Ig domain crystal structure [58]. Shown (as *sticks*) are also the glycosylation site Asn31 [101] and the Ser42 residue (at the hairpin of the MOG35-55 epitope), which when mutated to Pro, as in human MOG, produces a less encephalitogenic response [57]. **b** SRCD spectra of the human (*top*) and mouse (*bottom*) MOG35-55 peptides in the absence and presence of lipid vesicles. Similar results were also obtained in conventional CD at P/L ratios of 1:30 and 1:100. **c** TFE titration of the human (*left*) and mouse (*right*) peptides. **d** DPC titration. **e** SDS titration. Note the different behaviour of both peptides below and above the CMC

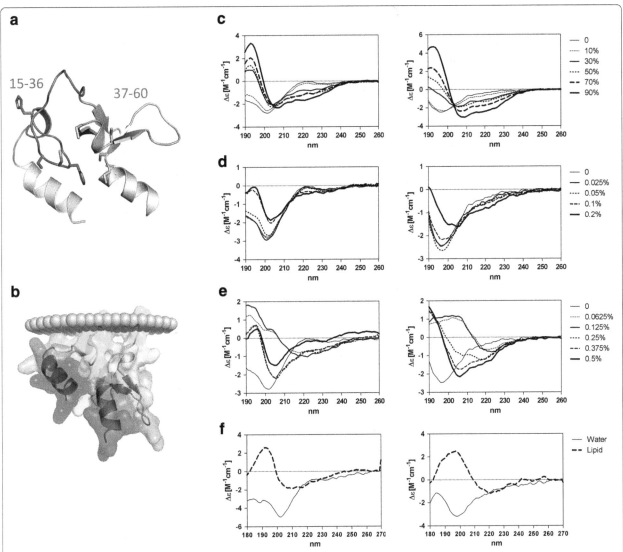

Fig. 5 Peptide epitopes from MOBP. **a** Predicted structure of the FYVE-like domain at the N terminus of MOBP. The regions corresponding to the peptides studied here are coloured, and potential metal ion-coordinating residues (Cys/His) are shown as *sticks*. **b** Predicted interaction [38] of the model with a membrane surface. **c** TFE titration of MOBP15-36 (*left*) and MOBP37-60 (*right*). **d** DPC titration. **e** SDS titration. Note the different behaviour below and above the CMC. **f** SRCD spectra in the absence and presence of DMPC/DMPG vesicles. The MOBP37-60 peptide has pronounced beta content, while MOBP15-36 is more helical

closely interact with the lipid membrane surface. So far, no high-resolution structural or functional studies with purified MOBP protein have been carried out. The *de novo* prediction suggested some β and α structures for the MOBP15-36 and 37–60 peptides, respectively, with disordered regions (Table 1), but in contrast to the MBP-mimicking and MOG35-55 peptides, models predicted by PEP-FOLD were not always consistent.

Both MOBP peptides (15–36, 37–60) showed hydrophobicity-induced folding (Fig. 5b–f). DPC induced some secondary structure formation at high concentrations (Fig. 5d), while both peptides behaved differently in SDS. Below the CMC of SDS, the CD spectra are reminiscent of β aggregates, while above the CMC, micelles of SDS induce significant helical components (Fig. 5e). The SRCD spectra of lipid vesicle-induced folding suggested a β sheet structure for MOBP37-60, while MOBP15-36 contains more helical structure (Fig. 5f). While these results differ somewhat from the other peptides in this study, which form α-helical structures under most conditions, they are logical and fit to the predicted FYVE domain structure of MOBP [43].

PLP-derived peptides fold in hydrophobic environments

The peptides from PLP were based on earlier studies on EAE models, and included both extra- and intracellular epitopes (Fig. 6a) shown to induce antibody responses related to demyelination in EAE [60, 61]. In the overlapping peptides PLP139-151 and PLPintra2, a region with strong propensity to fold into an amphipathic helix can be detected (Fig. 6b, c). Remarkably, all the PLP peptides also exhibited folding in membranous environments, although they are expected to represent loops between the transmembrane helices in the PLP protein (Fig. 6d, e). The result strongly suggests that these loops are able to interact directly with lipid membrane surfaces. In the case of compact myelin, this could lead to a single molecule of PLP acting as glue between three successive membrane layers. Interestingly, a C-terminal peptide

from PLP was also recently shown to fold upon membrane interaction, and the folding was affected by peptide concentration, the helices refolding into β sheet structure at high concentration on the lipid membrane – a process, which might play a role in myelin membrane stacking [62].

The peptides PLP139-151 and PLPintra2 overlap, PLPintra2 being an extended version of the widely used encephalitogenic PLP139-151 peptide. Furthermore, the region covered by PLPintra2 corresponds nearly exactly to the segment missing in the alternatively spliced DM20 isoform of PLP. DM20 is believed to be less adhesive in membrane multilayers than PLP [63]. The fact

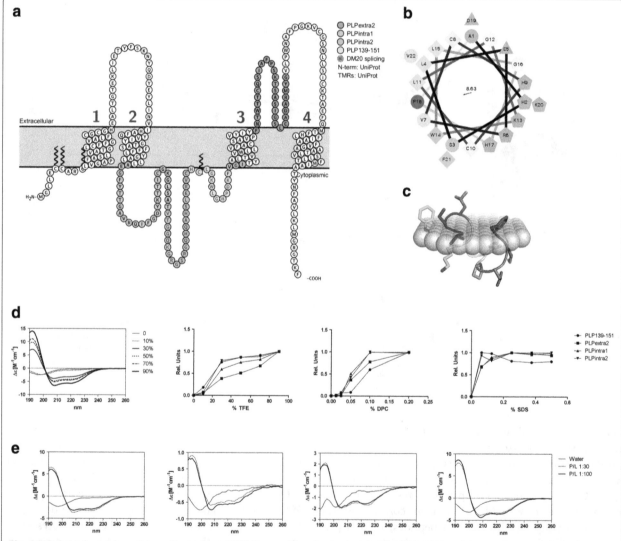

Fig. 6 PLP-derived peptides. **a** Schematic structure of PLP. The peptide colouring is shown in the legend, and the segment missing in DM20 is shown by *red sequence*. Potential palmitoylation sites are also indicated. **b** Helical wheel of a predicted amphipathic helix in the PLPintra2 (and PLP139-151) peptide. **c** Predicted membrane association of the C-terminal half of the PLPintra2 peptide, based on the PEP-FOLD model. **d** Behaviour of PLP peptides in membrane-mimicking conditions. From left to right: typical spectra for a TFE titration series (shown here for the PLPintra1 peptide), relative signals at 195 nm in the presence of TFE, DPC, and SDS for all peptides. **e** Conventional CD spectra of the PLP peptides (left to right: PLPintra1, PLPintra2, PLP139-151, PLPextra2) at different P/L ratios in the presence of DMPC/DMPG vesicles

that peptides corresponding to the region missing in DM20 show clear, strong folding events in membrane-like environments suggests that indeed, a membrane-binding site is removed from DM20 during alternative mRNA splicing. It is likely that this segment folds into an amphipathic helix onto the membrane surface (Fig. 6c); this propensity should be further strengthened by hydrophobic post-translational modifications (palmitoylation) on the two Cys residues, as suggested by a helical wheel representation (Fig. 6b).

The palmitoylation of the Cys residues has been observed to induce greater T cell and antibody responses in both EAE mice and MS patients compared to nonacylated peptides [64, 65]. This further supports the relevance of the hydrophobic surface of an amphipathic helix to the immunogenicity of PLP139-151 and PLPintra2 peptides. We believe that this segment is a strong membrane anchor in PLP. Whether it binds to the same or the apposing membrane surface in myelin, is currently unknown. Both scenarios would explain stronger adhesive properties of PLP in comparison to the DM20 isoform.

During evolution, the 35-residue segment distinguishing PLP from DM20 has been acquired in terrestrial vertebrates [63, 66]. Simultaneously, the expression of myelin protein zero (P0) in the CNS has been lost. This points towards a scenario, where the evolution of terrestrial vertebrates at the myelin molecular level has involved the loss of P0-mediated adhesion (which still is crucial in the PNS) and the acquirement of an additional adhesive segment in the cytoplasmic domain of PLP/DM20. PLP has a strong tendency to form dimers in transfected COS cells, primary oligodendrocytes, and in brain tissue, while DM20 exists mainly as a monomer. Cys108, located in the common part of intracellular loop of PLP/DM20, as well as in the PLPintra1 peptide, is involved in the dimerization of PLP [67].

Both the PLP139-151 and PLPintra2 peptides include a 'stop transfer signal' (residues HPDK^{150}), which restricts the ability of transmembrane helix 3 to shift in the cases of mutations in the second extracellular loop of PLP. These charged residues are omitted from DM20, enabling the movement of the transmembrane domain inside the membrane [68]. Thus, in some cases, the middle part of the PLPintra1 peptide (residues GLSAT^{115}) forms an extension of transmembrane helix 3 and can be embedded into the membrane. Several PLP139-151 epitope-mimicking peptides, not studied here, are also known e.g. from *Acanthamoeba castellanii* [69] and *Haemophilus influenza* [70]. Whether they share properties with PLP139-151 remains a subject for future research.

The second extracellular loop of PLP contains two disulphide bonds, located between Cys183-Cys227 and Cys200-Cys227, respectively. The membrane-proximal disulphide bond (Cys183-Cys227) is fundamental to the proper cell surface expression of PLP, and it is involved in Pelizaeus–Merzbacher disease [71]. The PLPextra2 peptide contains only two Cys residues (Cys183 and 200) and cannot form these disulphide bonds. However, all membrane-mimicking conditions induced an α-helical folding of the PLPextra2 peptide (Fig. 6d, e and Additional file 5: Table S2). Dhaunchak and Nave [71] also reported that the cell surface expression of PLP can be rescued if the cysteines in the second extracellular loop are mutated, indicating that the disulphide bonds are not crucial for the normal folding of the second extracellular loop.

The deconvolution of spectral data suggested 30–40% helical content in membrane vesicles for PLPextra2 and PLPintra1, which is consistent with the *de novo* predicted situation with partially folded and disordered state (Table 1). Although the change in spectrum indicated increased α-helical nature for PLPintra2, the calculated content of α helices was modest. This may be an underestimate due to putative aggregation, which is discussed below.

Membrane-induced folding of the GBS epitope from human peripheral nerve protein P2

P2 is one of the structurally best-characterized myelin proteins, being highly expressed in PNS myelin [72, 73]. It is a proposed target of autoimmune reactions in GBS, and P2 peptides can be used to induce EAN, the mouse model of human GBS [74, 75]. P2 is able to stack lipid bilayers together in an ordered manner in vitro [41, 76, 77], and the P2 knockout mouse has changes in myelin lipid composition and motor nerve conduction velocity during periods of active myelination [73].

The peptide studied here corresponds to the GBS epitope characterized earlier [78], and in the crystal structure, it comprises the first α helix of the lid of the 10-stranded β-barrel structure [44] (Fig. 7a). It is likely that the helical lid is centrally involved in membrane interactions during membrane stacking [79].

The P2gbs peptide showed helical folding at DPC and SDS concentrations above the CMC, and strong helical folding was present at 30% TFE (Fig. 7b–d). With lipid vesicles, a helical spectrum was observed in SRCD experiments, further indicating induction of α-helical folding of P2gbs in membrane-like conditions (Fig. 7e). While these results are not unexpected in light of *de novo* predictions (Table 1, Additional file 3: Figure S2) and the fact that the sequence is helical in the crystal structure and predicted to contact the membrane, they provide striking similarity to the CNS antigen peptides described above. Similar molecular mechanisms and principles could, thus, be involved in demyelination-related autoimmunity in the CNS and PNS.

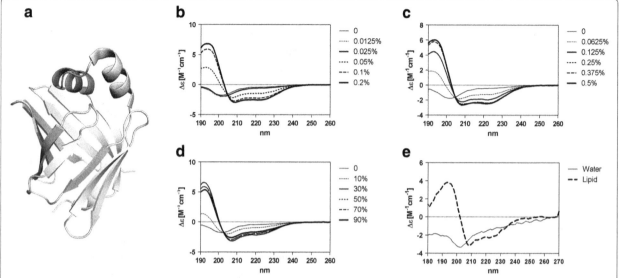

Fig. 7 The GBS epitope in P2. **a** The GBS epitope corresponds to the first α helix in the P2 crystal structure [44]. The two helices form a lid, proposed to interact with the myelin membrane and possibly open upon ligand entry and release [79]. **b** DPC titration. **c** SDS titration. **d** TFE titration. **e** SRCD spectra with and without lipid vesicles

Turbidimetry shows peptide-induced vesicle agglutination

In SRCD, one generally can use shorter pathlengths, and hence, much higher sample concentrations than in conventional CD, which has the problem of light intensity falling off at lower wavelengths. During SRCD experiments, peptide-induced aggregation was observed when lipid vesicles were added into solutions of high (0.5 mg/ml) concentrations of peptides. This was most severe for the EB-mimic, MOG35-55, and PLPintra2 peptides (data not shown). The problem could be circumvented by using lower peptide concentration (0.25 mg/ml) with a high (1:100) peptide:lipid ratio in SRCD experiments; this observation also triggered us to investigate the agglutination potency of the studied peptides more closely.

The monitoring of lipid vesicle aggregation was done by measuring absorption (turbidity) at 450 nm after mixing vesicles with increasing concentrations of peptides (Fig. 8a). Although the peptide-induced aggregation was modest compared to protein P2-induced agglutination (Fig. 8b), reproducible vesicle agglutination was detected for the EB-mimic, hMOG35-55, mMOG35-55, and PLPintra2 peptides, and occasionally also for IA-mimic and PA-mimic (Fig. 8 and data not shown). The observation of turbidity could indicate a propensity of the peptide to stack membrane bilayers together into multilayers (mimicking myelin); in the least, it is a sign of altered surface properties of the lipid membrane, promoting aggregation. Hence, we consider turbidity a functional assay for myelin membrane-stacking proteins/peptides. Having this property not only in myelin protein

peptides, but also in some of the molecular mimics, further indicates common properties for the studied encephalitogenic peptides.

Discussion

Despite huge efforts in the past decades, MS has so far evaded the deciphering of its pathogenesis. We know that in rodent EAE models, an active immunization with myelin antigens, or a passive adoptive transfer of myelin-specific autoreactive Th1/Th17 CD4 lymphocytes, phenocopies many features of MS [80–82]. There exists also understanding that the genetic susceptibility *via* the HLA-DR15 haplotype and certain environmental factors, such as infection by herpes viruses, especially by Epstein-Barr virus, are significant risk factors for MS [83]. However, we do not know whether induction of autoimmunity in MS takes place primarily in the periphery (like in EAE) or in the CNS. In the early stages of MS, the presence of infiltrated T lymphocytes predominates, while in later stages, CNS inflammation becomes self-sustainable, and the number of B cells in lesions increases [2]. However, we do not know the relative importance of CD4 and CD8 T cells or the exact roles of B cells and antibodies. Finally, although the structural similarity between the MHC II-bound MBP-derived peptides and their molecular mimics, like those from EBV polymerase, can explain how the mimic-specific TCRs in CD4 T cells can recognize self-antigens [84, 85], we lack structures of MBP/mimic-bound MHC I complexes. The latter are important, as cytotoxic CD8 T cells can directly attack the oligodendrocytes, which present peptides to them [86]. Neither do we know whether the

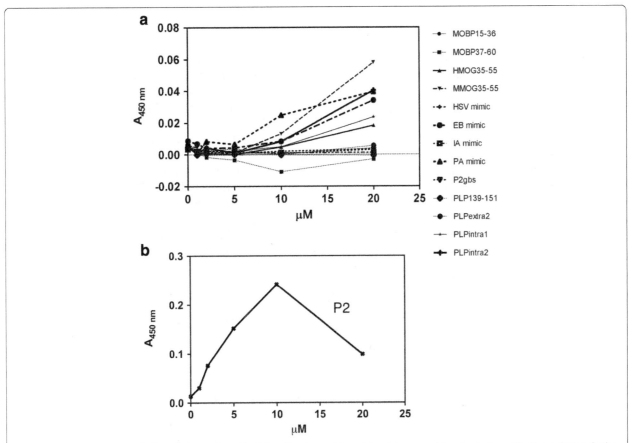

Fig. 8 Turbidimetric analysis of all studied peptides. **a** Turbidity of each peptide-vesicle mixture was determined after a 10-min incubation. **b** The human myelin protein P2 acts as a positive control for the assay. Note how concentrations above 10 μM decrease turbidity; this is caused by precipitation of the vesicle aggregates

autoantibodies, which recognize folded epitopes like those in MOG, may be induced by mimicking antigens.

MBP is the best-characterized myelin protein, both at the level of the full-length protein and as peptide segments. Much of the early research was carried out using MBP purified from tissue [20–25, 27], and more recently, recombinant MBP has also been intensively studied [29, 30, 48, 49]. According to the current view, MBP is intrinsically disordered in solution, but folds into short helical segments upon membrane binding [87]. The structure of MBP on membranes can be further affected by the lipid composition. Here, we did not assess the effects of different lipid compositions on peptide folding, but earlier research has shown that the helical structure of the autoimmune epitope of MBP does slightly change in different lipid membrane compositions [45, 88]. This is of interest because demyelination is linked to changes in lipid composition, and these changes may in turn alter the conformation, localization, and properties of MBP [89]. Furthermore, the epitope conformation may be affected by its presence in either a peptide or a full-length MBP protein [46, 47]. For obtaining detailed local

conformational information, we chose here to focus on short peptide segments. Even for the longest peptides, we believe that the membrane-binding segments will be short helices, as predicted *de novo* (Additional file 3: Figure S2).

How do our observations of the common membrane-induced folding of MBP mimics, and most other peptides studied here, fit into this big picture? It is possible that the propensity to adopt α-helical structure in the experiment merely illustrates similar biophysical properties. However, it is also possible that these peptides do adopt a helical structure in vivo, with relevance to the generation of autoimmunity *per se*. Two speculative hypotheses can be presented.

Firstly, the relatively low affinity and non-standard geometry in the binding of TCRs to MHC II-peptide complexes can explain the escape of self-reactive T cells from negative selection [90]. In the known MHC II-MBP/mimic structures, the peptide binds MHC in an extended conformation [84, 85]. Whether the peptide propensity to fold affects rescue from negative selection is not known. It can be speculated that during the generation of T cell tolerance, the amount of MHC-loadable non-folded self-peptides is low, but may become significant after inflammatory insult. Interestingly, the presence of autoantigenic MBP peptides in the spectrum of proteasomal products increases after MBP immunization [86]. Secondly, it is possible that mimic-specific, such as Epstein-Barr virus-infected and CNS-infiltrated, memory B cells [91] may have affinity against myelin neoepitopes that are exposed in degenerated/insulted myelin.

Neither scenario above suggests that membrane-induced folding universally leads to auto-immunogenicity, but it could be relevant in rare cases where both 1) the environment-induced conformational changes of myelin proteins can lead to changes in processing and/or peptide loading to affect negative selection of T cells or creation of neoepitopes for B cells and 2) the mimicking agent is present at the critical time. It is obvious that many hydrophobic self-sequences are strongly immunogenic [92, 93], but the corresponding T cells go to apoptosis in the thymus. An animal model with genetic or external exposure of myelin proteins/peptides, which do not significantly change the structure of the host protein, but alter membrane-induced conformational changes, might be useful to test these hypotheses.

Conclusions

The understanding of myelin autoimmunity at the molecular level is poor, also taking into account the fact that myelin protein epitopes in general are buried within the myelin sheath, a tightly packed multilayered membrane. On the other hand, these epitopes are hidden from the immune system in a healthy myelin environment, and might only be exposed in case of prior insult to the myelin membrane. All our experiments point towards highly similar properties for all the studied peptides. In this respect, it is of interest to note the possible potential of myelin protein-derived peptides in MS therapy; these include both cyclic and mutated variants of myelin antigen peptides, especially MBP85-99 [59, 94–98]; the design of such peptides could also take into account our observations on similar overall structural and membrane interaction properties of peptides with limited sequence similarity *per se*. While the link between membrane binding, membrane-induced folding, and autoimmune response is unclear, molecular mimicry possibly taking place in autoimmune demyelination may be based on 3D similarity of host and pathogen epitopes. In the case of MBP85-99 mimics, for example, while the peptides fold into amphipathic helices on lipid membranes, the extended conformation bound to the MHC shows the conserved residues being presented outwards, being important for immune response.

Our results give new insights into myelin protein-membrane interactions within short segments of the protein; the situation in the case of full-length proteins is of course more complex. For protein-peptide interactions, both electrostatic interactions and conformational flexibility are important factors in recognition and binding [99]. In the case of flexible proteins, such as MBP, a multitude of conformations are present [29, 87], and antibody binding might reflect a fortuitous capture of specific conformations that become more rigid. The conformations of MBP peptides on the membrane surface and when bound to MHC may reflect such a phenomenon. Similar properties between different peptide epitopes may provide means to multifaceted, but shared, recognition mechanisms, which in turn may relate to disease etiology. It is clear that more research in in vivo systems will be required to gain further answers to these questions in the case of autoimmune demyelination.

Additional files

> **Additional file 1: Table S1.** Details of peptide properties.
>
> **Additional file 2: Figure S1.** Helical wheel predictions of all peptides from this study.
>
> **Additional file 3: Figure S2.** PEP-FOLD model predictions for the studied peptides.
>
> **Additional file 4: Figure S3.** CD spectra for a negative control peptide from the *P. falciparum* formin display no folding under membrane-mimicking conditions. The peptide sequence is KKIPAPPPFLLKKK.
>
> **Additional file 5: Table S2.** Results from CD spectrum deconvolution of all 290 samples, with two different algorithms.

Abbreviations

CD: Circular dichroism; CMC: Critical micellar concentration; CNS: Central nervous system; DMPC: Dimyristoyl phosphatidylcholine; DMPG: Dimyristoyl phosphatidylglycerol; DPC: n-Dodecyl phosphocholine; EAE: Experimental autoimmune encephalomyelitis; EAN: Experimental autoimmune neuritis; GBS: Guillain-Barré syndrome; MBP: Myelin basic protein; MHC: Major histocompatibility complex; MOBP: Myelin-associated oligodendrocytic basic protein; MOG: Myelin-oligodendrocyte glycoprotein; MS: Multiple sclerosis; OCD: Oriented CD; PLP: Proteolipid protein; PNS: Peripheral nervous system; SDS: Sodium dodecyl sulfate; SRCD: Synchrotron radiation CD; TCR: T cell receptor; TFE: Trifluoroethanol

Acknowledgements

We extend our special thanks to the beamline staff at SOLEIL and ISA, as well as to staff at the Biocenter Oulu Proteomics and Protein Analysis Core Facility.

Funding

This study has been supported by the Emil Aaltonen Foundation (Finland), the Sigrid Juselius Foundation (Finland), the Academy of Finland, and the Research Council of Norway (SYNKNØYT program). The funders had no role in the design of the study, the collection, analysis, and interpretation of data, or in writing the manuscript.

Authors' contributions

JT planned and carried out experiments, analysed data, and was a major contributor in writing the manuscript. AR planned and carried out experiments, optimized methodologies, and participated in writing the manuscript. SR analysed data and participated in writing the manuscript. PK obtained funding for the study, planned experiments and analysed data, and was a major contributor in writing the manuscript. All authors read and approved the final manuscript.

Competing interests

The authors declare that they have no competing interests.

References

1. Compston A, Coles A. Multiple sclerosis. Lancet. 2008;372:1502–17.
2. Dendrou CA, Fugger L, Friese MA. Immunopathology of multiple sclerosis. Nat Rev Immunol. 2015;15:545–58.
3. Valli A, Sette A, Kappos L, Oseroff C, Sidney J, Miescher G, Hochberger M, Albert ED, Adorini L. Binding of myelin basic protein peptides to human histocompatibility leukocyte antigen class II molecules and their recognition by T cells from multiple sclerosis patients. J Clin Invest. 1993;91:616–28.
4. Bielekova B, Sung MH, Kadom N, Simon R, McFarland H, Martin R. Expansion and functional relevance of high-avidity myelin-specific CD4+ T cells in multiple sclerosis. J Immunol. 2004;172:3893–904.
5. Greer JM, Csurhes PA, Cameron KD, McCombe PA, Good MF, Pender MP. Increased immunoreactivity to two overlapping peptides of myelin proteolipid protein in multiple sclerosis. Brain. 1997;120:1447–60.
6. Mendel I, Kerlero de Rosbo N, Ben-Nun A. Delineation of the minimal encephalitogenic epitope within the immunodominant region of myelin oligodendrocyte glycoprotein: diverse V beta gene usage by T cells recognizing the core epitope encephalitogenic for T cell receptor V beta b and T cell receptor V beta a H-2b mice. Eur J Immunol. 1996;26:2470–9.
7. de Rosbo NK, Kaye JF, Eisenstein M, Mendel I, Hoeftberger R, Lassmann H, Milo R, Ben-Nun A. The myelin-associated oligodendrocytic basic protein region MOBP15-36 encompasses the immunodominant major encephalitogenic epitope(s) for SJL/J mice and predicted epitope(s) for multiple sclerosis-associated HLA-DRB1*1501. J Immunol. 2004;173:1426–35.
8. Holz A, Bielekova B, Martin R, Oldstone MB. Myelin-associated oligodendrocytic basic protein: identification of an encephalitogenic epitope and association with multiple sclerosis. J Immunol. 2000;164:1103–9.
9. Denic A, Johnson AJ, Bieber AJ, Warrington AE, Rodriguez M, Pirko I. The relevance of animal models in multiple sclerosis research. Pathophysiology. 2011;18:21–9.
10. Csurhes PA, Sullivan AA, Green K, Pender MP, McCombe PA. T cell reactivity to P0, P2, PMP-22, and myelin basic protein in patients with Guillain-Barré syndrome and chronic inflammatory demyelinating polyradiculoneuropathy. J Neurol Neurosurg Psychiatry. 2005;76:1431–9.
11. Hughes RA, Cornblath DR. Guillain-Barré syndrome. Lancet. 2005;366:1653–66.
12. Makowska A, Pritchard J, Sanvito L, Gregson N, Peakman M, Hayday A, Hughes R. Immune responses to myelin proteins in Guillain-Barré syndrome. J Neurol Neurosurg Psychiatry. 2008;79:664–71.
13. Loshaj-Shala A, Regazzoni L, Daci A, Orioli M, Brezovska K, Panovska AP, Beretta G, Suturkova L. Guillain Barré syndrome (GBS): new insights in the molecular mimicry between C. jejuni and human peripheral nerve (HPN) proteins. J Neuroimmunol. 2015;289:168–76.
14. Willison HJ, Jacobs BC, van Doorn PA. Guillain-Barré syndrome. Lancet. 2016;388:717–27.
15. Virtanen JO, Jacobson S. Viruses and multiple sclerosis. CNS Neurol Disord Drug Targets. 2012;11:528–44.
16. Virtanen JO, Wohler J, Fenton K, Reich DS, Jacobson S. Oligoclonal bands in multiple sclerosis reactive against two herpesviruses and association with magnetic resonance imaging findings. Mult Scler. 2014;20:27–34.
17. Wuest SC, Mexhitaj I, Chai NR, Romm E, Scheffel J, Xu B, Lane K, Wu T, Bielekova B. A complex role of herpes viruses in the disease process of multiple sclerosis. PLoS One. 2014;9:e105434.
18. Zheng MM, Zhang XH. Cross-reactivity between human cytomegalovirus peptide 981-1003 and myelin oligodendroglia glycoprotein peptide 35-55 in experimental autoimmune encephalomyelitis in Lewis rats. Biochem Biophys Res Commun. 2014;443:1118 23.
19. Wucherpfennig KW, Strominger JL. Molecular mimicry in T cell-mediated autoimmunity: viral peptides activate human T cell clones specific for myelin basic protein. Cell. 1995;80:695–705.
20. Anthony JS, Moscarello MA. A conformation change induced in the basic encephalitogen by lipids. Biochim Biophys Acta. 1971;243:429–33.
21. Chao LP, Einstein ER. Physical properties of the bovine encephalitogenic protein; molecular weight and conformation. J Neurochem. 1970;17:1121–32.
22. Epand RM, Moscarello MA, Zierenberg B, Vail WJ. The folded conformation of the encephalitogenic protein of the human brain. Biochemistry. 1974;13:1264–7.
23. Haas H, Oliveira CL, Torriani IL, Polverini E, Fasano A, Carlone G, Cavatorta P, Riccio P. Small angle x-ray scattering from lipid-bound myelin basic protein in solution. Biophys J. 2004;86:455–60.
24. Krigbaum WR, Hsu TS. Molecular conformation of bovine A1 basic protein, a coiling macromolecule in aqueous solution. Biochemistry. 1975;14:2542–6.
25. Mendz GL, Moore WJ, Brown LR, Martenson RE. Interaction of myelin basic protein with micelles of dodecylphosphocholine. Biochemistry. 1984;23:6041–6.
26. Polverini E, Fasano A, Zito F, Riccio P, Cavatorta P. Conformation of bovine myelin basic protein purified with bound lipids. Eur Biophys J. 1999;28:351–5.
27. Wood DD, Moscarello MA, Epand RM. Studies on chemically modified forms of the myelin basic protein: requirements for encephalitogenicity. FEBS Lett. 1976;66:290–2.
28. Vassall KA, Bessonov K, De Avila M, Polverini E, Harauz G. The effects of threonine phosphorylation on the stability and dynamics of the central molecular switch region of 18.5-kDa myelin basic protein. PLoS One. 2013;8:e68175.
29. Vassall KA, Jenkins AD, Bamm VV, Harauz G. Thermodynamic analysis of the disorder-to-alpha-helical transition of 18.5-kDa myelin basic protein reveals an equilibrium intermediate representing the most compact conformation. J Mol Biol. 2015;427:1977–92.
30. Wang C, Neugebauer U, Bürck J, Myllykoski M, Baumgärtel P, Popp J, Kursula P. Charge isomers of myelin basic protein: structure and interactions with membranes, nucleotide analogues, and calmodulin. PLoS One. 2011;6:e19915.
31. Muruganandam G, Bürck J, Ulrich AS, Kursula I, Kursula P. Lipid membrane association of myelin proteins and peptide segments studied by oriented and synchrotron radiation circular dichroism spectroscopy. J Phys Chem B. 2013;117:14983–93.
32. Musse AA, Boggs JM, Harauz G. Deimination of membrane-bound myelin basic protein in multiple sclerosis exposes an immunodominant epitope. Proc Natl Acad Sci U S A. 2006;103:4422–7.
33. Aggarwal S, Snaidero N, Pähler G, Frey S, Sánchez P, Zwckstetter M, Janshoff A, Schneider A, Weil MT, Schaap IA, Görlich D, Simons M. Myelin membrane assembly is driven by a phase transition of myelin basic proteins into a cohesive protein meshwork. PLoS Biol. 2013;11:e1001577.
34. von Budingen HC, Hauser SL, Ouallet JC, Tanuma N, Menge T, Genain CP. Frontline: Epitope recognition on the myelin/oligodendrocyte glycoprotein differentially influences disease phenotype and antibody effector functions in autoimmune demyelination. Eur J Immunol. 2004;34:2072–83.
35. Lees JG, Smith BR, Wien F, Miles AJ, Wallace BA. CDtool-an integrated software package for circular dichroism spectroscopic data processing, analysis, and archiving. Anal Biochem. 2004;332:285–9.
36. Shen Y, Maupetit J, Derreumaux P, Tuffery P. Improved PEP-FOLD Approach for Peptide and Miniprotein Structure Prediction. J Chem Theory Comput. 2014;10:4745–58.
37. Thevenet P, Shen Y, Maupetit J, Guyon F, Derreumaux P, Tuffery P. PEP-FOLD: an updated de novo structure prediction server for both linear and disulfide bonded cyclic peptides. Nucleic Acids Res. 2012;40:W288–93.
38. Lomize MA, Pogozheva ID, Joo H, Mosberg HI, Lomize AL. OPM database and PPM web server: resources for positioning of proteins in membranes. Nucleic Acids Res. 2012;40:D370–6.
39. Whitmore L, Wallace BA. DICHROWEB, an online server for protein secondary structure analyses from circular dichroism spectroscopic data. Nucleic Acids Res. 2004;32:W668–73.
40. Micsonai A, Wien F, Kernya L, Lee YH, Goto Y, Refregiers M, Kardos J. Accurate secondary structure prediction and fold recognition for circular dichroism spectroscopy. Proc Natl Acad Sci U S A. 2015;112:E3095–103.
41. Ruskamo S, Yadav RP, Sharma S, Lehtimäki M, Laulumaa S, Aggarwal S, Simons M, Bürck J, Ulrich AS, Juffer AH, Kursula I, Kursula P. Atomic resolution view into the structure-function relationships of the human

myelin peripheral membrane protein P2. Acta Crystallogr D Biol Crystallogr. 2014;70:165–76.

42. Jo E, Boggs JM. Aggregation of acidic lipid vesicles by myelin basic protein: dependence on potassium concentration. Biochemistry. 1995;34:13705–16.

43. Kursula P. Structural properties of proteins specific to the myelin sheath. Amino Acids. 2008;34:175–85.

44. Majava V, Polverini E, Mazzini A, Nanekar R, Knoll W, Peters J, Natali F, Baumgärtel P, Kursula I, Kursula P. Structural and functional characterization of human peripheral nervous system myelin protein P2. PLoS One. 2010;5:e10300.

45. Ahmed MA, Bamm VV, Harauz G, Ladizhansky V. Solid-state NMR spectroscopy of membrane-associated myelin basic protein—conformation and dynamics of an immunodominant epitope. Biophys J. 2010;99:1247–55.

46. Ahmed MA, De Avila M, Polverini E, Bessonov K, Bamm VV, Harauz G. Solution nuclear magnetic resonance structure and molecular dynamics simulations of a murine 18.5 kDa myelin basic protein segment (S72–S107) in association with dodecylphosphocholine micelles. Biochemistry. 2012;51:7475–87.

47. Farès C, Libich DS, Harauz G. Solution NMR structure of an immunodominant epitope of myelin basic protein. Conformational dependence on environment of an intrinsically unstructured protein. FEBS J. 2006;273:601–14.

48. Libich DS, Harauz G. Solution NMR and CD spectroscopy of an intrinsically disordered, peripheral membrane protein: evaluation of aqueous and membrane-mimetic solvent conditions for studying the conformational adaptability of the 18.5 kDa isoform of myelin basic protein (MBP). Eur Biophys J. 2008;37:1015–29.

49. Libich DS, Ahmed MA, Zhong L, Bamm VV, Ladizhansky V, Harauz G. Fuzzy complexes of myelin basic protein: NMR spectroscopic investigations of a polymorphic organizational linker of the central nervous system. Biochem Cell Biol. 2010;88:143–55.

50. Myllykoski M, Baumgärtel P, Kursula P. Conformations of peptides derived from myelin-specific proteins in membrane-mimetic conditions probed by synchrotron radiation CD spectroscopy. Amino Acids. 2012;42:1467–74.

51. Li Y, Li H, Martin R, Mariuzza RA. Structural basis for the binding of an immunodominant peptide from myelin basic protein in different registers by two HLA-DR2 proteins. J Mol Biol. 2000;304:177–88.

52. Katsara M, Yuriev E, Ramsland PA, Deraos G, Tselios T, Matsoukas J, Apostolopoulos V. A double mutation of MBP(83–99) peptide induces IL-4 responses and antagonizes IFN-gamma responses. J Neuroimmunol. 2008;200:77–89.

53. Potamitis C, Matsoukas MT, Tselios T, Mavromoustakos T, Golič GS. Conformational analysis of the MBP83-99 (Phe91) and MBP83-99 (Tyr91) peptide analogues and study of their interactions with the HLA-DR2 and human TCR receptors by using molecular dynamics. J Comput Aided Mol Des. 2011;25:837–53.

54. Lu X, Qi J, Shi Y, Wang M, Smith DF, Heimburg-Molinaro J, Zhang Y, Paulson JC, Xiao H, Gao GF. Structure and receptor binding specificity of hemagglutinin H13 from avian influenza A virus H13N6. J Virol. 2013;87:9077–85.

55. Mendel I, Kerlero de Rosbo N, Ben-Nun A. A myelin oligodendrocyte glycoprotein peptide induces typical chronic experimental autoimmune encephalomyelitis in H-2b mice: fine specificity and T cell receptor V beta expression of encephalitogenic T cells. Eur J Immunol. 1995;25:1951–9.

56. Moreno M, Guo F, Mills Ko E, Bannerman P, Soulika A, Pleasure D. Origins and significance of astrogliosis in the multiple sclerosis model, MOG peptide EAE. J Neurol Sci. 2013;333:55–9.

57. Rich C, Link JM, Zamora A, Jacobsen H, Meza-Romero R, Offner H, Jones R, Burrows GG, Fugger L, Vandenbark AA. Myelin oligodendrocyte glycoprotein-35-55 peptide induces severe chronic experimental autoimmune encephalomyelitis in HLA-DR2-transgenic mice. Eur J Immunol. 2004;34:1251–61.

58. Clements CS, Reid HH, Beddoe T, Tynan FE, Perugini MA, Johns TG, Bernard CC, Rossjohn J. The crystal structure of myelin oligodendrocyte glycoprotein, a key autoantigen in multiple sclerosis. Proc Natl Acad Sci U S A. 2003;100:11059–64.

59. Tselios T, Aggelidakis M, Tapeinou A, Tseveleki V, Kanistras I, Gatos D, Matsoukas J. Rational design and synthesis of altered peptide ligands based on human myelin oligodendrocyte glycoprotein 35-55 epitope: inhibition of chronic experimental autoimmune encephalomyelitis in mice. Molecules. 2014;19:17968–84.

60. Recks MS, Grether NB, van der Broeck F, Ganscher A, Wagner N, Henke E, Ergun S, Schroeter M, Kuerten S. Four different synthetic peptides of proteolipid protein induce a distinct antibody response in MP4-induced experimental autoimmune encephalomyelitis. Clin Immunol. 2015;159:93–106.

61. Kennedy MK, Tan LJ, Dal Canto MC, Tuohy VK, Lu ZJ, Trotter JL, Miller SD. Inhibition of murine relapsing experimental autoimmune encephalomyelitis by immune tolerance to proteolipid protein and its encephalitogenic peptides. J Immunol. 1990;144:909–15.

62. Appadu A, Jelokhani-Niaraki M, DeBruin L. Conformational Changes and Association of Membrane-Interacting Peptides in Myelin Membrane Models: A Case of the C-Terminal Peptide of Proteolipid Protein and the Antimicrobial Peptide Melittin. J Phys Chem B. 2015;119:14821–30.

63. Stecca B, Southwood CM, Gragerov A, Kelley KA, Friedrich VLJ, Gow A. The evolution of lipophilin genes from invertebrates to tetrapods: DM-20 cannot replace proteolipid protein in CNS myelin. J Neurosci. 2000;20:4002–10.

64. Greer JM, Denis B, Sobel RA, Trifilieff E. Thiopalmitoylation of myelin proteolipid protein epitopes enhances immunogenicity and encephalitogenicity. J Immunol. 2001;166:6907–13.

65. Pfender NA, Grosch S, Roussel G, Koch M, Trifilieff E, Greer JM. Route of uptake of palmitoylated encephalitogenic peptides of myelin proteolipid protein by antigen-presenting cells: importance of the type of bond between lipid chain and peptide and relevance to autoimmunity. J Immunol. 2008;180:1398–404.

66. Inouye H, Kirschner DA. Evolution of myelin ultrastructure and the major structural myelin proteins. Brain Res. 2016;1641:43–63.

67. Daffu G, Sohi J, Kamholz J. Proteolipid protein dimerization at cysteine 108: Implications for protein structure. Neurosci Res. 2012;74:144–55.

68. Dhaunchak AS, Colman DR, Nave KA. Misalignment of PLP/DM20 transmembrane domains determines protein misfolding in Pelizaeus-Merzbacher disease. J Neurosci. 2011;31:14961–71.

69. Massilamany C, Steffen D, Reddy J. An epitope from Acanthamoeba castellanii that cross-react with proteolipid protein 139-151-reactive T cells induces autoimmune encephalomyelitis in SJL mice. J Neuroimmunol. 2010;219:17–24.

70. Olson JK, Croxford JL, Calenoff MA, Dal Canto MC, Miller SD. A virus-induced molecular mimicry model of multiple sclerosis. J Clin Invest. 2001;108:311–8.

71. Dhaunchak AS, Nave KA. A common mechanism of PLP/DM20 misfolding causes cysteine-mediated endoplasmic reticulum retention in oligodendrocytes and Pelizaeus-Merzbacher disease. Proc Natl Acad Sci U S A. 2007;104:17813–8.

72. Trapp BD, McIntyre LJ, Quarles RH, Sternberger NH, Webster HD. Immunocytochemical localization of rat peripheral nervous system myelin proteins: P2 protein is not a component of all peripheral nervous system myelin sheaths. Proc Natl Acad Sci U S A. 1979;76:3552–6.

73. Zenker J, Stettner M, Ruskamo S, Domènech-Estévez E, Baloui H, Médard JJ, Verheijen MH, Brouwers JF, Kursula P, Kieseier BC, Chrast R. A role of peripheral myelin protein 2 in lipid homeostasis of myelinating Schwann cells. Glia. 2014;62:1502–12.

74. Abramsky O, Teitelbaum D, Webb C, Arnon R. Neuritogenic and encephalitogenic properties of the peripheral nerve basic proteins. J Neuropathol Exp Neurol. 1975;34:36–45.

75. Uyemura K, Suzuki M, Kitamura K, Horie K, Ogawa Y, Matsuyama H, Nozaki S, Muramatsu I. Neuritogenic determinant of bovine P2 protein in peripheral nerve myelin. J Neurochem. 1982;39:895–8.

76. Sedzik J, Blaurock AE, Hoechli M. Reconstituted P2/myelin-lipid multilayers. J Neurochem. 1985;45:844–52.

77. Suresh S, Wang C, Nanekar R, Kursula P, Edwardson JM. Myelin basic protein and myelin protein 2 act synergistically to cause stacking of lipid bilayers. Biochemistry. 2010;49:3456–63.

78. Taylor WA, Brostoff SW, Hughes RA. P2 specific lymphocyte transformation in Guillain-Barré syndrome and chronic idiopathic demyelinating polyradiculoneuropathy. J Neurol Sci. 1991;104:52–5.

79. Laulumaa S, Nieminen T, Lehtimäki M, Aggarwal S, Simons M, Koza MM, Vattulainen I, Kursula P, Natali F. Dynamics of the peripheral membrane protein P2 from human myelin measured by neutron scattering–a comparison between wild-type protein and a hinge mutant. PLoS One. 2015;10:e0128954.

80. Constantinescu CS, Farooqi N, O'Brien K, Gran B. Experimental autoimmune encephalomyelitis (EAE) as a model for multiple sclerosis (MS). Br J Pharmacol. 2011;164:1079–106.

81. Pettinelli CB, McFarlin DE. Adoptive transfer of experimental allergic encephalomyelitis in SJL/J mice after in vitro activation of lymph node cells by myelin basic protein: requirement for Lyt 1+ 2- T lymphocytes. J Immunol. 1981;127:1420–3.

82. Reboldi A, Coisne C, Baumjohann D, Benvenuto F, Bottinelli D, Lira S, Uccelli A, Lanzavecchia A, Engelhardt B, Sallusto F. C-C chemokine receptor 6-regulated entry of TH-17 cells into the CNS through the choroid plexus is required for the initiation of EAE. Nat Immunol. 2009;10:514–23.

83. Sospedra M, Zhao Y, zur Hausen H, Muraro PA, Hamashin C, de Villiers EM, Pinilla C, Martin R. Recognition of conserved amino acid motifs of common viruses and its role in autoimmunity. PLoS Pathog. 2005;1:e41.

84. Sethi DK, Schubert DA, Anders AK, Heroux A, Bonsor DA, Thomas CP, Sundberg EJ, Pyrdol J, Wucherpfennig KW. A highly tilted binding mode by a self-reactive T cell receptor results in altered engagement of peptide and MHC. J Exp Med. 2011;208:91–102.

85. Yin Y, Li Y, Mariuzza RA. Structural basis for self-recognition by autoimmune T-cell receptors. Immunol Rev. 2012;250:32–48.

86. Belogurov A, Kuzina E, Kudriaeva A, Kononikhin A, Kovalchuk S, Surina Y, Smirnov I, Lomakin Y, Bacheva A, Stepanov A, Karpova Y, Lyupina Y, Kharybin O, Melamed D, Ponomarenko N, Sharova N, Nikolaev E, Gabibov A. Ubiquitin-independent proteosomal degradation of myelin basic protein contributes to development of neurodegenerative autoimmunity. FASEB J. 2015;29:1901–13.

87. Vassall KA, Bamm VV, Harauz G. MyelStones: the executive roles of myelin basic protein in myelin assembly and destabilization in multiple sclerosis. Biochem J. 2015;472:17–32.

88. Bates IR, Feix JB, Boggs JM, Harauz G. An immunodominant epitope of myelin basic protein is an amphipathic alpha-helix. J Biol Chem. 2004;279:5757–64.

89. Shaharabani R, Ram-On M, Avinery R, Aharoni R, Arnon R, Talmon Y, Beck R. Structural Transition in Myelin Membrane as Initiator of Multiple Sclerosis. J Am Chem Soc. 2016;138:12159–65.

90. Harkiolaki M, Holmes SL, Svendsen P, Gregersen JW, Jensen LT, McMahon R, Friese MA, van Boxel G, Etzensperger R, Tzartos JS, Kranc K, Sainsbury S, Harlos K, Mellins ED, Palace J, Esiri MM, van der Merwe PA, Jones EY, Fugger L. T cell-mediated autoimmune disease due to low-affinity crossreactivity to common microbial peptides. Immunity. 2009;30:348–57.

91. Fernández-Menéndez S, Fernández-Morán M, Fernández-Vega I, Pérez-Álvarez A, Villafani-Echazú J. Epstein-Barr virus and multiple sclerosis. From evidence to therapeutic strategies. J Neurol Sci. 2016;361:213–9.

92. Chowell D, Krishna S, Becker PD, Cocita C, Shu J, Tan X, Greenberg PD, Klavinskis LS, Blattman JN, Anderson KS. TCR contact residue hydrophobicity is a hallmark of immunogenic CD8+ T cell epitopes. Proc Natl Acad Sci U S A. 2015;112:E1754–62.

93. Huang L, Kuhls MC, Eisenlohr LC. Hydrophobicity as a driver of MHC class I antigen processing. EMBO J. 2011;30:1634–44.

94. Apostolopoulos V, Deraos G, Matsoukas MT, Day S, Stojanovska L, Tselios T, Androutsou ME, Matsoukas J. Cyclic citrullinated MBP87-99 peptide stimulates T cell responses: Implications in triggering disease. Bioorg Med Chem. 2017;25:528–38.

95. Day S, Tselios T, Androutsou ME, Tapeinou A, Frilligou I, Stojanovska L, Matsoukas J, Apostolopoulos V. Mannosylated Linear and Cyclic Single Amino Acid Mutant Peptides Using a Small 10 Amino Acid Linker Constitute Promising Candidates Against Multiple Sclerosis. Front Immunol. 2015;6:136.

96. Deraos G, Rodi M, Kalbacher H, Chatzantoni K, Karagiannis F, Synodinos L, Plotas P, Papalois A, Dimisianos N, Papathanasopoulos P, Gatos D, Tselios T, Apostolopoulos V, Mouzaki A, Matsoukas J. Properties of myelin altered peptide ligand cyclo(87–99)(Ala91, Ala96)MBP87-99 render it a promising drug lead for immunotherapy of multiple sclerosis. Eur J Med Chem. 2015;101:13–23.

97. Grigoriadis N, Tselios T, Deraos S, Orologas A, Deraos G, Matsoukas J, Mavromatis I, Milonas I. Animal models of central nervous system immune-mediated diseases: therapeutic interventions with bioactive peptides and mimetics. Curr Med Chem. 2005;12:1513–9.

98. Katsara M, Deraos G, Tselios T, Matsoukas J, Apostolopoulos V. Design of novel cyclic altered peptide ligands of myelin basic protein MBP83-99 that modulate immune responses in SJL/J mice. J Med Chem. 2008;51:3971–8.

99. Dagliyan O, Proctor EA, D'Auria KM, Ding F, Dokholyan NV. Structural and dynamic determinants of protein-peptide recognition. Structure. 2011;19:1837–45.

100. Lunemann JD, Ruckert S, Kern F, Wendling U, van der Zee R, Volk HD, Zipp F. Cross-sectional and longitudinal analysis of myelin-reactive T cells in patients with multiple sclerosis. J Neurol. 2004;251:1111–20.

101. Carotenuto A, D'Ursi AM, Nardi E, Papini AM, Rovero P. Conformational analysis of a glycosylated human myelin oligodendrocyte glycoprotein peptide epitope able to detect antibody response in multiple sclerosis. J Med Chem. 2001;44:2378–81.

8

Cytokine profiles in pediatric multiple sclerosis

Vikram Bhise[1,4*], Konstantin Balashov[1], Marc Sturgill[2], Lauren Krupp[3] and Suhayl Dhib-Jalbut[1]

Abstract

Background: The immunopathogenesis of pediatric multiple sclerosis (MS) is not well understood.

Methods: We studied the cytokine profile in pre-treatment serum specimens of 19 pediatric MS patients, 25 adult MS patients, and 22 age- and gender-matched pediatric healthy controls. In addition to IL-2, IL-12p40, IL-12p70, IL-18, IL-23, IL-6, TNF-α, TGF-β-1, IFN-γ, IL-17A, IL-21, IL-10, IL-4, IL-5, IL-13, and GM-CSF, we measured osteopontin and soluble VCAM-I.

Results: In children with MS, significantly lower levels of IL-6 were present compared to age- and gender-matched healthy control children ($p < 0.05$). Moreover, significantly higher levels of osteopontin ($p < 0.02$) and sVCAM-1 ($p < 0.02$) and lower levels of IL-6 ($p < 0.01$) were present, with trends toward lower levels of IL-12p70 ($p = 0.074$) and IL-17a ($p = 0.05$) compared to adults with MS.

Conclusions: These findings indicate important differences in cytokine signatures in children with MS and suggest an unexpected possible lower inflammatory cytokine profile in children with MS.

Keywords: Multiple sclerosis, Child, Cytokines, Interleukin-6, Osteopontin, Soluble vascular cell adhesion molecule

Background

The pathophysiology of multiple sclerosis (MS) is orchestrated by an array of molecular messengers known as cytokines. These signaling molecules are produced by or modulate the activity of T-cells and other immune cells. Many studies in adult MS have examined individual cytokines or their profiles to better characterize the pathogenesis of this disease, but only a limited number of studies have examined pediatric patients with MS.

Studies in experimental autoimmune encephalomyelitis (EAE), the animal model of MS, and in adult MS patients have identified disease-associated cytokines that are thus characterized as pro-inflammatory and conversely anti-inflammatory for those associated with disease remission or amelioration. In serum and CSF studies of adult MS patients, elevations of pro-inflammatory IL-2, IL-12, IL-6, TNF-α, and IFN-γ, as well as anti-inflammatory/regulatory IL-10, IL-4, and

TGF-β-1 cytokines, are identified [1]. A recent study by Martins et al of 833 adult subjects with MS and 117 healthy controls using a protocol similar to our study found elevations in pro-inflammatory IFN-γ, IL-2, IL-1B, and TNF-α, and anti-inflammatory IL-4, IL-10, and IL-13 [2]. Higher levels of IL-18, IL-23, and IL-17 are also seen in the serum of MS patients compared to healthy controls [3].

Pediatric MS has distinct features from adult MS insinuating important differences are to be found in the immune profile. The vast majority of patients (over 95 %) present with a relapsing-remitting course. Compared to adults with MS, pediatric-onset individuals have higher relapse rates and shorter times to their second attack, but better recovery from relapses [4, 5]. CSF studies in younger children possess more inflammatory features with greater neutrophilic counts than older children, and are less likely to demonstrate oligoclonal banding [6]. Additionally, for these younger patients, MRI lesions may resolve entirely over the course of a few months [7]. Disability milestones take on average 5 years longer to reach in children compared to adults

* Correspondence: bhisevi@rwjms.rutgers.edu
[1]Rutgers University-Robert Wood Johnson Medical School, New Brunswick, USA
[4]Child Health Institute, 89 French Street, Suite 2200, New Brunswick, NJ 08901, USA
Full list of author information is available at the end of the article

with MS [8]. These features collectively imply a greater inflammatory pathophysiology in childhood MS.

Published studies in pediatric MS pathophysiology have focused on humoral and cellular aspects of the disease. Children with central demyelinating disease demonstrate increased peripheral T-cell proliferation responses to myelin-based and dietary antigens when compared to healthy controls [9]. Additionally, there may be elevated myelin oligodendrocyte glycoprotein (MOG) antibodies, particularly in patients under 10 years of age [10, 11], and higher affinity antibodies present for myelin-basic protein in children [12]. A recent study identified elevated CSF complement anaphylatoxins C5a, C4a, and C3a, and CSF IL-6 levels in children with either monophasic central demyelination or MS, higher in the former, when compared to other neurological diseases [13]. In addition, plasma MOG antibodies in monophasic disease and MS both correlated with CSF IL-6 levels. These differences confirm evidence of abnormal immune physiology in children with demyelinating disease, but lack comparison to adult cohorts.

Our specific aims in this study were to establish a baseline cytokine profile in pediatric MS patients and to compare this profile to that in age- and gender-matched healthy controls and adults with MS to identify cytokine signatures unique to pediatric-onset MS.

Methods
MS patients were enrolled in the study at the time of an outpatient clinic visit to the MS Comprehensive Care Center at RWJMS, the Child Health Institute of NJ, and the Pediatric MS Center at Stony Brook, NY and met 2010 McDonald [14] and/or International Pediatric MS Study Group (IPMSSG) consensus criteria for MS [15]. Peripheral pre-treatment serum samples were collected from 19 pediatric MS patients, 25 adult MS patients, and 22 age- and gender-matched pediatric healthy controls, centrifuged at 1500 rpm for 15-20 minutes and then stored as serum in a -70 ° C freezer. Cytokine analysis was performed using the Cytometric Bead Array immunoassay at a commercial laboratory center (Millipore). The MILLIPLEX™ MAP technology uses microspheres color coded with two fluorescent dyes each and coated with specific antibodies. Following capture, an analyte is bound by a biotinylated detection antibody and then incubated with a Streptavidin-Phycoerythrin conjugate, completing the reaction. The microspheres then pass through two lasers, the first exciting the internal dye, the second, the conjugate dye. High-speed digital processors quantify the fluorescent signals. Multiple microspheres may be used to detect multiple analytes in a single ultra low volume sample.

The following cytokines were tested: IL-2, IL-12p40, IL-12p70, IL-18, IL-23, IL-6, TNF-α, IFN-γ, IL-17A, IL-21,

and osteopontin as measures of pro-inflammatory activity, and IL-10, IL-4, IL-5, IL-13, GM-CSF, sVCAM-I, and TGF-β-1as measures of anti-inflammatory activity.

All enrolled pediatric MS patients were post-pubertal. Clinical data for pediatric MS subjects collected included most recent prior brain MRI lesion count, contrast-enhancing lesion number, T1 hypointense black hole number, time from first event, time from last event, total number of prior attacks, time to next clinical attack, CSF oligoclonal bands, CSF IgG index, CSF white blood cell (WBC) count, and nearest serum vitamin D level. Patients did not receive IV steroids within the 30 days prior to the specimen collection and were naïve to disease-modifying therapy. Adult MS patients had fewer overall relapses and longer disease durations on average.

Statistical analysis was performed using SigmaPlot. Results classified as below laboratory detection standards were scored as 0. Data was analyzed for normality testing followed by application of the Mann-Whitney rank sum test, except for unpaired two-tailed T-test on sVCAM data which was normally distributed with equal variances. Statistical significance was determined by p-value <0.05. Fisher's exact test and student T-test were used to compare patient demographic data. Post hoc-analyses were conducted for vitamin D level, number of attacks, CSF WBC count, time from last clinical attack to blood draw, time from first clinical attack to blood draw (i.e. disease duration), baseline MRI T2 lesion number, and presence of gadolinium-enhancing lesions on baseline MRI.

Results
Mean age and gender distribution were not significantly different between healthy controls and pediatric MS patients (see Table 1), nor gender distribution between adult and pediatric MS. Differences in several cytokines were identified.

Comparison to healthy controls
Lower levels of IL-6 were seen in patients with pediatric MS compared to pediatric healthy controls (p = 0.046) (see Table 2). Patients with pediatric MS also had lower levels of GM-CSF, IFN-γ, IL-12p70, and IL-17A compared to healthy controls, but these differences were not identified as significantly different. A non-significant elevation in IL-23 was also observed in pediatric MS patients compared to pediatric healthy controls (p = 0.11).

Comparison to adult MS
Levels of interferon (IFN)-gamma were lower in pediatric MS patients compared to both adult MS patients and healthy pediatric controls, though not significant. IL-12p70 was also lower in pediatric MS patients compared to adults with MS but not significant (p = 0.074).

Table 1 Demographics

	Untreated Pediatric MS	Untreated Adult MS	Pediatric Healthy Controls
Female	12 (63 %)*	19 (76 %)***	16 (73 %)
Male	7 (37 %)	6 (24 %)	6 (27 %)
Age mean (SD)	16.0 years (1.4)**	37.9 years (10.5)	15.6 years (1.7)
Age range (y)	13.4-18.0	19.0-54.7	12.3-17.9
No. attacks mean	2.1	1.4****	
Disease duration mean (months)	6.9	54.5	

* $p = 0.74$ HC vs PMS, ** $p = 0.33$ HC vs PMS, *** $p = 0.51$ HC vs AMS, **** $p = 0.08$ PMS vs AMS (in past 2 years)

Similarly, levels of IL-17A and IL-6 were lower compared to adults with MS ($p = 0.050$ and $p = 0.004$ respectively). Adult MS patients had lower sVCAM-1 levels than patients with pediatric MS ($p = 0.015$). However, no difference in sVCAM-1 was noted between pediatric healthy controls and patients with pediatric MS.

Clinical correlation

No significant correlations were present for patients with vs without contrast-enhancing brain MRI lesions, number of clinical attacks prior to sample collection, total CSF WBCs, or MRI total brain lesion count with serum levels of cytokines. Testing for CSF oligoclonal bands was positive in all but one patient but the number of unique bands was listed for only a few. CSF IgG index on the other hand was only available for 6 patients. Serum levels of TGF-β-1 negatively correlated (-0.69) with serum vitamin D levels ($p < 0.01$). Serum IL-17F levels had a modest positive correlation (0.47) with time from first clinical attack ($p < 0.05$).

Discussion

Serum levels of IL-6 were significantly lower in children with MS compared to healthy controls ($p = 0.046$) and adults with MS ($p = 0.004$). In contrast, serum IL-6 appears to correlate positively with disease activity in other inflammatory childhood diseases such as Kawasaki disease, juvenile inflammatory arthritis (JIA), and ulcerative colitis [16–18]. Indeed, anti-IL-6 therapy is currently in use for JIA [19]. IL-6 is a multifunctional cytokine produced by many cell types in response to infection, but

also plays a pro-inflammatory role in incurring EAE [20–22]. These actions are mediated by the soluble form of the IL-6 receptor (IL-6R) that may be induced by up-regulation of ICAM-1 and VCAM-1, which allows T_H1 cell entry into the CNS. Previous studies have shown elevated IL-6 levels in the CSF of patients with ADEM which correlates with the presence of anti-MOG antibodies. [13, 23, 24] In MS lesions, T-cells, microglia, and activated astrocytes secrete IL-6 in the setting of augmented receptor responses [25]. This cytokine also appears to stimulate T_H17 differentiation and inhibits TGF-β Treg cell formation [25]. IL-6 also maintains a separate anti-inflammatory and neuroprotective function through oligodendrocyte differentiation, neurotropism, and peripheral nerve regeneration mediated by the membrane-bound IL-6R on select cells such as microglia [26]. Human monocytes are directed away from differentiation into dendritic cells and toward macrophages which have increased anti-inflammatory IL-4 and IL-10 and decreased IL-1β production [27]. Given the dual roles of IL-6, it is possible the relative balance between the two pathways shifts with age. Further studies could examine prepubertal patients with MS to search for even starker differences.

Cytokine levels for IL-6 were found to be significantly lower in patients with pediatric MS than adults with MS, as were IFN-γ, IL-12p70, and IL-17A (though not statistically significant), while osteopontin and sVCAM were higher. These findings are somewhat surprising, as all the markers save for osteopontin and sVCAM that were identified as significantly different indicate a greater inflammatory

Table 2 Select mean serum cytokine values

	IL-6	sVCAM-1	Osteopontin	IL-17A	GM-CSF	IFN-γ	IL-12p70	IL-23
Peds MS ($n = 19$)	2.1 (8)	479,253 (120,408)	16,506 (8913)	19.3 (28)	10.2 (40)	41.6 (64)	11.9 (28)	1599 (4809)
Adult MS ($n = 24$)	12.5 (22)	408,110 (118,417)	10,557 (5336)	40.9 (44)	7.3 (19)	72.1 (91)	33.3 (57)	490 (1307)
Pediatric Healthy Controls ($n = 22$)	18.2 (31)	497,982 (128,890)	14,240* (10,718)**	41.0 (54)	40.1 (109)	74.6 (91)	39.6 (86)	820 (1499)
HC vs Peds MS (p)	**0.046**	0.637	0.255	0.454	0.302	0.408	0.112	0.108
Adult MS vs Peds MS (p)	**0.004**	**0.015**	**0.022**	**0.050**	0.742	0.248	0.074	0.334

* Mean value of cytokine concentration in serum in pg/ml
** Standard deviation values are listed in parentheses ()
Significant findings listed in bold

profile in adults. Given the seemingly greater inflammatory clinical nature of patients with pediatric MS, it was anticipated that that all these markers would be elevated instead relative to adults with MS. This may represent a substantial finding which challenges the little-known pathophysiology in early-onset MS. These results highlight that these particular cytokines may be useful markers of disease activity. Alternatively, given the small sample size, these findings may be driven by chance (Type 1 error), for example by inadvertent selection of patients with relatively low disease activity.

Soluble vascular cell adhesion molecule-I (sVCAM-I) is elevated in MS patients and correlates with clinical and MRI disease activity [28–30]. Five samples were found to be erroneously collected from post-treatment patients, 3 with Rebif and 2 with Copaxone all started a few months prior to sample collection. These patients were not included (original $n = 24$) in the statistical analysis. The sample size of 5 patients may be too low to support meaningful findings, but we did note elevated mean levels of osteopontin and sVCAM-1 in the treated patients compared to untreated patients (as well as controls), which was significant for sVCAM-1 ($p = 0.011$). In line with prior studies, interferon-β increases sVCAM levels [31–33], but rather is noted to downregulate osteopontin [34]. It is unclear if osteopontin represents a variant pathway in pediatric MS.

The negative correlation identified between serum levels of TGF-β-1 and serum vitamin D levels ($p < 0.01$) highlights other studies in MS and findings that vitamin D supplementation may increase TGF-β expression, which may play a role in its mechanism of action [35–37]. TGF-β-1 is an anti-inflammatory cytokine produced by regulatory T-cells. In mouse models of EAE, vitamin D administration induces TGF-β-1 production, [38], while exogenous TGF-β-1 ameliorates the disease [39]. Human derived T-cell lines from active MS patients produce less TGF-β-1 than stable patients [40]. Other studies indicate effects on TGF-β-2 instead [41]. In our pretreatment cohort, we may be seeing compensatory efforts to elevate TGF-β where vitamin D is lacking.

The correlation between serum IL-17 F levels and time from first clinical attack ($p < 0.05$) may explain the lack of certain significant findings in cytokine profiles if time from clinical attack is relevant. Thus, acquiring samples at the time of relapse may be informative as well and a useful goal for future studies. Lower levels of IL-17 at the time of attack and lower levels of IL-6 in children compared to adults may implicate pediatric MS as a more T_H1 mediated disease. Possibly T_H17 activity becomes a more prominent feature with disease chronicity or is simply not well developed in early MS. Nevertheless, IL-17 responses do appear to play a role, but may explain why concomitant responses in IL-6 and TGF-β are not seen [42].

Osteopontin is classified as a T_H1 cytokine, as it has diverse effects on inflammation, cell survival, cell-mediated immunity, bone mineralization, and more [43, 44]. Various cells produce this cytokine which induces IL-12 and IFN-γ and inhibits IL-10 expression from monocytes. OPN-deficient EAE mice show milder disease [45]. Elevated levels are seen in CSF and plasma of MS patients, even greater at times of relapses [46, 47].

Conclusions

A panel of inflammatory markers, namely IL-6, sVCAM-1, osteopontin, and IL-17A, have been found differentially expressed in serum samples of children with MS compared to pediatric healthy controls and adults with MS. The combination of findings suggests a lower inflammatory profile in children with MS compared to adult MS, contrary to clinical expectations. Future prospective studies with larger samples sizes and cohorts including prepubertal patients are needed to validate this pilot data and assess if they are prognostic of disease outcome. The absence of longitudinal samples in this study limits further interpretation. Such studies would also benefit from serial samples including post-treatment assessment. Additional investigations should also focus on cell types that express or are targeted by the cytokines identified in this study as well as broader examination of CSF.

Acknowledgements
We would like to thank Yaritza Rosario, APN-C, MSCN and Lisa Cerracchio, BSN, RN, CCRC for their kind assistance in helping conduct the study.

Funding
Supported by a grant from the New Jersey Health Foundation, Inc to Vikram Bhise, MD.

Authors' contributions
VB conceived the project, recruited and consented pediatric patients, performed statistical analysis, and composed the manuscript. KB recruited and consented adult MS patients, and was a major contributor in writing the manuscript. MS performed statistical analysis on the data. LK assisted with project design and recruited and consented pediatric MS patients. SDJ assisted with project design and was a major contributor in writing the manuscript. All authors have read and approved the final manuscript.

Competing interests
The authors declare that they have no competing interests.

Description
This study reports differences found in serum cytokine signatures in pretreatment children with multiple sclerosis (MS) compared to age- and gender-matched pediatric healthy controls and pretreatment adults with MS.

Author details
[1]Rutgers University-Robert Wood Johnson Medical School, New Brunswick, USA. [2]Rutgers University-Ernest Mario School of Pharmacy, Piscataway, USA. [3]New York University Langone Medical Center, New York City, USA. [4]Child Health Institute, 89 French Street, Suite 2200, New Brunswick, NJ 08901, USA.

References

1. Imitola J, Chitnis T, Khoury SJ. Cytokines in multiple sclerosis: from bench to bedside. Pharmacol Ther. 2005;106(2):163–77.
2. Martins TB, Rose JW, Jaskowski TD, Wilson AR, Husebye D, Seraj HS, et al. Analysis of proinflammatory and anti-inflammatory cytokine serum concentrations in patients with multiple sclerosis by using a multiplexed immunoassay. Am J Clin Pathol. 2011;136(5):696–704.
3. Chen YC, Chen SD, Miao L, Liu ZG, Li W, Zhao ZX, et al. Serum levels of interleukin (IL)-18, IL-23 and IL-17 in Chinese patients with multiple sclerosis. J Neuroimmunol. 2012;243(1-2):56–60.
4. Trojano M, Liguori M, Bosco Zimatore G, Bugarini R, Avolio C, Paolicelli D, et al. Age-related disability in multiple sclerosis. Ann Neurol. 2002;51(4):475–80.
5. Gorman MP, Healy BC, Polgar-Turcsanyi M, Chitnis T. Increased relapse rate in pediatric-onset compared with adult-onset multiple sclerosis. Arch Neurol. 2009;66(1):54–9.
6. Chabas D, Ness J, Belman A, Yeh EA, Kuntz N, Gorman MP, et al. Younger children with MS have a distinct CSF inflammatory profile at disease onset. Neurology. 2010;74(5):399–405.
7. Chabas D, Castillo-Trivino T, Mowry EM, Strober JB, Glenn OA, Waubant E. Vanishing MS T2-bright lesions before puberty: a distinct MRI phenotype? Neurology. 2008;71(14):1090–3.
8. Renoux C, Vukusic S, Mikaeloff Y, Edan G, Clanet M, Dubois B, et al. Natural history of multiple sclerosis with childhood onset. N Engl J Med. 2007;356(25):2603–13.
9. Banwell B, Bar-Or A, Cheung R, Kennedy J, Krupp LB, Becker DJ, et al. Abnormal T-cell reactivities in childhood inflammatory demyelinating disease and type 1 diabetes. Ann Neurol. 2008;63(1):98–111.
10. McLaughlin KA, Chitnis T, Newcombe J, Franz B, Kennedy J, McArdel S, et al. Age-dependent B cell autoimmunity to a myelin surface antigen in pediatric multiple sclerosis. J Immunol. 2009;183(6):4067–76.
11. Brilot F, Dale RC, Selter RC, Grummel V, Kalluri SR, Aslam M, et al. Antibodies to native myelin oligodendrocyte glycoprotein in children with inflammatory demyelinating central nervous system disease. Ann Neurol. 2009;66(6):833–42.
12. O'Connor KC, Lopez-Amaya C, Gagne D, Lovato L, Moore-Odom NH, Kennedy J, et al. Anti-myelin antibodies modulate clinical expression of childhood multiple sclerosis. J Neuroimmunol. 2010;223(1-2):92–9.
13. Horellou P, Wang M, Keo V, Chretien P, Serguera C, Waters P, et al. Increased interleukin-6 correlates with myelin oligodendrocyte glycoprotein antibodies in pediatric monophasic demyelinating diseases and multiple sclerosis. J Neuroimmunol. 2015;289:1–7.
14. Polman CH, Reingold SC, Banwell B, Clanet M, Cohen JA, Filippi M, et al. Diagnostic criteria for multiple sclerosis: 2010 revisions to the McDonald criteria. Ann Neurol. 2011;69(2):292–302.
15. Krupp LB, Tardieu M, Amato MP, Banwell B, Chitnis T, Dale RC, et al. International Pediatric Multiple Sclerosis Study Group criteria for pediatric multiple sclerosis and immune-mediated central nervous system demyelinating disorders: revisions to the 2007 definitions. Mult Scler. 2013;19(10):1261–7.
16. de Benedetti F, Massa M, Robbioni P, Ravelli A, Burgio GR, Martini A. Correlation of serum interleukin-6 levels with joint involvement and thrombocytosis in systemic juvenile rheumatoid arthritis. Arthritis Rheum. 1991;34(9):1158–63.
17. Tan Z, Yuan Y, Chen S, Chen Y, Chen TX. Plasma Endothelial Microparticles, TNF-a and IL-6 in Kawasaki Disease. Indian Pediatr. 2013;50(5):501–3.
18. Wine E, Mack DR, Hyams J, Otley AR, Markowitz J, Crandall WV, et al. Interleukin-6 is associated with steroid resistance and reflects disease activity in severe pediatric ulcerative colitis. J Crohns Colitis. 2013;7(11):916–22.
19. Frampton JE. Tocilizumab: a review of its use in the treatment of juvenile idiopathic arthritis. Paediatr Drugs. 2013;15(6):515–31.
20. Eugster HP, Frei K, Kopf M, Lassmann H, Fontana A. IL-6-deficient mice resist myelin oligodendrocyte glycoprotein-induced autoimmune encephalomyelitis. Eur J Immunol. 1998;28(7):2178–87.
21. Gijbels K, Brocke S, Abrams JS, Steinman L. Administration of neutralizing antibodies to interleukin-6 (IL-6) reduces experimental autoimmune encephalomyelitis and is associated with elevated levels of IL-6 bioactivity in central nervous system and circulation. Mol Med. 1995;1(7):795–805.
22. Diab A, Zhu J, Xiao BG, Mustafa M, Link H. High IL-6 and low IL-10 in the central nervous system are associated with protracted relapsing EAE in DA rats. J Neuropathol Exp Neurol. 1997;56(6):641–50.
23. Dale RC, Morovat A. Interleukin-6 and oligoclonal IgG synthesis in children with acute disseminated encephalomyelitis. Neuropediatrics. 2003;34(3):141 5.
24. Ishizu T, Minohara M, Ichiyama T, Kira R, Tanaka M, Osoegawa M, et al. CSF cytokine and chemokine profiles in acute disseminated encephalomyelitis. J Neuroimmunol. 2006;175(1-2):52–8.
25. Janssens K, Slaets H, Hellings N. Immunomodulatory properties of the IL-6 cytokine family in multiple sclerosis. Ann N Y Acad Sci. 2015;1351:52–60.
26. Rothaug M, Becker-Pauly C, Rose-John S. The role of interleukin-6 signaling in nervous tissue. Biochim Biophys Acta. 2016;1863(6 Pt A):1218–27.
27. Frisdal E, Lesnik P, Olivier M, Robillard P, Chapman MJ, Huby T, et al. Interleukin-6 protects human macrophages from cellular cholesterol accumulation and attenuates the proinflammatory response. J Biol Chem. 2011;286(35):30926–36.
28. Calabresi PA, Tranquill LR, Dambrosia JM, Stone LA, Maloni H, Bash CN, et al. Increases in soluble VCAM-1 correlate with a decrease in MRI lesions in multiple sclerosis treated with interferon beta-1b. Ann Neurol. 1997;41(5):669–74.
29. Rieckmann P, Altenhofen B, Riegel A, Baudewig J, Felgenhauer K. Soluble adhesion molecules (sVCAM-1 and sICAM-1) in cerebrospinal fluid and serum correlate with MRI activity in multiple sclerosis. Ann Neurol. 1997;41(3):326–33.
30. Matsuda M, Tsukada N, Miyagi K, Yanagisawa N. Increased levels of soluble vascular cell adhesion molecule-1 (VCAM-1) in the cerebrospinal fluid and sera of patients with multiple sclerosis and human T lymphotropic virus type-1-associated myelopathy. J Neuroimmunol. 1995;59(1-2):35–40.
31. Rieckmann P, Kruse N, Nagelkerken L, Beckmann K, Miller D, Polman C, et al. Soluble vascular cell adhesion molecule (VCAM) is associated with treatment effects of interferon beta-1b in patients with secondary progressive multiple sclerosis. J Neurol. 2005;252(5):526–33.
32. Graber J, Zhan M, Ford D, Kursch F, Francis G, Bever C, et al. Interferon-beta-1a induces increases in vascular cell adhesion molecule: implications for its mode of action in multiple sclerosis. J Neuroimmunol. 2005;161(1-2):169–76.
33. Bitsch A, Bahner D, Wachter C, Elitok E, Bogumil T, Dressel A, et al. Interferon beta-1b modulates serum sVCAM-1 levels in primary progressive multiple sclerosis. Acta Neurol Scand. 2004;110(6):386–92.
34. Hong J, Hutton GJ. Regulatory effects of interferon-beta on osteopontin and interleukin-17 expression in multiple sclerosis. J Interferon Cytokine Res. 2010;30(10):751–7.
35. Mahon BD, Gordon SA, Cruz J, Cosman F, Cantorna MT. Cytokine profile in patients with multiple sclerosis following vitamin D supplementation. J Neuroimmunol. 2003;134(1-2):128–32.
36. Mosayebi G, Ghazavi A, Ghasami K, Jand Y, Kokhaei P. Therapeutic effect of vitamin D3 in multiple sclerosis patients. Immunol Invest. 2011;40(6):627–39.
37. Mann EH, Chambers ES, Chen YH, Richards DF, Hawrylowicz CM. 1alpha,25-dihydroxyvitamin D3 acts via transforming growth factor-beta to up-regulate expression of immunosuppressive CD73 on human CD4+ Foxp3- T cells. Immunology. 2015;146(3):423–31.
38. Cantorna MT, Woodward WD, Hayes CE, DeLuca HF. 1,25-dihydroxyvitamin D3 is a positive regulator for the two anti-encephalitogenic cytokines TGF-beta 1 and IL-4. J Immunol. 1998;160(11):5314–9.
39. Racke MK, Cannella B, Albert P, Sporn M, Raine CS, McFarlin DE. Evidence of endogenous regulatory function of transforming growth factor-beta 1 in experimental allergic encephalomyelitis. Int Immunol. 1992;4(5):615–20.
40. Mokhtarian F, Shi Y, Shirazian D, Morgante L, Miller A, Grob D. Defective production of anti-inflammatory cytokine, TGF-beta by T cell lines of patients with active multiple sclerosis. J Immunol. 1994;152(12):6003–10.
41. Shirvani-Farsani Z, Behmanesh M, Mohammadi SM, Naser MA. Vitamin D levels in multiple sclerosis patients: Association with TGF-beta2, TGF-betaRI, and TGF-betaRII expression. Life Sci. 2015;134:63–7.
42. Vargas-Lowy D, Kivisakk P, Gandhi R, Raddassi K, Soltany P, Gorman MP, et al. Increased Th17 response to myelin peptides in pediatric MS. Clin Immunol. 2013;146(3):176–84.
43. O'Regan A, Berman JS. Osteopontin: a key cytokine in cell-mediated and granulomatous inflammation. Int J Exp Pathol. 2000;81(6):373–90.
44. Ashkar S, Weber GF, Panoutsakopoulou V, Sanchirico ME, Jansson M, Zawaideh S, et al. Eta-1 (osteopontin): an early component of type-1 (cell-mediated) immunity. Science. 2000;287(5454):860–4.
45. Jansson M, Panoutsakopoulou V, Baker J, Klein L, Cantor H. Cutting edge: Attenuated experimental autoimmune encephalomyelitis in eta-1/osteopontin-deficient mice. J Immunol. 2002;168(5):2096–9.
46. Braitch M, Nunan R, Niepel G, Edwards LJ, Constantinescu CS. Increased osteopontin levels in the cerebrospinal fluid of patients with multiple sclerosis. Arch Neurol. 2008;65(5):633–5.

9

Pediatric versus adult MS: similar or different?

Angelo Ghezzi[1*], Damiano Baroncini[1], Mauro Zaffaroni[1] and Giancarlo Comi[2]

Abstract

In this review the most important aspects of pediatric multiple sclerosis are presented and compared with the adult form. Some findings appear peculiar of pediatric MS:

a. Clinical manifestations are similar in adolescents and adults with MS, however in very young subjects MS frequency at onset is similar in males and females, with a higher frequency of brainstem/cerebellar involvement and acute polysymptomatic/ADEM like onset;
b. The course is relapsing-remitting in the large majority of patients, with a high relapse rate;
c. Mild or severe disability is reached after a longer interval, but at a lower age compared to adult MS;
d. The frequency of cognitive dysfunction is relatively high, with a quick deterioration but also the capability to partially recover with time;
e. MRI is fundamental for diagnosis and prognosis: the pattern of MRI has some peculiar aspects in pediatric MS patients: i) the classic diagnostic criteria cannot be fulfilled, ii) lesion load is more relevant, iii) lesions are less destructive, have a more pronounced inflammatory pattern and have enhanced capability to recover with time;
f. Diagnostic criteria of adults can be applied to patients with less than 18 years, but with limitations for subjects with less than 12 years and ADEM-like onset;
g. The approach in differential diagnosis is particular complex and many disorders with clinical manifestations in the pediatric age must be considered: in this context it is important to pay attention to clinical, MRI and CSF red flags. Anti-MOG abs syndrome has been recently identified and should be carefully considered in patients with Acquired Demyelinating Syndrome;
h. CSF oligoclonal bands are less frequent in pediatric MS patients, their presence in patients with Acquired Demyelinating Syndrome is strongly correlated to the risk of MS;
i. The interplay between genetic and environmental factors determine the risk of developing MS;
j. MS has a more pronounced inflammatory pattern (as suggested by the high relapse rate and the most relevant inflammatory pattern at brain MRI);
k. The treatment is based on the approach used for adults: as MS has a strong impact on patients and their family the model of care should involve a team with specialized neurologists, pediatricians and neuro-pediatricians, nurses, psychologists, social workers and specialists of rehabilitative medicine.

Keywords: Pediatric multiple sclerosis, Acquired Demyelinating Syndrome, Cognitive dysfunction, Diagnosis, Differential diagnosis, MRI, CSF, Genetic factors, Environmental factors, Therapy

* Correspondence: angelo.ghezzi@asst-valleolona.it
[1]Centro Studi Sclerosi Multipla, ASST Valleolona, Via Pastori 4, Gallarate 21013, Italy
Full list of author information is available at the end of the article

Background

Multiple sclerosis (MS) typically starts between 20–40 years of age, but it is increasingly recognized in young subjects, before 18 years of age: according to literature data about 3–10% of all MS cases have their first manifestations in childhood or adolescence [1, 2]. According to the definition of the International Pediatric MS Study Group, the pediatric onset applies to patients with less than 18 years of age, having in mind that children (arbitrarily defined as aged less than 10–12 years) can present some different clinical and laboratory features, requiring a particular care when applying diagnostic criteria and planning treatment interventions [1–3].

The incidence of cases with a first acute episode of presumed inflammatory cause (otherwise called Acquired Demyelinating Syndrome –ADS-) per year varies from 0.6 to 1.9 per 100,000, in relation to different geographic areas (Holland [4], Canada [5], USA [6]) and probably to the methods of cases ascertainment. Some recent studies [7, 8] have reported a higher incidence, up to 2.85/100,000 for pediatric-MS (ped-MS) cases in Sardinia (Italy) [7].

Many factors have contributed to increase the interest towards pediatric MS, mainly: the closer collaborations among specialists (neurologists, neuropediatricians, pediatricians), the definition of shared diagnostic criteria, the possibility to use effective medications, and, from a scientific point of view, the possibility to better explore risk factors as pediatric patients are closer to the real onset of the disease, compared to adults.

In addition to numerous studies carried out in North-America and Europe, recent studies have been published on pediatric cohorts of selected populations (Hispanic North-Americans) [9] or from other countries such as Turkey, Kuwait, Iran, Brazil, Marroch, Korea and Japan [10–17], indicating an increased interest in this area of clinical research. Many papers have been recently published giving a better definition of incidence, clinical aspects, pathophysiology, immunology, neuroimaging and treatment: a summary of these studies is provided by a recent publication of the International Pediatric MS Study Group [18].

The objective of this presentation is to summarize the most important advances on ped-MS research and to offer a guidance among the most meaningful contributions, with a focus on the basic question, whether ped-MS form is the same disease of the adult form or not.

Clinical aspects: how similar to adult MS?

Many reviews are available describing clinical features of ped-MS [1, 2, 4, 19, 20]; the objective here is to highlight the peculiar and distinctive aspects of this form compared to the adult one.

As in adult MS, females are more frequently affected than males with a ratio of about 3:1, but in subjects less than 10–12 years f/m ratio is about 1:1 [19, 21–25], suggesting that sex hormones can have a role in facilitating MS onset during puberty [26–28]. Hormones can also facilitate the development of relapses, as they are more frequent during the peri-menarche compared to post-menarche period [28]. Experimental studies have confirmed the role of sex hormones in the development of EAE [26].

Symptoms at presentation are in general similar to those observed in adults [1, 19, 20] but two findings are described as typical of ped-MS:

-   the ADEM-like onset (acute polysymptomatic onset with encephalopathy) especially in children [1, 29, 30];
-   the frequent initial presentation with symptoms indicating cerebellar or brainstem involvement [10, 17, 19, 21].

In addition, very young patients, in general with age < 12, are likely to present a polysymptomatic onset, a high number of relapses, a more severe clinical involvement, and a worse prognosis [10, 17, 19, 21].

The course is progressive in about 10% of patients with adult-MS but this evolution is exceptional in ped-MS [1]. Typically ped-MS patients present a relapsing-remitting (RR) course with an high relapse rate, at least in the initial phase of disease, about twice higher than that of the adult form [31, 32], although this finding has not been confirmed in all studies [10, 11, 21]. Relapse rate as well accumulation of disability and early shift to progression have been recognized as factors correlated to a negative prognosis [1, 19, 33, 34].

In spite of the high relapse rate, the time to reach mild or severe disability is longer in ped-MS than in adult-MS, with a delay of about 10 year; as a counterpart the age when these levels of disability are reached is about 10 years lower [10, 19, 21, 33–35], raising the question whether ped-MS is more benign or not with respect to the adult form; it could be considered more benign if the time to reach disability is considered, but more severe if the actual age is taken into account. This issue will also be discussed further on Conclusions.

In the late years there has been an increasing interest in exploring the presence and the pattern of cognitive dysfunction (CD) in ped-MS. Some reviews have recently summarized the most outstanding aspects of this issue [36–38], which are summarized below. Briefly:

-   CD is found in about 30–50% of cases, some of them with a low IQ [38–40], and also in 18% of subjects at MS onset [40];

- Patients with a younger age at MS onset [39, 41, 42], a longer disease duration [41, 42] and a higher disability [40, 42] are more at risk of CD;
- the most frequently affected functions are attention, language (receptive, verbal fluency and naming); visual-spatial and motor functions, spatial memory, executive functions and abstract reasoning.
- Language impairment [39] and impairment in information-processing speed are more pronounced in pediatric than in adult MS [43];
- fatigue, affective disorders (anxiety, depression), behavioural problems (somatization, attention problems) are commonly observed [38, 39, 44, 45];
- psychological and behavioural problems have a negative impact on executive function [45], and are strongly associated with CD [46];
- CD has a negative effect on quality of life and is related to limitations in social, academic and recreational activities [38, 39];
- social cognition (the capability of inferring another's mental state, knowledges, beliefs and emotions) is also affected, compromising social relationships and contributing to mental decline [47];
- stable in the short term [48], CD increases in frequency and severity with time [49–51]. A study has demonstrated a partial recovery after a phase of deterioration, anyway remaining more severe compared to baseline [49], suggesting a better capability of the brain of children to compensate brain damage, compared to adults;
- CD is correlated with brain MRI structural (lesion load, location of lesions) and functional alterations, detectable with non-conventional techniques [52–55];
- The cognitive background (the so called "cognitive reserve") has a significant role in protecting against cognitive decline [56];

The latest findings (increased severity of CD with time, effects on social functioning) indicate how severe is the effect of MS on subjects [57, 58]. Nevertheless, in spite of this severity, the brain of pediatric patients exibits an high capability to compensate the damage: this finding is supported by the possibility to partially reduce the extent of CD in the long-term, and by studies with functional and non-conventional MRI demonstrating an higher plasticity of the brain. It has been demonstrated that the activation of brain areas after a simple movement of the hand, that is progressively more widespread with progression of MS, is more restricted in pediatric compared to adult MS [59], indicating a relatively preserved functional organization of the brain; moreover the pattern of connectivity among brain areas is more efficient in children, compared to adults (see also Differential diagnosis: can clinical manifestations and ancillary investigations make the difference? section).

The issue of cognitive reserve, together with the positive effect of physical activity on brain plasticity [60, 61] (see MRI: a true distinctive pattern in ped-MS? section), underlines the concept of an higher brain plasticity in ped-MS, indicating that the enrichment and reinforcement of brain activity help the brain to better compensate the damage caused by MS [62].

In clinical practice it is advisable to explore the cognitive function in patients with ped-MS: short batteries have been proposed [63, 64], the Symbol Digit Modality Test has the advantage to be effective and easy to use [63].

Diagnosis: are diagnostic criteria of MS applicable to the pediatric form?

The pediatric form of MS has been included in the last revision of the McDonald diagnostic criteria of MS [65] on the consideration that most patients presenting a clinically isolated syndrome (CIS) before 18 years of age have the same pattern of adult-MS (>2 lesions in 2 of the 4 specific CNS locations). However 15–20% of pediatric patients, mostly aged < 11 years, can present with the so called acute disseminated encephalomyelitis (ADEM) pattern, suggesting caution in applying adult diagnostic criteria in these subjects, who are required to present 2 or more subsequent non-ADEM like attacks, or 1 non-ADEM like attack plus accrual of clinically silent lesions on MRI during the follow up, for the final diagnosis of MS.

The International Pediatric MS Study Group [3] has incorporated the revised McDonald criteria in the current classification of pediatric demyelinating disorders, that includes: patients with ADEM and its multiphasic form, clinically isolated syndrome (CIS), ped-MS, neuromyelitis optica (NMO). The Krupp's new diagnostic criteria are summarized in Table 1 [29]. Diagnosis of NMO has been recently revised according to new criteria [30].

The revised McDonald's criteria have been validated in cohorts of patients with less than 18 years, confirming their high sensitivity and specificity, meanwhile confirming the limitations when applied in patients with less than 11 years [66, 67].

It is worthy to remind that the pattern of MRI lesions typical of the adult form cannot always be found in children and adolescents with suspected (and sometimes confirmed) MS, a finding that has led to investigate whether a more specific pattern of lesions can be recognised in patients with suspected MS (Table 2). At present none of these proposals has been validated.

Spinal cord MRI can also provide further evidence of dissemination in time and space, although this aspect has not been systematically evaluated in young patients [68].

Brain MRI helps define the risk of developing MS after a first demyelinating episode: in a cohort of patients with ADS Verhey's criteria (simultaneous presence of one or more T2 periventricular lesions and one or more T1

Table 1 Diagnostic criteria for Acquired Demyelinating Syndromes [2, 3]

CIS	A first monofocal or multifocal CNS demyelinating event; encephalopathy is absent, unless due to fever
Monophasic ADEM	• A first polyfocal clinical CNS event with presumed inflammatory cause • Encephalopathy that cannot be explained by fever is present • MRI typically shows diffuse, poorly demarcated, large, >1-2 cm lesions involving predominantly the cerebral white matter; TI hypointense white matter lesions are rare; Deep grey matter lesions (e.g. thalamus or basal ganglia) can be present • No new symptoms, signs or MRI findings after 3 months of the incident ADEM
Multiphasic ADEM	• New event of ADEM 3 months or more after the initial event that can be associated with new or re-emergence of prior clinical and MRI findings. Timing in relation to steriods is no longer pertinent.
MS	Any of the following: • Two or more nonencephalopathic CNS clinical events separated by more than 30 days, involving more than one area of the CNS • Single clinical event and MRI features rely on 2010 Revised McDonald criteria[b] for DIS and DIT [4] (but criteria relative for DIT for a single attack and single MRI only apply to children ≥12 years and only apply to cases without an ADEM onset) • ADEM followed 3 months later by a nonencephalopathic clinical event with new lesions on brain MRI consistent with MS
NMO	All are required: • Optic neuritis • Acute myelitis • At least two of three supportive criteria: • Contiguous spinal cord MRI lesion ≥3 vertebral segments • Brain MRI not meeting diagnostic criteria for MS • Anti-aquaporin-4 IgG seropositive status

Table 2 Different MRI criteria for diagnosis of MS in pediatric patients

KIDMUS criteria	Callen's criteria	Verhey's criteria
1 of 2: - Lesions perpendicular to long axis of the corpus callosum - Sole presence of well defined lesions	Diagnosis: 2 of 3 - ≥2 T2 weighted lesions - 2 periventricular lesions - ≥1 Brain stem lesion MS vs ASEM, 2 of 3: - Absence of a diffuse bilateral lesion pattern - Presence of black holes - ≥2 periventricular lesions	2 of 2: - 1 periventricular lesions - 1 hypointense lesions on T1 images

hypointense lesions) were associated with an increased likelihood of MS diagnosis, with an high sensitivity and specificity; conversely the presence of contrast enhancement, cerebral white matter, intracallosal and brainstem lesions was not associated with an increased risk of MS [69]. The predictive role of Verhey's criteria has been validated in a large cohort of children with ADS [70]. Anyway, meeting or not the 2010 McDonald criteria at onset does not correlate with subsequent clinical course [71].

CSF examination, to detect intrathecal IgG synthesis, is not formally included among diagnostic criteria, nevertheless it can give an additional considerable contribution for diagnosis in patients at their first clinical episode, in addition to MRI [29, 72, 73].

Differential diagnosis: can clinical manifestations and ancillary investigations make the difference?

The differential diagnosis is particularly complex in children and adolescents with suspected MS as many diseases with onset in the pediatric age must be considered. As for adult form the criterion of "no better explanation" is required for the final diagnosis of MS.

Many conditions can mimic MS clinically, such as systemic lupus erythematosus (SLE), Bechet disease, neurosarcoidosis, angiitis of the CNS, tumors, infections, neurometabolic, hereditary disorders and many others: a complete list is reported and discussed in the work of Rostasy et al. [74].

Atypical manifestations or symptoms such as seizures, headache, psychosis, cranial neuropathy, persistent or recurrent visual loss, retinopathy, peripheral neuropathy, progressive or recurrent encephalopathy, spastic paraplegia should induce to consider diagnostic alternatives as summarized in Table 3 [75].

The course of ped-MS is typically relapsing-remitting, the progressive evolution being exceptional. So far, an atypical presentation with an hyperacute, or subacute or progressive onset should advice to explore alternative diagnoses [1] (Table 4), although the final diagnosis of MS cannot be excluded if supported by appropriate laboratory findings.

In clinical practice ADEM is a frequent diagnostic problem as it can be difficult to differentiate from MS, and possibly being the first presentation of MS in some patients, especially the youngest. The demographic, clinical and laboratory findings summarized in Table 5 (from Krupp et al. modified) can help to differentiate the two disorders, having in mind that patients ADEM must be carefully followed for the possible risk of a subsequent MS.

Serum autoantibodies to myelin peptides could be helpful to distinguish ADEM from relapsing-remitting MS. In a study [76] ADEM was associated to IgG autoantibodies targeting epitopes derived from myelin basic

Table 3 Clinical red flags for alternative diagnosis [74, 85]

Red flags	Diagnosis to consider
Seizures	- Vasculitis - tumor - infection - NMDA-receptor encephalitis
Headache	- Vasculitis - Susac syndrome (visual/hearing loss) - infection - venous thrombosis - cerebral edema - idiopathic intracranial hypertension
Psychosis	- vasculitis - SLE - GM2 gangliosidosis - Susac syndrome - corticosteroid therapy
Cranial neuropathy	- neuroborelliosis - neurosarcoidosis - Bechet disease
Visual loss	- LHON - Psychogenic
Recurrent optic neuropathy	- NMO - LHON - CRION
retinopathy	- Susac syndrome - Mitochondrial encephalopathy
Peripheral neuropathy	- Charcot Marie-Tooth disease - neuroborelliosis - Guillain-Barré Syndrome
Progressive/relapsing encephalopathy	- Leukodystrophies - Mitochondrial encephalopathy - CADASIL
Spastic paraplegia	- NMO - Tumor, vascular disorders - SLE - neurosarcoidosis - Hereditary spastic paraplegia

SLE systemic lupus erythematosus, *NMO* neuromyelitis optica, *LHON* Leber hereditary optic neuropathy, *CRION*, chronic inflammatory optic neuropathy, *CADASIL* cerebral autosomal dominant arteriopathy with subcortical infarcts and leukoencephalopathy

Table 4 Diagnostic alternatives in relation to clinical evolution (from ref [1], modified)

ONSET	CONSIDER also
Hyperacute	- Vascular disorders - Trauma - Toxic/infectious aetiologies
Acute or subacute	- Infectious aetiologies - Vascular/reumatological diseases - Malignancies - Macrophage-activation syndrome
Insidious, progressive	- Inherited metabolic disorders - Nutritional deficiencies (B12) - Vascular disorders

protein, proteolipid protein, myelin-associated oligodendrocyte basic glycoprotein and alpha-B-crystallin; by contrast, IgM autoantibodies targeting myelin basic protein, proteolipid protein, myelin-associated oligodendrocyte basic glycoprotein and oligodendrocyte-specific protein resulted associated to MS.

MRI, with the technique of susceptibility-weighted imaging, can also help discriminate ADEM from ped-MS [77].

Antibodies (Abs) to myelin oligodendrocytes glycoprotein (anti MOG Abs) have been detected in patients with ADEM, ADEM followed by attacks of optic neuritis, recurrent optic neuritis, transverse myelitis, ADS and could define a particular subset of patients with ADS [78–83]. They were present in about 35% of cases in a large cohort of patients with ADS, across all its clinical phenotypes [78]; anti-MOG positive patients rarely showed CSF oligoclonal bands (OBs) and MRI abnormalities, and had a lower risk of progression to MS after 1 year (13% vs 38%). In this study the risk of MS in the follow up was 4 fold higher in negative vs positive anti-MOG Abs patients, particularly if positive for CSF OBs. Other 2 studies have found anti-MOG Abs in about 18% of patients with ADS, in some NMO seronegative patients, in patients with ADEM/encephalopathy and in subjects with isolated ON [81, 82]. So far, anti-MOG positive patients seem to have a distinct clinical phenotype, with lower progression to MS.

A complete review on autoantibodies in ADS was published in a recent issue of this journal [83].

CSF examination provides meaningful data for differential diagnosis. OBs are rarely observed in conditions such as ADEM and NMO, that more frequently show increased cells pleocytosis. Determination of lactate and lactate/pyruvate ratio is recommended if suspicion of mitochondrial encephalopathy, CSF culture, viral/bacterial antibobies, cytology if suspicion of infections, neoplasms [75].

CSF analysis can show an increased white blood cells count, especially in children [84].

Whilst OBs are detected in more than 90% of adults with MS, they are less frequent in patients with ped-MS (in 40–70% of cases), particularly in children [2].

Two recent studies, one including patients with ON at presentation, the other one including patients with ADS, have shown that OBs are linked to a higher risk of subsequent MS, in addition and independently from the presence of lesions at brain MRI [72, 73].

As already stated, brain MRI has an irreplaceable role in diagnosis and prognosis, but it also provides helpful information for differential diagnosis. Cases of transverse myelitis, spinal infarction, acute disseminated encephalomyelitis, fever-induced refractory epileptic encephalopathy in school-aged children, small-vessel vasculitis, Griscelli

Table 5 Criteria to differentiate ADEM from MS (from ref. [29] modified)

Typical features	ADEM	MS
Demographic	More frequent in young subjects (<10–12 years); no gender predilection	More frequent in adolescents; girls more affected than boys
Prior flu-like illness	Very frequent	Variable
Symptoms		
▪ Seizures	Variable	Rare
▪ Encephalopathy	Required in definition	Rare early in the disease
▪ Discrete event	A single event can fluctuate over the course of 12 weeks	Discrete events separated by at least 4 weeks
MRI:		
▪ Large lesions involving gray and white matter	Frequent	Rare
▪ Enhancement	Frequent	Frequent
▪ Longitudinal MRI findings	Lesions typically either resolve or show only residual findings	Typically associated with development of new lesions
CSF		
▪ Pleocytosis	Variable	rare, white blood cell count almost always < 50
▪ Oligoclonal bands	Variable	Frequent

syndrome type 2, cysticercosis, vitamin B12 deficiency and chronic relapsing inflammatory optic neuropathy have been described highlighting the unusual clinical and radiologic features that should be considered in differential diagnosis of ped-MS [85]. Other relevant red flags are: absence of T2 weighted lesions, failure to document T2 lesion accrual, presence of meningeal gadolinium enhancement, visible cortical lesions, focal cortical volume loss, long extending spinal cord lesions in spinal MRI [2]. In relation to the prevalent site of white matter involvement or the selective involvement of white matter tracts, or to spinal cord involvement, other alternative conditions should be considered [74] (Table 6).

Extensive lesions, greater than 3 spinal cord segments, are more likely related to ADEM or NMO.

MRI: a true distinctive pattern in ped-MS?

Brain MRI offers the possibility to study in vivo the characteristics of lesions, their structure and evolution, with insights on the pathological substratum. Studies with conventional and non-conventional MRI have shown some peculiar aspects of lesions of ped-MS patients:

- lesions are more frequently found in the cerebellum/brainstem [86, 87], leading to an impaired age-expected cerebellar growth [88];
- lesions have more pronounced inflammatory aspects suggested by the large edematous aspect of lesions, and by the frequent enhancement after gadolinium injection, especially in children, with a frequent capability to recover and disappear with time [86, 87, 89, 90];

- lesions are less destructive and/or have a greater reparative capacity, as they show a greater recovery of T1 intensity with time [86];
- studies with non-conventional MRI have shown a less severe structural damage and a better capability to compensate brain damage and to promote remyelination [91–95];
- gray matter involvement is lower and cortical lesions are less, at least initially, in pediatric compared to adult MS, but thalamus is typically involved bilaterally [96–101];
- lesions at brain MRI correlate with CD and clinical outcome [52, 97];
- demyelinating lesions have a severe effect on brain development, reducing brain volume and skull size [102, 103];

Pathobiology and pathophysiology: common risk factors for a fairly rare disease?

With respect to adult MS, the pediatric form offers the unique possibility to better explore environmental factors associated to the risk of developing MS and relapses, as confounding factors occurring along the course of MS are less present [104].

Studies in children and adolescents have pointed out that an increased risk of MS is related to previous exposure to passive smoking [105], to Epstein-Barr virus (demonstrated by two independent studies [106, 107]), and to BMI [108]. Obesity in childhood or at 20 years of age has been confirmed as a risk factor in a cohort of 1235 adult MS patients [109], and further increases the risk in patients with previous EBV infection [110] and

Table 6 Diagnostic alternatives in relation to the pattern of lesions on brain MRI (from ref. [74], modified)

Region of white matter involvement	Clinical conditions	Letter: It permits to identify the occurrence of the same disease in other rows
Frontal	- Alexander disease - metachromatic leukodystrophy - megalencephalic leukoencephalopathy with subcortical cysts - variant adrenoleukodystrophy	a b
Parieto-occipital	- Adrenoleukodystrophy - Krabbe disease - paroxisomal disorders - mitochondrial disorders	c d e
Temporal	- CADASIL - Aicardi-Goutières syndrome - Cytomegalovirus encephalitis - megalencephalic leukoencephalopathy with subcortical cysts	f g
Periventricular	- Hemophagocitic lymphohisiocytosis - metachromatic leukodystrophy - leukoencephalopathy with brainstem-spinal cord involvement and elevated lactate - vanishing white matter disease - CADASIL	b h f
Basal ganglia	- mitochondrial disorders - biotinidase deficiency - Wilson disease - Bilateral striatal necrosis - Biotin-responsive basal ganglia disease - Aicardi-Goutières syndrome	e g
Thalamus	- Malignancies - Hepatic encephalopathy - Acute necrotizing encephalopathy - leukoencephalopathy with thalamus and brainstem involvement and elevated lactate - Fabry disease	i l m n
Brainstem	- Malignancies - Rhombencephalitis - Tuberculosis - Bechet disease - Alexander disease - leukoencephalopathy with thalamus and brainstem involvement and elevated lactate - leukoencephalopathy with brainstem-spinal cord involvement and elevated lactate	i a m h
Involvement of white matter tracts		
Corticospinal	- adrenoleukodystrophy - adrenomyeloneuropathy - Krabbe disease - adult-onset leukoencephalopathy with axonal spheroids and pigmental glia	c d
Dorsal column	- leukoencephalopathy with thalamus and brainstem involvement and elevated lactate - vitamin B12/copper deficiency	m
Subcortical U-fibers	- Canavan disease - Kearns-Sayre syndrome	
External capsule/insula	- Acute necrotizing encephalopathy - CADASIL	l f
Corpus callosum	- Susac syndrome, - Krabbe disease	d
Spinal cord		
Hyperintensity	- Sarcoidosis - Systemic lupus erythematosus - CLIPPERS (chronic lymphocytic inflammation with pontine perivascular enhancement responsive to steroids) - infections	
Atrophy	- leukoencephalopathy with thalamus and brainstem involvement and elevated lactate - Alexander disease - adult polyglucosan body disease	m a

carrying the HLA-DRB1*15 allele [111]. Diet has been investigated as a possible risk factor: in this context the role of salt-intake has been investigated in a recent publication, but no correlation was found [112].

Low levels of vitamin D were linked to an increased risk of MS in two independent studies. However the supplementation with vitamin D has only a marginal effect in adult MS patients whose increase in blood level is lower compared with controls [113].

Life-style and physical activity should be included among modifiable risk factors. A reduced physical activity per se [61], or as consequence of factors related to MS such as ongoing disease activity, perceived limitations, depression and fatigue [60], has found to be related a higher level of disease activity (more relapses, more MRI T2 lesions), suggesting a potential protective effect of strenuous physical activity in this population. This finding has lead to develop an agenda for promoting further studies on this topic, and to plan interventions for enhancing physical activity in subjects with ped-MS [61]. Surprisingly, there is a strong analogy with the approach to cognitive dysfunction management: both strategies have the objective to reinforce the physical and mental background (functional reserve) to better protect from brain loss and to improve brain plasticity.

Hormonal changes during puberty can also facilitate MS onset as already discussed in Background section. Female sex involves a risk of MS about twice higher in patients with ADS [106].

The genetic background has a well known important role to determine the risk of MS. HLA-DRB1 alleles were characterized in 266 children presenting with ADS, 64 of them with a final diagnosis of MS [114]: children harboring DRB1*15 alleles were more likely to be diagnosed with MS (OR = 2.7), supporting a fundamental similar genetic contribution to MS risk in both pediatric- and adult-onset disease. In a large-scale genome-wide association study 57 genetic risk loci have been identified in adult patients with MS: the same pattern has been found in a cohort of 53 MS patients from a cohort of 188 children with ADS, indicating that the combined effect of 57 SNPs exceeded the effect of HLA-DRB1*15 alone [115], conferring an increased susceptibility to pediatric-onset MS compared to monophasic ADS.

The genetic predisposition further enhances the risk of developing MS in combination with other factors such as obesity, previous infections, vitamin D status [110, 111, 116], the latter factor also with a possible effect on disease activity [117].

At present it is not known whether ped-MS patients have a higher genetic burden, studies are ongoing to better evaluate this aspect.

Many alterations of the immune response have been documented in ped-MS, with findings not so far different from those observed in adult MS in spite of the more immature immune system [2, 118–120].

To conclude, the genetic background plays an important role, combined with physical and environmental factors, to determine the risk of MS (see also Table 7), with pathogenetic mechanisms not so different form the adult form.

Treatment: borrowing from adulthood, but still many obstacles to overcome

Differently from adult form, medications for MS have not been tested in children and adolescents with randomized controlled trials. Data are only available from open label observational studies, providing information on safety and, in some extent, on effectiveness. It is desirable to better evaluate the effects of medications in pediatric MS patients [121], nevertheless many factors limit the possibility to perform clinical trials in this population [122]:

- the use of placebo, required by Regulatory Authorities in some studies,
- the difficulty to propose a trial with a medication that has been already approved for adults,
- the difficulty, in some cases, to obtain the informed consent,
- the difficulty to have access to hospital, with loss of days of school or work (for parents),
- the relative rarity of ped-MS,
- the competition among drugs now available in the market.

In spite of their intrinsic limitations, observational studies have provided data on the effect of some first and second line disease modifying drugs (DMDs); their indications and limitations have been defined in two documents of experts [123, 124].

- For the treatment of acute attacks high dose corticosteroids are recommended (Methylprednisolone 10–40 mg/kg e.v. for 3–5 consecutive days). For severe cases with poor recovery in spite of corticosteroids, plasma exchange can be considered.
- To prevent relapses and progression the use of DMDs is strongly recommended. IFNB-1a and Glatiramer acetate are standard treatment, as used for many years without signals of consistent adverse events [124–126]. A common and shared approach is summarized in Fig. 1 (ref 124, modified).
- Among second line therapies, Natalizumab has been tested in many cohorts of patients with less than 18 years; it is an option for subjects with a very active evolution or no response to IFNB-1a or GA

Table 7 Factors related to the risk of developing MS in children and adolescents

Author	Study population	Risk factor	Change in risk
Langer-Gould et al.	n. 75, MS onset < 18 years	BMI	- Overweight x 1.58 - Moderately obese x 1.78 - Extremely obese x 3.76
Mikaeloff et al.	n.90, MS onset 10 to <16 years	Passive smoking	x 2.49
Banwell et al.	n. 49, MS onset < 16 years	Remote EBV infection	x 2.58
Waubant et al.	n. 189, MS onset < 18 years	Remote EBV infection	x 3.72
Disanto et al.	n. 64, MS onset < 16 years	≥1 HLA-DRB1 alleles	x 3.2
McDonald et al.	n. 170, MS onset < 18 years	Salt intake	No effect
Banwell et al.	n. 63, MS onset < 16 years	Vitamin D increase + 10 nmol/L	10% reduction
Monry et al.	n. 110, MS onset ≤ 18 years	Vitamin D increase + 10 nmol/L	30% reduction
Waubant et al.	n. 189, MS onset < 18 years	VCM seropositivity	73% reduction

[123, 124, 127–130]. A limitation in its use is represented by the risk of a rare but severe adverse events, the occurrence of progressive multifocal leukoencephalopathy (PML) due to reactivation of JCV virus, however this risk can be properly assessed checking anti-JCV antibodies [121]: the risk of PML increases closely with the antibodies titre and the duration of exposure to Natatizumab. In patients negative for anti-JCV antibodies the risk is close to 0. Natalizumab has shown a very strong effect in reducing disease activity and putting patients in the condition of NEDA (No Evidence of Disease Activity – patients free from relapses, disease progression, T2 and Gd + lesions at brain MRI) in the large majority of cases and for a long time [130].
- Trials are ongoing testing the effect new oral medications [129], with different study design and

different endpoints: i) Fingolimod (PARADIGMS study) in a double blind trial vs an active comparator (this trial has recently closed the enrollment of patients), having annualized relapse rate as primary endpoint ii) Dimetylfumarate in a single blind controlled study vs active comparator (CONNECT Study), evaluating the proportion of patients free of new or newly enlarging T2 lesions iii) Teriflunomide in a double blind trial vs placebo having the time to first relapse as primary endpoint (TERIKIDS Study).

Fingolimod and Dimetylfumarate have been evaluated in two small observational trials [131, 132]: they resulted well tolerated, but data are not sufficient for long term assessment of effectiveness and safety.

Cyclophosphamide, rituximab, mitoxantrone could be used in selected cases with aggressive MS. Alemtuzumab

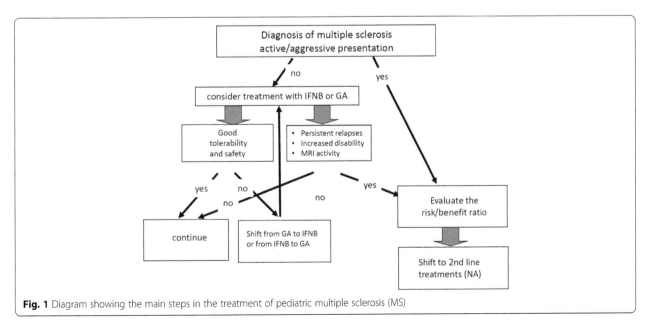

Fig. 1 Diagram showing the main steps in the treatment of pediatric multiple sclerosis (MS)

has been recently approved for adults with active MS [121, 123, 124], hemopoietic stems cells transplantation [133] is proposed for active non-responder patients: however data are not available in children and adolescents with MS.

As already discussed, diagnosis of MS per se as well as the possible physical disability have a strong psychological effect on patients, their parents and family. Model of care should be centered on patients and their families, in specialized centers involving neurologists expert of MS, pediatricians or pediatric neurologists, specialized nurses, psychologists, social workers and specialists of rehabilitative medicine, as highlighted in a recent document of the IPMSSG [134].

The knowledge of a protective role of cognitive reserve and the evidence that physical activity improves brain functioning opens new perspectives in the field of rehabilitation.

Conclusions

There is large body of evidence that MS evolution is age-dependent, more relapsing in young subjects, more progressive in older ones, with a different speed to progress [135].

In ped-MS the basic pathophysiological findings are similar to those of the adult form, but differently modulated due to the immaturity of the nervous and immunological systems.

Some aspects seem to be peculiar of ped-MS:

– clinical manifestations are similar in adolescents and adults with MS; however, in younger subjects male to female ratio tends to be 1:1, with frequent brainstem/cerebellar involvement and an acute polysymptomatic/ADEM-like onset;
– the course is relapsing-remitting in the large majority of patients, with an high relapse rate;

– the interval to reach mild or severe disability is more prolonged but the age is lower in ped-MS patients compared to adults;
– the frequency of cognitive dysfunction is relatively high, with a quick deterioration but also the capability to recover partially in the long-term follow-up;
– diagnostic criteria can be applied to patients with less than 18 years, but with limitations for subjects with less than 12 years and ADEM-like onset;
– the approach in differential diagnosis is particular complex and many disorders with clinical manifestations in the pediatric age must be considered: in this context it is important to pay attention to clinical, MRI and CSF red flags;
– anti-MOG Ab syndrome has been recently identified and should be carefully considered in patients with ADS;
– CSF OBs are less frequent in ped-MS patients, their presence in patients with ADS being strongly correlated to risk of MS;
– MRI is fundamental for diagnosis and prognosis;
– the pattern of MRI has some peculiar aspects in ped-MS patients: i) the classic diagnostic criteria cannot be fulfilled, ii) lesion load is more relevant, iii) lesions more frequently involve the brainstem/cerebellum, have a more pronounced inflammatory pattern, iii) lesions can disappear with time, less frequently evolve to T1 hypo intense lesions, indicating less structural damage, iiii) lesions are less destructive, and have enhanced capability to recover with time;
– ped-MS has a more pronounced inflammatory pattern (as suggested by clinical evolution – predominant RR evolution with high relapse rate- and MRI data), nevertheless axonal damage is also considerable [136].

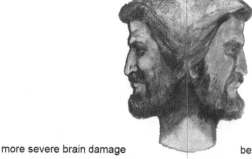

more severe brain damage

more prominent inflammation

better capability to recover and to compensate brain damage

Fig. 2 pediatric MS: more or less benign with respect to the adult form?

Some findings such as the high relapse rate, the acute onset with severe symptoms in some patients, the presence of cognitive dysfunction, the lower age to reach mild and severe disability, the effect of lesions on brain tissue and skull size are compatible with a more severe evolution.

On the contrary some other findings, such as the longer interval to reach mid/severe disability, the capability of the brain to recover and compensate brain damage, seem to suggest a more favorable evolution.

These findings lead to the conclusion that ped-MS is a more severe disease, compared to the adult form, but this higher severity is mitigated by the higher capability of the brain to compensate brain damage and to partially recover with time (Fig. 2).

Acknowledgements
None.

Funding
None.

Authors' contributions

Dr. AG conceived the work, collected and revised literature data, wrote the first and the final version of the manuscript. Dr. DB and Dr. MZ helped to collect and revise literature data, revised and contributed to the final version of the manuscript. Prof. GC critically revised the manuscript. All authors have read the manuscript, the paper has not been previously published and is not under simultaneous consideration by another journal. No ghost writing by authors not named on the list. All authors read and approved the final manuscript.

Competing interests

Angelo Ghezzi serves on scientific advisory boards for Merck Serono and Teva Pharmaceutical Industries ltd; received honoraria for speaking form Merck Serono, Biogen Idec, Bayer Schering Pharma and Novartis; serves as a consultant for Novartis, receives research support from Sanofi Aventis, Biogen Idec and Merck Serono.
Damiano Baroncini received honoraria from Almirall for creation of editorial publication and travel grants for participation to national and international congresses/courses from Genzyme, Merck and Novartis.
Mauro Zaffaroni has received honoraria for consulting or lecturing or travel grants for attending meetings from Almirall, Biogen Idec, Genzyme, Medtronic, Merck Serono, Novartis and Teva.
Giancarlo Comi serves on scientific advisory boards for Bayer Schering Pharma, Merck Serono, Teva Pharmaceutical Industries Ltd, Sanofi Aventis, Novartis and Biogen-Idec; has received speaker honoraria from Teva Pharmaceutical Industries Ltd, Sanofi Aventis, Serono Sumposia International Foundation, Biogen-Idec, Merck Serono, Novartis, Bayer Schering and Sanofi Aventis.

Author details
[1]Centro Studi Sclerosi Multipla, ASST Valleolona, Via Pastori 4, Gallarate 21013, Italy. [2]Department of Neurology, Scientific Institute H.S. Raffaele, Milan, Italy.

References
1. Banwell B, Ghezzi A, Bar-Or A, Mikaeloff Y, Tardieu M. Multiple sclerosis in children: clinical diagnosis, therapeutic strategies, and future directions. Lancet Neurol. 2007;6:887–902.
2. Waldman A, Ghezzi A, Bar-Or A, Mikaeloff Y, Tardieu M, Banwell B. Multiple sclerosis in children: an update on clinical diagnosis, therapeutic strategies, and research. Lancet Neurol. 2014;13:936–48.
3. Krupp LB, Tardieu M, Amato MP, et al. International Pediatric Multiple Sclerosis Study Group criteria for pediatric multiple sclerosis and immune-mediated central nervous system demyelinating disorders: revisions to the 2007 definitions. Mult Scler. 2013;19:1261–7.
4. Ketelslegers IA, Catsman-Berrevoets CE, Neuteboom RF, et al. Incidence of acquired demyelinating syndromes of the CNS in Dutch children: a nationwide study. J Neurol. 2012;259:1929–35.
5. Langer-Gould A, Zhang JL, Chung J, Yeung Y, Waubant E, Yao J. Incidence of acquired CNS demyelinating syndromes in a multiethnic cohort of children. Neurology. 2011;77:1143–8.
6. Banwell B, Kennedy J, Sadovnick D, et al. Incidence of acquired demyelination of the CNS in Canadian children. Neurology. 2009;72:232–9.
7. Dell'Avvento S, Sotgiu MA, Manca S, Sotgiu G, Sotgiu S. Epidemiology of multiple sclerosis in the pediatric population of Sardinia, Italy. Eur J Pediatr. 2016;175:19–29.
8. Reinhardt K, Weiss S, Rosenbauer J, Gartner J, von Kries R. Multiple sclerosis in children and adolescents: incidence and clinical picture - new insights from the nationwide German surveillance (2009–2011). Eur J Neurol. 2014;21:654–9.
9. Langille MM, Islam T, Burnett M, Amezcua L. Clinical characteristics of pediatric-onset and adult-onset multiple sclerosis in hispanic americans. J Child Neurol. 2016;31:1068–73.
10. Alroughani R, Ahmed SF, Al-Hashel J. Pediatric-onset multiple sclerosis disease progression in Kuwait: a retrospective analysis. Pediatr Neurol. 2015;53:508–12.
11. Alroughani R, Akhtar S, Ahmed SF, Behbehani R, Al-Abkal J, Al-Hashel J. Incidence and prevalence of pediatric onset multiple sclerosis in Kuwait: 1994–2013. J Neurol Sci. 2015;353:107–10.
12. Etemadifar M, Nourian SM, Nourian N, et al. Early-onset multiple sclerosis in Isfahan, Iran: report of the demographic and clinical features of 221 patients. J Child Neurol. 2016;31:932–7.
13. Fragoso YD, Ferreira ML, Morales Nde M, et al. Multiple sclerosis starting before the age of 18 years: the Brazilian experience. Arq Neuropsiquiatr. 2013;71:783–7.
14. Araqi-Houssaini A, Dany F, Sekkat Z, et al. Pediatric multiple sclerosis: is it different from the adult form? Rev Neurol. 2014;170:531–5.
15. Kim YM, Kim HY, Cho MJ, et al. Optic neuritis in Korean children: Low risk of subsequent multiple sclerosis. Pediatr Neurol. 2015;53:221–5.
16. Yamaguchi Y, Torisu H, Kira R, et al. A nationwide survey of pediatric acquired demyelinating syndromes in Japan. Neurology. 2016;87:2006–15.
17. Derle E, Kurne AT, Konuskan B, Karabudak R, Anlar B. Unfavorable outcome of pediatric onset multiple sclerosis: Follow-up in the pediatric and adult neurology departments of one referral center, in Turkey. Mult Scler Relat Disord. 2016;9:1–4.
18. Tanuja Chitnis and Daniela Pohl, On behalf of the International Pediatric MS Study Group (IPMSSG) Steering Committee Pediatric demyelinating disorders: Global updates, controversies, and future directions Neurology 2016;1-S116.
19. Ghezzi A. Clinical characteristics of multiple sclerosis with early onset. Neurol Sci. 2004;25(Suppl 4):S336–9.
20. Waldman A, Ness J, Pohl D, et al. Pediatric multiple sclerosis: Clinical features and outcome. Neurology. 2016;87:S74–81.
21. Huppke B, Ellenberger D, Rosewich H, Friede T, Gartner J, Huppke P. Clinical presentation of pediatric multiple sclerosis before puberty. Eur J Neurol. 2014;21:441–6.
22. Duquette P, Murray TJ, Pleines J, et al. Multiple sclerosis in childhood: clinical profile in 125 patients. J Pediatr. 1987;111:359–63.

23. Ruggieri M, Polizzi A, Pavone L, Grimaldi LM. Multiple sclerosis in children under 6 years of age. Neurology. 1999;53:478–84.

24. Ruggieri M, Iannetti P, Polizzi A, Pavone L, Grimaldi LM, Italian Society of Paediatric Neurology Study Group on Childhood Multiple S. Multiple sclerosis in children under 10 years of age. Neurol Sci. 2004;25(Suppl 4):S326–35.

25. Haliloglu G, Anlar B, Aysun S, et al. Gender prevalence in childhood multiple sclerosis and myasthenia gravis. J Child Neurol. 2002;17:390–2.

26. Ahn JJ, O'Mahony J, Moshkova M, et al. Puberty in females enhances the risk of an outcome of multiple sclerosis in children and the development of central nervous system autoimmunity in mice. Mult Scler. 2015;21:735–48.

27. Chitnis T. Role of puberty in multiple sclerosis risk and course. Clin Immunol (Orlando, Fla). 2013;149:192–200.

28. Lulu S, Graves J, Waubant E. Menarche increases relapse risk in pediatric multiple sclerosis. Mult Scler. 2016;22:193–200.

29. Krupp LB, Banwell B, Tenembaum S, International Pediatric MSSG. Consensus definitions proposed for pediatric multiple sclerosis and related disorders. Neurology. 2007;68:S7–12.

30. Tenembaum S, Chitnis T, Nakashima I, et al. Neuromyelitis optica spectrum disorders in children and adolescents. Neurology. 2016;87:S59–66.

31. Benson LA, Healy BC, Gorman MP, et al. Elevated relapse rates in pediatric compared to adult MS persist for at least 6 years. Mult Scler Relat Disord. 2014;3:186–93.

32. Gorman MP, Healy BC, Polgar-Turcsanyi M, Chitnis T. Increased relapse rate in pediatric-onset compared with adult-onset multiple sclerosis. Arch Neurol. 2009;66:54–9.

33. Boiko A, Vorobeychik G, Paty D, Devonshire V, Sadovnick D, University of British Columbia MSCN. Early onset multiple sclerosis: a longitudinal study. Neurology. 2002;59:1006–10.

34. Simone IL, Carrara D, Tortorella C, et al. Course and prognosis in early-onset MS: comparison with adult-onset forms. Neurology. 2002;59:1922–8.

35. Renoux C, Vukusic S, Mikaeloff Y, et al. Natural history of multiple sclerosis with childhood onset. N Engl J Med. 2007;356:2603–13.

36. Cardoso M, Olmo NR, Fragoso YD. Systematic review of cognitive dysfunction in pediatric and juvenile multiple sclerosis. Pediatr Neurol. 2015;53:287–92.

37. Suppiej A, Cainelli E. Cognitive dysfunction in pediatric multiple sclerosis. Neuropsychiatr Dis Treat. 2014;10:1385–92.

38. Amato MP, Krupp LB, Charvet LE, Penner I, Till C. Pediatric multiple sclerosis: Cognition and mood. Neurology. 2016;87:S82–7.

39. Amato MP, Goretti B, Ghezzi A, et al. Cognitive and psychosocial features of childhood and juvenile MS. Neurology. 2008;70:1891–7.

40. Julian L, Serafin D, Charvet L, et al. Cognitive impairment occurs in children and adolescents with multiple sclerosis: results from a United States network. J Child Neurol. 2013;28:102–7.

41. Banwell BL, Anderson PE. The cognitive burden of multiple sclerosis in children. Neurology. 2005;64:891–4.

42. MacAllister WS, Belman AL, Milazzo M, et al. Cognitive functioning in children and adolescents with multiple sclerosis. Neurology. 2005;64:1422–5.

43. Baruch NF, O'Donnell EH, Glanz BI, et al. Cognitive and patient-reported outcomes in adults with pediatric-onset multiple sclerosis. Mult Scler. 2016;22:354–61.

44. Charvet L, Cersosimo B, Schwarz C, Belman A, Krupp LB. Behavioral symptoms in pediatric multiple sclerosis: relation to fatigue and cognitive impairment. J Child Neurol. 2016;31:1062–7.

45. Holland AA, Graves D, Greenberg BM, Harder LL. Fatigue, emotional functioning, and executive dysfunction in pediatric multiple sclerosis. Child Neuropsychol. 2014;20:71–85.

46. Weisbrot D, Charvet L, Serafin D, et al. Psychiatric diagnoses and cognitive impairment in pediatric multiple sclerosis. Mult Scler. 2014;20:588–93.

47. Charvet LE, Cleary RE, Vazquez K, Belman AL, Krupp LB, MS USNfP. Social cognition in pediatric-onset multiple sclerosis (MS). Mult Scler. 2014;20:1478–84.

48. Charvet LE, O'Donnell EH, Belman AL, et al. Longitudinal evaluation of cognitive functioning in pediatric multiple sclerosis: report from the US Pediatric Multiple Sclerosis Network. Mult Scler. 2014;20:1502–10.

49. Amato MP, Goretti B, Ghezzi A, et al. Neuropsychological features in childhood and juvenile multiple sclerosis: five-year follow-up. Neurology. 2014;83:1432–8.

50. Amato MP, Goretti B, Ghezzi A, et al. Cognitive and psychosocial features in childhood and juvenile MS: two-year follow-up. Neurology. 2010;75:1134–40.

51. Till C, Racine N, Araujo D, et al. Changes in cognitive performance over a 1-year period in children and adolescents with multiple sclerosis. Neuropsychology. 2013;27:210–9.

52. Maghzi AH, Revirajan N, Julian LJ, et al. Magnetic resonance imaging correlates of clinical outcomes in early multiple sclerosis. Mult Scler Relat Disord. 2014;3:720–7.

53. Rocca MA, Absinta M, Amato MP, et al. Posterior brain damage and cognitive impairment in pediatric multiple sclerosis. Neurology. 2014;82:1314–21.

54. Rocca MA, Morelli ME, Amato MP, et al. Regional hippocampal involvement and cognitive impairment in pediatric multiple sclerosis. Mult Scler. 2016;22:628–40.

55. Weier K, Till C, Fonov V, et al. Contribution of the cerebellum to cognitive performance in children and adolescents with multiple sclerosis. Mult Scler. 2016;22:599–607.

56. Pasto L, Portaccio E, Goretti B, et al. The cognitive reserve theory in the setting of pediatric-onset multiple sclerosis. Mult Scler. 2016;22:1741–9.

57. Krysko KM, O'Connor P. Quality of life, cognition and mood in adults with pediatric multiple sclerosis. Can J Neurol Sci. 2016;43:368–74.

58. Till C, Udler E, Ghassemi R, Narayanan S, Arnold DL, Banwell BL. Factors associated with emotional and behavioral outcomes in adolescents with multiple sclerosis. Mult Scler. 2012;18:1170–80.

59. Rocca MA, Absinta M, Ghezzi A, Moiola L, Comi G, Filippi M. Is a preserved functional reserve a mechanism limiting clinical impairment in pediatric MS patients? Hum Brain Mapp. 2009;30:2844–51.

60. Grover SA, Aubert-Broche B, Fetco D, et al. Lower physical activity is associated with higher disease burden in pediatric multiple sclerosis. Neurology. 2015;85:1663–9.

61. Yeh EA, Kinnett-Hopkins D, Grover SA, Motl RW. Physical activity and pediatric multiple sclerosis: Developing a research agenda. Mult Scler. 2015;21:1618–25.

62. Hubacher M, DeLuca J, Weber P, et al. Cognitive rehabilitation of working memory in juvenile multiple sclerosis-effects on cognitive functioning, functional MRI and network related connectivity. Restor Neurol Neurosci. 2015;33:713–25.

63. Charvet LE, Beekman R, Amadiume N, Belman AL, Krupp LB. The Symbol Digit Modalities Test is an effective cognitive screen in pediatric onset multiple sclerosis (MS). J Neurol Sci. 2014;341:79–84.

64. Portaccio E, Goretti B, Lori S, et al. The brief neuropsychological battery for children: a screening tool for cognitive impairment in childhood and juvenile multiple sclerosis. Mult Scler. 2009;15:620–6.

65. Polman CH, Reingold SC, Banwell B, et al. Diagnostic criteria for multiple sclerosis: 2010 revisions to the McDonald criteria. Ann Neurol. 2011;69:292–302.

66. Kornek B, Schmitl B, Vass K, et al. Evaluation of the 2010 McDonald multiple sclerosis criteria in children with a clinically isolated syndrome. Mult Scler. 2012;18:1768–74.

67. Sadaka Y, Verhey LH, Shroff MM, et al. 2010 McDonald criteria for diagnosing pediatric multiple sclerosis. Ann Neurol. 2012;72:211–23.

68. Hummel HM, Bruck W, Dreha-Kulaczewski S, Gartner J, Wuerfel J. Pediatric onset multiple sclerosis: McDonald criteria 2010 and the contribution of spinal cord MRI. Mult Scler. 2013;19:1330–5.

69. Verhey LH, Branson HM, Shroff MM, et al. MRI parameters for prediction of multiple sclerosis diagnosis in children with acute CNS demyelination: a prospective national cohort study. Lancet Neurol. 2011;10:1065–73.

70. Verhey LH, van Pelt-Gravesteijn ED, Ketelslegers IA, et al. Validation of MRI predictors of multiple sclerosis diagnosis in children with acute CNS demyelination. Mult Scler Relat Disord. 2013;2:193–9.

71. Bigi S, Marrie RA, Verhey L, Yeh EA, Banwell B. 2010 McDonald criteria in a pediatric cohort: is positivity at onset associated with a more aggressive multiple sclerosis course? Mult Scler. 2013;19:1359–62.

72. Heussinger N, Kontopantelis E, Gburek-Augustat J, et al. Oligoclonal bands predict multiple sclerosis in children with optic neuritis. Ann Neurol. 2015;77:1076–82.

73. Neuteboom RF, Boon M, Catsman Berrevoets CE, et al. Prognostic factors after a first attack of inflammatory CNS demyelination in children. Neurology. 2008;71:967–73.

74. Rostasy K, Bajer-Kornek B, Venkateswaran S, Hemingway C, Tardieu M. Differential diagnosis and evaluation in pediatric inflammatory demyelinating disorders. Neurology. 2016;87:S28–37.

75. O'Mahony J, Bar-Or A, Arnold DL, et al. Masquerades of acquired demyelination in children: experiences of a national demyelinating disease program. J Child Neurol. 2013;28:184–97.

76. Van Haren K, Tomooka BH, Kidd BA, et al. Serum autoantibodies to myelin peptides distinguish acute disseminated encephalomyelitis from relapsing-remitting multiple sclerosis. Mult Scler. 2013;19:1726–33.

77. Kelly JE, Mar S, D'Angelo G, Zhou G, Rajderkar D, Benzinger TL. Susceptibility-weighted imaging helps to discriminate pediatric multiple sclerosis from acute disseminated encephalomyelitis. Pediatr Neurol. 2015;52:36–41.

78. Hacohen Y, Absoud M, Deiva K, et al. Myelin oligodendrocyte glycoprotein antibodies are associated with a non-MS course in children. Neurol Neuroimmunol Neuroinflamm. 2015;2:e81.

79. Rostasy K, Mader S, Hennes EM, et al. Persisting myelin oligodendrocyte glycoprotein antibodies in aquaporin-4 antibody negative pediatric neuromyelitis optica. Mult Scler. 2013;19:1052–9.

80. Rostasy K, Mader S, Schanda K, et al. Anti-myelin oligodendrocyte glycoprotein antibodies in pediatric patients with optic neuritis. Arch Neurol. 2012;69:752–6.

81. Fernandez-Carbonell C, Vargas-Lowy D, Musallam A, et al. Clinical and MRI phenotype of children with MOG antibodies. Mult Scler. 2016;22:174–84.

82. Ketelslegers IA, Van Pelt DE, Bryde S, et al. Anti-MOG antibodies plead against MS diagnosis in an Acquired Demyelinating Syndromes cohort. Mult Scler. 2015;21:1513–20.

83. Armangue T, Yeshokumar A, Sepúlveda M, et al. Antibodies in acquired demyelinating disorders in children. Mult Scler Demyelinating Disord. 2016;1:5.

84. Chabas D, Ness J, Belman A, et al. Younger children with MS have a distinct CSF inflammatory profile at disease onset. Neurology. 2010;74:399–405.

85. O'Mahony J, Shroff M, Banwell B. Mimics and rare presentations of pediatric demyelination. Neuroimaging Clin N Am. 2013;23:321–36.

86. Ghassemi R, Narayanan S, Banwell B, et al. Quantitative determination of regional lesion volume and distribution in children and adults with relapsing-remitting multiple sclerosis. PLoS One. 2014;9:e85741.

87. Waubant E, Chabas D, Okuda DT, et al. Difference in disease burden and activity in pediatric patients on brain magnetic resonance imaging at time of multiple sclerosis onset vs adults. Arch Neurol. 2009;66:967–71.

88. Weier K, Fonov V, Aubert-Broche B, Arnold DL, Banwell B, Collins DL. Impaired growth of the cerebellum in pediatric-onset acquired CNS demyelinating disease. Mult Scler. 2016;22:1266–78.

89. Chabas D, Castillo-Trivino T, Mowry EM, Strober JB, Glenn OA, Waubant E. Vanishing MS T2-bright lesions before puberty: a distinct MRI phenotype? Neurology. 2008;71:1090–3.

90. Nunan-Saah J, Paulraj SR, Waubant E, Krupp LB, Gomez RG. Neuropsychological correlates of multiple sclerosis across the lifespan. Mult Scler. 2015;21:1355–64.

91. Rocca MA, Valsasina P, Absinta M, et al. Intranetwork and internetwork functional connectivity abnormalities in pediatric multiple sclerosis. Hum Brain Mapp. 2014;35:4180–92.

92. Ghassemi R, Brown R, Banwell B, Narayanan S, Arnold DL, Canadian Pediatric Demyelinating Disease Study G. Quantitative Measurement of tissue damage and recovery within new T2w lesions in pediatric- and adult-onset multiple sclerosis. Mult Scler. 2015;21:718–25.

93. Rocca MA, Absinta M, Moiola L, et al. Functional and structural connectivity of the motor network in pediatric and adult-onset relapsing-remitting multiple sclerosis. Radiology. 2010;254:541–50.

94. Akbar N, Banwell B, Sled JG, et al. Brain activation patterns and cognitive processing speed in patients with pediatric-onset multiple sclerosis. J Clin Exp Neuropsychol. 2016;38:393–403.

95. Akbar N, Giorgio A, Till C, et al. Alterations in functional and structural connectivity in pediatric-onset multiple sclerosis. PLoS One. 2016;11:e0145906.

96. Donohue K, Cox JL, Dwyer MG, et al. No regional gray matter atrophy differences between pediatric- and adult-onset relapsing-remitting multiple sclerosis. J Neuroimaging. 2014;24:63–7.

97. Rocca MA, De Meo E, Amato MP, et al. Cognitive impairment in paediatric multiple sclerosis patients is not related to cortical lesions. Mult Scler. 2015;21:956–9.

98. Absinta M, Rocca MA, Moiola L, et al. Cortical lesions in children with multiple sclerosis. Neurology. 2011;76:910–3.

99. Tortorella P, Rocca MA, Mezzapesa DM, et al. MRI quantification of gray and white matter damage in patients with early-onset multiple sclerosis. J Neurol. 2006;253:903–7.

100. Brown RA, Narayanan S, Banwell B, Arnold DL, Canadian Pediatric Demyelinating Disease N. Magnetization transfer ratio recovery in new lesions decreases during adolescence in pediatric-onset multiple sclerosis patients. Neuroimage Clin. 2014;6:237–42.

101. Mesaros S, Rocca MA, Absinta M, et al. Evidence of thalamic gray matter loss in pediatric multiple sclerosis. Neurology. 2008;70:1107–12.

102. Aubert-Broche B, Fonov V, Narayanan S, et al. Onset of multiple sclerosis before adulthood leads to failure of age-expected brain growth. Neurology. 2014;83:2140–6.

103. Kerbrat A, Aubert-Broche B, Fonov V, et al. Reduced head and brain size for age and disproportionately smaller thalami in child-onset MS. Neurology. 2012;78:194–201.

104. Waubant E, Ponsonby AL, Pugliatti M, Hanwell H, Mowry EM, Hintzen RQ. Environmental and genetic factors in pediatric inflammatory demyelinating diseases. Neurology. 2016;87:S20–7.

105. Mikaeloff Y, Caridade G, Tardieu M, Suissa S, group Ks. Parental smoking at home and the risk of childhood-onset multiple sclerosis in children. Brain. 2007;130:2589–95.

106. Banwell B, Bar-Or A, Arnold DL, et al. Clinical, environmental, and genetic determinants of multiple sclerosis in children with acute demyelination: a prospective national cohort study. Lancet Neurol. 2011;10:436–45.

107. Waubant E, Mowry EM, Krupp L, et al. Common viruses associated with lower pediatric multiple sclerosis risk. Neurology. 2011;76:1989–95.

108. Langer-Gould A, Brara SM, Beaber BE, Koebnick C. Childhood obesity and risk of pediatric multiple sclerosis and clinically isolated syndrome. Neurology. 2013;80:548–52.

109. Gianfrancesco MA, Acuna B, Shen L, et al. Obesity during childhood and adolescence increases susceptibility to multiple sclerosis after accounting for established genetic and environmental risk factors. Obes Res Clin Pract. 2014;8:e435–47.

110. Hedstrom AK, Lima Bomfim I, Hillert J, Olsson T, Alfredsson L. Obesity interacts with infectious mononucleosis in risk of multiple sclerosis. Eur J Neurol. 2015;22:578–e38.

111. Hedstrom AK, Lima Bomfim I, Barcellos L, et al. Interaction between adolescent obesity and HLA risk genes in the etiology of multiple sclerosis. Neurology. 2014;82:865–72.

112. McDonald J, Graves J, Waldman A, et al. A case–control study of dietary salt intake in pediatric-onset multiple sclerosis. Mult Scler Relat Disord. 2016;6:87–92.

113. Bhargava P, Steele SU, Waubant E, et al. Multiple sclerosis patients have a diminished serologic response to vitamin D supplementation compared to healthy controls. Mult Scler. 2016;22:753–60.

114. Disanto G, Magalhaes S, Handel AE, et al. HLA-DRB1 confers increased risk of pediatric-onset MS in children with acquired demyelination. Neurology. 2011;76:781–6.

115. van Pelt ED, Mescheriakova JY, Makhani N, et al. Risk genes associated with pediatric-onset MS but not with monophasic acquired CNS demyelination. Neurology. 2013;81:1996–2001.

116. Waubant E, Mowry EM, Krupp L, et al. Antibody response to common viruses and human leukocyte antigen-DRB1 in pediatric multiple sclerosis. Mult Scler. 2013;19:891–5.

117. Graves JS, Barcellos LF, Shao X, et al. Genetic predictors of relapse rate in pediatric MS. Mult Scler. 2016;22:1528–35.

118. Quintana FJ, Patel B, Yeste A, et al. Epitope spreading as an early pathogenic event in pediatric multiple sclerosis. Neurology. 2014;83:2219–26.

119. Vargas-Lowy D, Kivisakk P, Gandhi R, et al. Increased Th17 response to myelin peptides in pediatric MS. Clin Immunol Rev (Orlando, Fla). 2013;146:176–84.

120. Bar-Or A, Hintzen RQ, Dale RC, Rostasy K, Bruck W, Chitnis T. Immunopathophysiology of pediatric CNS inflammatory demyelinating diseases. Neurology. 2016;87:S12–9.

121. Chitnis T, Tardieu M, Amato MP, et al. International Pediatric MS Study Group Clinical Trials Summit: meeting report. Neurology. 2013;80:1161–8.

122. Ghezzi A. Randomized clinical trial in pediatric multiple sclerosis: are they really necessary? Mult. Scler. J. 2016. doi:10.1177/1352458516684025.

123. Chitnis T, Tenembaum S, Banwell B, et al. Consensus statement: evaluation of new and existing therapeutics for pediatric multiple sclerosis. Mult Scler. 2012;18:116–27.

124. Ghezzi A, Banwell B, Boyko A, et al. The management of multiple sclerosis in children: a European view. Mult Scler. 2010;16:1258–67.

125. Ghezzi A, Amato MP, Makhani N, Shreiner T, Gartner J, Tenembaum S. Pediatric multiple sclerosis: Conventional first-line treatment and general management. Neurology. 2016;87:S97–S102.

126. Krupp LB, Pohl D, Ghezzi A, et al. Subcutaneous interferon beta-1a in pediatric patients with multiple sclerosis: Regional differences in clinical features, disease management, and treatment outcomes in an international retrospective study. J Neurol Sci. 2016;363:33–8.

127. Ghezzi A, Pozzilli C, Grimaldi LM, et al. Natalizumab in pediatric multiple sclerosis: results of a cohort of 55 cases. Mult Scler. 2013;19:1106–12.

128. Kornek B, Aboul-Enein F, Rostasy K, et al. Natalizumab therapy for highly active pediatric multiple sclerosis. JAMA Neurol. 2013;70:469–75.

129. Chitnis T, Ghezzi A, Bajer-Kornek B, Boyko A, Giovannoni G, Pohl D. Pediatric multiple sclerosis: Escalation and emerging treatments. Neurology. 2016;87:S103–9.

130. Ghezzi A, Moiola L, Pozzilli C, et al. Natalizumab in the pediatric MS population: results of the Italian registry. BMC Neurol. 2015;15:174.

131. Fragoso YD, Alves-Leon SV, Barreira AA, et al. Fingolimod prescribed for the treatment of multiple sclerosis in patients younger than age 18 years. Pediatr Neurol. 2015;53:166–8.

132. Makhani N, Schreiner T. Oral dimethyl fumarate in children with multiple sclerosis: a dual-center study. Pediatr Neurol. 2016;57:101–4.

133. Muraro PA, Pasquini M, Atkins HL, et al. Long-term Outcomes After Autologous Hematopoietic Stem Cell Transplantation for Multiple Sclerosis. JAMA Neurol. 2017. doi:10.1001/jamaneurol.2016.5867. [Epub ahead of print].

134. Krupp LB, Rintell D, Charvet LE, Milazzo M, Wassmer E. Pediatric multiple sclerosis: perspectives from adolescents and their families. Neurology. 2016;87:S4–7.

135. Scalfari A, Lederer C, Daumer M, Nicholas R, Ebers GC, Muraro PA. The relationship of age with the clinical phenotype in multiple sclerosis. Mult Scler. 2016;22:1750–8.

136. Pfeifenbring S, Bunyan RF, Metz I, et al. Extensive acute axonal damage in pediatric multiple sclerosis lesions. Ann Neurol. 2015;77:655–67.

10

The link of inflammation and neurodegeneration in progressive multiple sclerosis

Fernando Pérez-Cerdá[*], María Victoria Sánchez-Gómez and Carlos Matute

Abstract

Progressive multiple sclerosis (MS) is characterized clinically by the accumulation of neurological disability without unequivocal recovery. Understanding the mechanisms that determine entering in this stage of the disease is a great challenge in order to identify potential therapeutic targets. Recent advances in defining more accurately the progressive phenotype of MS, have concluded that differences between primary and secondary progressive forms of disease are relatively quantitative rather than qualitative. In both cases, a large number of molecular and cellular events that might lead to neurodegeneration have been suggested. These include microglia activation, chronic oxidative injury, accumulation of mitochondrial damage in axons, age-related disturbances and dysfunctional axonal transport among others. Commonly, these pathological mechanisms have been considered as a result of inflammatory demyelination but a primary degenerative condition has also been argued. It is now clear that both events contribute to the progression of the disease, however their temporal sequence is still a matter of debate. A detailed knowledge of progressive MS pathogenesis will allow to develop effective treatments for both progression and symptom management that should be based on a combination of anti-inflammatory, regenerative and neuroprotective strategies. In this review, we summarize current data and recent hypothesis about pathological forces that drive progression of damage in MS, i.e. cumulative cortical demyelination and neurodegeneration as well as diffuse alterations (microglia activation, axonal injury and atrophy) throughout white and grey matter in the brain and spinal cord. Finally, we discuss the potential of the aforementioned proposed disease mechanisms with regard to developing suitable therapies to halt the progression in MS pathology.

Keywords: Inflammation, Microgliosis, Mitochondria, Energy failure, Axonal damage, Iron accumulation

Background

Multiple sclerosis (MS) is a chronic inflammatory, demyelinating and neurodegenerative disorder of the central nervous system (CNS) and it is the most common cause of non-traumatic neurological disability in young adults [1–7]. The diagnostic criteria for MS are the clinical course of disease supported by paraclinical laboratory assessments and the demonstration by magnetic resonance imaging (MRI) of dissemination of lesions in space and time. The initial clinical phenotype of MS is frequently characterized by episodes of neurological disturbances followed with residual deficits or full recovery (relapsing-remitting MS, RRMS) and in a minority (10–20 %) by a

* Correspondence: fernando.perez@ehu.eus
Achucarro Basque Center for Neuroscience, Departamento de Neurociencias and CIBERNED, Universidad del País Vasco (UPV/EHU), 48940 Leioa, Spain

slowly accumulation of disability from the onset (primary progressive MS, PPMS). Usually with time, a majority of RRMS patients (up to 70 %) transitions into a predominant gradual worsening over exacerbations or relapses (secondary progressive MS, SPMS) [8].

Recently, the classification of the MS phenotypes has been reorganized into categories according to the presence/absence of activity and/or gradual illness progression [9]. Disease activity is defined by clinical relapses and/or lesion activity in CNS imaging and is related to episodes of tissue injury associated with inflammation. Progression is linked to increasing neurologic dysfunction which by current understanding reflects neurodegenerative processes. Progression and activity are very close to one another but conceptually four phenotypes are possible: progression with/without activity; no progression but with activity;

and no progression and no activity (stable disease). Thus, SPMS and PPMS are considered parts of the spectrum of progressive MS (PMS) phenotypes and differences between them are relative rather than absolute. Almost no treatment options are available for PMS patients (more than 50 % of people with MS), so a good clinical classification of patients is very important to better design trials for study the value of new therapies [10, 11]. However, the most fundamental issue in developing new treatments for PMS is to understand the pathological events that underpin the disease process.

The pathological mechanisms that drive neurodegeneration in PMS are poorly understood though a large range of disease processes have been proposed as discussed here. Commonly, neurodegeneration has been regarded as a result of inflammatory demyelination due to peripheral immune system activation (the outside-in hypothesis). Recently an explanation of disease progression suggests that inflammatory demyelinating processes in early MS trigger a cascade of events (among others microglia activation, chronic oxidative injury, mitochondrial damage in axons) that lead to neurodegeneration and are amplified by pathogenic mechanisms related to brain ageing and accumulated disease burden [2, 12–14]. Alternatively, MS can be regarded as a primary degenerative condition which initiates in the myelinating unit (oligodendroglia, their processes and myelin) and results in neuroinflammation (the inside-out hypothesis) [15, 16]. It is highly likely that immune-triggered inflammation in turn drives further damage and degeneration of CNS elements, creating a vicious circle. According to this hypothesis, progression in MS would be present from the beginning of illness and progressive cytodegeneration would underlie all disease processes. Resolution of these conflicting ideas is unresolved, nonetheless both suggest that treatment of PMS, preferable at the early stages of disease, should be based on a combination of anti-inflammatory, regenerative and neuroprotective strategies [11, 17, 18]. Nevertheless, although inflammatory and neurodegenerative events act in concert to induce MS-specific brain damage their relevance changes during the course of chronic disease evolution.

Review

The pathology of MS is defined by a spectrum of tissue alterations in the CNS [2, 6, 19]. Classically include plaques of primary demyelination with oligodendrocyte loss and profound axonal degeneration surrounded by an astrocytic scar formation in the white and gray matter of the brain and spinal cord. These plaques are typically inactive and very frequent in all stages of MS. In contrast, active lesions display a focal disruption of the blood-brain-barrier (BBB) together with inflammatory cells (lymphocytes, macrophages and activated microglia)

which are present throughout the lesion or at the periphery in acute or chronic active plaques respectively. In PMS half of focal plaques are characterized by a peripheral small rim composed of a small number of inflammatory cells (slowly expanding pre-existing lesions) whereas damage to BBB is less obvious. In addition to focal plaques, diffuse alterations affecting the normal-appearing CNS with a low-grade on-going inflammation are seen in patients with PMS (Table 1). These changes include microglial activation mild demyelination and axonal-neuronal loss in the context of an inflammatory process partly compartmentalized behind an intact BBB.

There is an increasing recognition in the MS field [6, 12, 14, 19–22] that progression of disease that finally result in CNS atrophy, is related with the accumulation over time of the following lesions:

- grey matter demyelination, particularly with a subpial location, largely irrespective of immune cell infiltration and lesion load in white matter tracts; and that is associated with both a very limited remyelination capacity and destruction and loss of nerve cells.
- diffuse tissue loss in the normal-appearing CNS, that are only weakly correlated with the number, size and destructive changes in classical focal white matter lesions.

Assuming that SPMS and PPMS share the same pathologic basis implies that in SPMS patients neurodegeneration occurs from the beginning of disease, even before symptoms of relapses (clinically active inflammation) appear. Likewise, there will be an ongoing chronic "below the radar" subclinical inflammation in PPMS patients, prior to onset of progressive neurodegenerative symptoms. Accordingly, it has been recently proposed that a cascade of immunological and neurodegenerative

Table 1 Key aspects of progressive multiple sclerosis (PMS) distinguishing it from relapsing-remitting multiple sclerosis (RRMS)

- Time to disability progression is not driven by relapse rate, frequency or severity
- Fewer active plaques (less inflammation and peripheral immune cell activation and fewer gadolinium enhancing lesions [signifying fewer blood-brain barrier breaches])
- Compartmentalised inflammation within the central nervous system (CNS): meningeal inflammatory aggregates (lymphatic follicles-like)
- More neurodegeneration: more demyelination and axonal loss in gray matter; more cortical pathology (subpial lesions are almost specific of PMS) and CNS atrophy
- More diffuse abnormalities and tissue loss in the normal appearing CNS
- Universal progressive spinal cord disease
- Anti-inflammatory therapies less effective or ineffective

events act in concert to induce MS specific CNS damage [12]. Key elements driving neurodegeneration include microglia activation, chronic oxidative injury, accumulation of mitochondrial damage in axons, and age-related iron accumulation in the human CNS [5, 13, 14, 21, 23, 24]. Altered mitochondrial damage in axons might be of particular importance since it leads to chronic cell stress and imbalance of ionic homeostasis, resulting in axonal and neuronal death.

Loss of the symbiotic relationship between the axon and myelin sheath after persistent demyelination in MS causes progressive axonal damage providing a logical explanation for continuous and irreversible neurological decline in PMS. Chronic deprivation of myelin-derived trophic support of axons, results in a slowly development of axonopathy manifested by axonal swelling, reduction in axonal calibre and ultimately axonal degeneration. Current hypotheses indicate that the compensatory plasticity of the CNS delays the onset and progression of neurological decline in MS patients. Adaptive and neuroprotective mechanisms that may compensate for initial dysfunction include activation of cortical areas, neurogenesis, remyelination, redistribution of sodium channels on demyelinated axons, increases in mitochondrial content and respiratory functions in axons and enhanced production of neurotrophic factors by CNS resident cells [22, 25]. However, once a threshold of axonal loss is reached the exhaustion of the functional reservoir results in a steady progression of MS.

Neuropathological features of progressive multiple sclerosis

How do chronically demyelinated axons and neurons degenerate? It has been suggested that failure of remyelination is the pathological substrate for disease progression in MS [1, 26]. In fact, the pattern of tissue injury in PMS is quite homogeneous and it is characterized by oligodendrocyte loss, demyelination and lack of remyelination, as well as preferential destruction of small-calibre axons and astrocytic gliosis. Characteristics of PMS pathology are focal lesions of demyelination, strips or bands of cortical demyelination and diffuse pathology in the normal appearing white and grey matter (Table 1).

- An absence of focal new inflammatory demyelinating lesions as measured by MRI and histopathology is predominant in the course of PMS [2]. Inactive or slowly spanding pre-existing MS plaques are usually seen, latter characterized by a rim of microglia and a low-grade myelin and axonal destruction at the lesion edge. But "inactivity" does not mean stability of disease lesions. Most axons can survive acute demyelination, and some grade of remyelination is possible if active lesions are resolved, but chronically demyelinated axons degenerate. Dynamics of axonal loss are not well documented but this is a prominent feature of PMS that can explain partly the concomitant CNS atrophy observed and is the major cause of irreversible neurological disability.

- Cortical and deep grey matter demyelination is very common in MS and exceeds white matter demyelination. However, little is known about its dynamics because lesion load measures have been difficult both by MRI and by histopathology [26–28]. In PMS strips or bands of subpial cortical demyelination, which differ in appearance from intracortical and leukocortical focal lesions ones, are by far the biggest contributors to total cortical lesion load, and do not occur in other inflammatory or non-inflammatory human CNS diseases. In addition to demyelination and oligodendrocyte loss, cortical lesions show neuritic transections, neuronal death and synaptic loss and when active are linked to local inflammation in the meninges and activation of microglia. Similar alterations also occur in spinal cord and other CNS locations of grey matter.

- On the other hand, macroscopically normal appearing CNS of patients with MS also show diffuse and global changes that are already present from the beginning of disease [19, 21]. They include microglial activation, astrocytic gliosis and mild inflammation, demyelination, and axonal injury. With time there is an increasing and progressive loss of axons in the normal-appearing white matter and of neurons in gray matter which correlates with the CNS atrophy that appear in advanced PMS. This atrophy does not correlate with focal lesions load suggesting that diffuse neurodegeneration is at least partly, an independent process from anterograde Wallerian degeneration and/or retrograde neuronal dying back started in white and gray plaques.

Molecular mechanisms underlying progression in multiple sclerosis

They are summarized in Table 2 and detailed in the following subsections.

Inflammation and microglial activation

In all forms of MS, inflammation is always present when active demyelination and neurodegeneration occur [3, 12, 20]. Inflammatory released products as reactive oxygen or nitric oxide species (ROS and RNS), excitotoxins as glutamate, and cytotoxic cytokines alter myelin sheaths and cellular metabolism in neurons and their axons. However inflammation declines with disease duration while neurodegeneration proceeds and activated microglia persists in all lesions in PMS [29].

Table 2 Mechanisms and amplification factors for neurodegeneration in progressive multiple sclerosis (PMS)

- Chronic microglial activation and low-grade inflammation: excitotoxicity, and chronic oxidative stress which leads to mitochondrial injury

- Mitochondrial dysfunction (energy failure; ionic imbalance) that might underlie features of Multiple Sclerosis lesions: demyelination, oligodendrocyte apoptosis and lack of remyelination; and axonal injury

- Accumulation of lesion burden: retrograde and anterograde degeneration of demyelinated axons due to lack of trophic support and abnormal axonal excitability (altered expression of ion channels) and amplification of microglia activation

- Mitochondrial DNA deletion over time and with age as in other classical neurodegenerative diseases: increased energy deficiency and amplification of oxidative injury

- Iron accumulation with ageing in the brain cells and release of iron in demyelinating lesions (more oxidative injury)

- Progression of age-related neurodegeneration and exhaustion of central nervous system functional reserve capacity

Whether inflammation in PMS, as in other stages of disease, is a cause (the outside-in theory: immune dysregulation) or result of neurodegeneration (inside-out model: governed by released immunogenic material after cytodegeneration) remains to be determined [15]. Also, a key unresolved question is if the inflammatory response is qualitatively the same in PMS as in other stages of disease where different patterns of inflammatory processes occur [30, 31]. Quantitatively, PMS inflammation becomes, at least in part, trapped within the CNS behind an unaffected BBB forming lymph follicle-like aggregates in the meninges. Demyelination and neurodegeneration in the cortex of PMS patients are more pronounced when these structures are present [32].

Microglial activation, probably due to a chronically inflammatory milieu, is invariably seen in the CNS of patients with PMS [33]. However this is common in many other CNS diseases in absence of selective primary demyelination. Perhaps the "specific" contribution of chronically activated microglia to the induction of demyelination and progressive axonal injury in MS is the generation of chronic oxidative stress, by xanthine and NADPH (nicotinamide-adenine dinucleotide phosphate) oxidases as well as myeloperoxidase, and subsequent mitochondrial injury in axons and oligodendrocytes. In addition, activated microglia impairs glutamate transport in astrocytes, and thus, promote neuronal and oligodendrocyte excitotoxicity [5, 12, 33].

Mitochondrial injury and axonal energy failure

Several lines of evidence have led to the hypothesis that mitochondrial injury is a primary phenomenon in MS [24, 34]. Remarkably, mitochondria and mitochondrial DNA, essential for oxidative phosphorylation, are highly susceptible to oxidative injury. In fact, chronic increased local levels of ROS and RNS by activated microglia are pronounced in PMS despite low levels of inflammation and can promote mitochondrial dysfunction. Moreover, the mechanisms of axonal degeneration in MS are similar to those occurring in ischemic/hypoxic insults. Thus, it has been hypothesized that energy deficiency or "virtual hypoxia" might have also a pathogenic role in MS. Demyelination has a substantial effect on axonal mitochondria and renders the demyelinated axon susceptible to chronic environmental conditions that eventually result in axon transection and degeneration. Key features related to mitochondrial dysfunction [2, 5, 12, 13, 19, 22, 34] are the following:

- After demyelination, aberrant expression of Na^+ channels along the entire length of the demyelinated axon increases energy demands of nerve conduction, and ATP production by mitochondria might become compromised causing axoplasmic ionic imbalance and intracellular Ca^{2+} accumulation. In conditions of energy deficiency and mitochondrial "functional overload", the ATP-dependent Na^+ pump does not remove Na^+, which accumulates in the axon an is replaced by Ca^{2+} through reverse operation of the Na^+/Ca^{2+} exchanger. Additional Ca^{2+} enters the axon via glutamate receptors and voltage-gated Ca^{2+} channels present in the axolemma. If mitochondrial damage passes a certain threshold, reduced local energy production might precipitate axonal demise. In that way, thin-calibre axons with proportionally less mitochondria in relation to the surface area of axolemma than thick ones, are more severely affected.

- When axoplasmic Ca^{2+} accumulation exceeds the buffering capacity by mitochondria, initiates a vicious cycle of deleterious and finally fatal effects on the axon characterized by activation of degradative enzymes that compromise axonal transport, impaired mitochondrial operation, reduced energy production, and more axoplasmic Ca^{2+}. In fact, cytoskeletal disturbances as fragmentation of neurofilaments by Ca^{2+} activated degradative enzymes as calpain, appear in chronic MS lesions, altering the turnover and redistribution of mitochondria and fast axonal transport. Also, in patients with PMS, a lost or impaired functional activity of mitochondrial respiratory chain complexes has been described in neurons. Therefore, chronic mitochondrial injury amplifies chronic oxidative stress present in MS and viceversa. Additionally, oxidative injury causes mitochondrial DNA deletions in both the white matter and grey matter. Accumulation of mitochondrial dysfunctions in patients with PMS as a final result of the demyelination, could partly explain their increased susceptibility of brain tissue to neurodegeneration through enhancement of oxidative injury, energy failure and altered calcium homeostasis.

- In oligodendrocytes, mitochondrial injury results in the release of apoptosis-inducing factor, its translocation into the nucleus and induction of DNA damage which ultimately leads to cell death.

Age-dependent iron accumulation amplifies injury in PMS

Iron accumulation in patients with MS can further amplify ROS and RNS mediated injury, by generating toxic reactants [2, 5, 12]. Iron loading in the brain increases with age and is predominantly stored in oligodendrocytes in the non-toxic ferric (Fe^{3+}) form bound to ferritin. Importantly, injury of these cells during MS releases iron into the extracellular space where it is converted into Fe^{2+}, which might further amplify oxidative damage in axons and other cells. Released iron is then taken up by activated microglia, which becomes dystrophic and degenerate, releasing a second way of Fe^{2+} and increasing the susceptibility of the surrounding tissue to free-radical-driven demyelination and neurodegeneration. It is worth noting that although iron accumulation is an age-dependent process, and for that reason likely more pronounced in PMS than previously in the disease, the pathogenic role of iron in MS is on discussion. In fact, in chronic MS, a significant decrease in iron levels is observed in normal appearing CNS [35]. Also it must be taken into account that previous disease history also influences the development of neurodegenerative amplification damage. In fact, the earlier and/or higher relapse rates, the shorter time to onset of PMS [9].

Advances in imaging in progressive multiple sclerosis

Pathological assessment is the gold standard to identify MS lesions, but there are intrinsic limitations due to the very limited availability of biopsy tissue and additionally, tissue evaluation only provides one snapshot in time, not allowing observation of the evolution of pathological changes over time. Because of that, MRI and related techniques with higher specificity are promising tools for a better understanding of the pathophysiology of the PMS "in vivo" [8]. Although conventional T1-weighted images show less sensitivity than T2-weighted MRI images, they are more specific to MS pathology and probably T1 hypointense signals are reflecting tissue lesions with oedema, demyelination, neuroaxonal loss and gliosis [36]. In clinical practice, it is difficult to differentiate a case of PMS from RRMS using MRI [8, 37–39], but studies have found some population-based differences between these two groups. In PMS, there is somehow a

preponderance of spinal cord/brainstem lesions and relative paucity of new gadolinium-enhancing brain lesions over time. A decrease in their occurrence is related to the clinical transition from RRMS to SPMS. Also there are differences in brain atrophy localization, mainly due to loss of white matter in RRMS as seen by ventricular enlargement, while in PMS atrophy tends to be more a cortical phenomenon, particularly common in PPMS. However conventional MRI approaches are basically unable to detect cortical lesions and diffuse tissue damage in the normal appearing CNS. As a consequence, they correlate only weakly with clinical manifestations and evolution of PMS.

On the contrary, advanced MRI techniques that are far away of being integrated into routine clinical practice at present, have shown greater sensitivity and specificity for assessing the pathological substrates of MS, in particular demyelination and neuroaxonal loss, providing better prognostic information [13, 40–42]. These include magnetization transfer (MT) imaging and its quantitative index MT ratio which has been proposed as a marker of brain myelin content, also in the cerebral cortex; diffusion tensor MRI tractography for axonal loss; and proton MR spectroscopy that records signals from metabolites as N-acetyl aspartate, a marker of neuroaxonal integrity, or choline and lactate, biochemical correlates of inflammation and demyelination. Additional insights into the characteristics of MS lesions have been obtained from iron-sensitive MRI sequences, especially at very high field strengths (7.0 Tesla) where its accumulation shows a close match to neurodegeneration. These quantitative MR techniques by measuring the disease burden within focal lesions and in the normal-appearing CNS instead volume changes are contributing significantly to the understanding of the pathological mechanisms underlying the irreversible accumulation of disability in PMS. However, and despite their potential, most of the new MR techniques still require future research and validation.

Potential therapies

Oligodendrocytes and axons express neurotransmitter receptors to glutamate so it may act as a potential excitotoxin under acute and chronic insults, and ultimately contribute to neurodegeneration in PMS. Thus, numerous studies conducted in cellular and animal models of MS, as well as in post-mortem brain and in patients, indicate that excitotoxicity mediated by Ca^{2+}-permeable glutamate receptors contributes to oligodendrocyte death, demyelination, and tissue damage in MS [43]. In particular, experimental MS is alleviated by α-amino-3-hydroxy-5-methyl-4-isoxazolepropionate (AMPA) and kainate receptor antagonists, but not N-methyl-d-aspartate receptor blockade, and combination with anti-inflammatory agents expands neuroprotection even at advanced disease stages [44]. Moreover, genome-wide association screening associated alleles in AMPA receptor genes in MS patients to brain volume loss in patients with high glutamate levels [45]. In turn, glutamate levels are increased in the brain in MS as a consequence of reduced expression of the glutamate transporters (excitatory amino acid transporters 1 and 2) and upregulation of the cystine/glutamate antiporter in the monocyte-macrophage-microglia lineage is associated with immune activation in both MS and experimental autoimmune encephalomyelitis (EAE) [43, 46]. Like glutamate, ATP, when in excess, is a potent endogenous toxin that can directly kill oligodendrocytes via activation of purinergic P2X7 receptors whose blockade during the chronic phase of EAE attenuates the symptoms and tissue damage [47]. Interestingly, P2X7 variants are associated with a reduced or increased risk to suffer from MS [48, 49]. All in all, these studies in MS animal models and in the disease proper offer new ideas to develop novel therapies to treat PMS.

Recently, results of clinical trials have challenged the long-held belief that pathogenesis of PMS is more neurodegenerative than inflammatory, and distinct from these aspects in RRMS. Indeed, ocrelizumab, a humanized monoclonal antibody targeting CD20 B cells, has significant efficacy in both forms of MS reducing the relapse rate in RRMS and delaying the risk of clinical disability progression in RRMS and, although modestly, also for the first time in primary PMS [50]. Pivotal ocrelizumab trials [51, 52] had showed that mature B cells, which express the antigen CD20 on their surface, played a central role in the pathophysiology of RRMS traditionally considered to be driven by T cells due to the observations of activated T lymphocytes in MS plaques [2, 3, 6, 19]. This idea is now extended to PMS where lymphoid follicles containing B cells are present in the meninges [32]. Although the mechanisms whereby anti-CD20 exerts its beneficial effects are not well understood, there is evidence that CD20 B cells, which represent a few percent of the total B-cell pool, are involved in progressive aspects of MS [53]. Moreover, clinical trials have shown that CD20 B-cell depletion is effective without significant compromise of the normal immune reactivity. Further stratification of disease subtypes will be needed for a better understanding of the complex roles of B cells in MS [54–56]. Also, if the presence of disease activity measured as T1 gadolinium-enhancing lesions favours the response to ocrelizumab as suggested by recent data [57]. However, the lack of biomarkers predicting the level of activity and/or progression in MS, namely active demyelination and neurodegeneration, hinders the stratification of disease types [11, 18]. In this regard, further promising developments in PMS therapies with targeted disease-modifying drugs may contribute to better understanding the underlying molecular and cellular pathology of MS. Lastly, but not least, global research collaboration will be needed to overcome the challenges of understanding and treating efficiently PMS [23, 58].

Conclusions

In MS, the progression of disease is the consequence of a pathogenic cascade of events caused and/or related to long-lasting accumulation of CNS damage which initiated earlier, even when clinical symptoms were not present. Chronic inflammation and neurodegeneration are interlinked in MS from early stages of disease course and there are multiple potential mechanisms that trigger and sustain damage in PMS [59, 60]. Oxidative damage, severe ion channel dysfunction, mitochondrial injury, microglial activation without obvious disruption of the BBB, and age related changes in CNS, are mechanisms that also contribute to other neurodegenerative diseases. Unlike in other neurodegenerative conditions, there is no evidence of a primary trigger in MS for myelin and oligodendrocytic injury, and it is unknown why usually it has not a monophasic course from its beginning. Perhaps the absence of remission in PMS is a sign of exhaustion of CNS compensatory mechanisms rather than a change in the disease process. Moreover, there is no imaging, pathological, or biomarker characteristics that reliably distinguish between first episodes of MS and progressive MS. Although the molecular and cellular mechanisms driving the cyclic course and/or progression of disease are incompletely understood, widespread and diffuse loss of neurons and axons in the white and grey matter with resultant atrophy has a key role in disability progression in MS. In fact, subpial cortical demyelination appears to be exquisitely specific for MS, since it is not present in any other inflammatory, neurodegenerative or metabolic CNS disease. Despite the unknowns, from a therapeutic point of view, a combination of immunomodulatory and neuroprotective strategies introduced earlier in the development of disease appear to be the most promising strategy to limit the progression of MS. Also appropriate animal models, good biomarkers and imaging measures remain indispensable to understand the disease and test novel potential treatments.

Abbreviations

AMPA, α-amino-3-hydroxy-5-methyl-4-isoxazolepropionate; ATP, Adenosine triphosphate; BBB, Blood brain barrier; Ca^{2+}, Calcium ion; CNS, Central nervous system; DNA, Deoxyribonucleic acid; EAE, Experimental autoimmune encephalomyelitis; Fe^{2+}; Fe^{3+}, Ferrous ion; Ferric ion; MRI, Magnetic resonance imaging; MS, Multiple sclerosis; Na^{+}, Sodium ion; NADPH, Nicotinamide-adenine dinucleotide phosphate (reduced form); PMS, Progressive multiple sclerosis; PPMS, Primary progressive multiple sclerosis; RNS, Reactive nitric oxide species; ROS, Reactive oxygen species; RRMS, Relapsing-remitting multiple sclerosis; SPMS, Secondary progressive multiple sclerosis

Acknowledgements

Work in our laboratory is funded by CIBERNED, Gobierno Vasco (EJ/GV) and MINECO (SAF2013-45084-R).

Authors' contributions

FP-C designed and coordinated the review and drafted the manuscript. MVS-G revised it critically for important intellectual content. CM conceived the review, participated in its design and coordination and helped to draft the manuscript. All authors read and approved the final manuscript.

Competing interests

The authors declare that they have no competing interests.

Search strategy and selection criteria

We searched PubMed with the terms "progressive multiple sclerosis", "magnetic resonance imaging" and "clinical trials" in papers published in English. References were also identified through searches of unloaded articles and of our own files. We focused on the previous decade of research and on reviews with a great influence in the understanding of PMS. Final list of publications was selected on the basis of relevance to the aims of this review.

References

1. Trapp BD, Nave KA. Multiple sclerosis: an immune or neurodegenerative disorder? Annu Rev Neurosci. 2008;31:247–69.
2. Lassmann H, van Horssen J, Mahad D. Progressive multiple sclerosis: pathology and pathogenesis. Nat Rev Neurol. 2012;8:647–56.
3. Stadelmann C, Wegner C, Brück W. Inflammation, demyelination, and degeneration - recent insights from MS pathology. Biochim Biophys Acta. 1812;2011:275–82.
4. Ellwardt E, Zipp F. Molecular mechanisms linking neuroinflammation and neurodegeneration in MS. Exp Neurol. 2014;262:8–17.
5. Friese MA, Schattling B, Fugger L. Mechanisms of neurodegeneration and axonal dysfunction in multiple sclerosis. Nat Rev Neurol. 2014;10:225–38.
6. Kutzelnigg A, Lassmann H. Pathology of multiple sclerosis and related inflammatory demyelinating diseases. In: Goodin DS, editor. Handbook of clinical neurology (vol 122): Multiple sclerosis and related disorders. Amsterdam: Elsevier; 2014. p. 15–58.
7. Schaeffer J, Cossetti C, Mallucci G, Pluchino S. Multiple sclerosis. In: Zigmond MJ, Rowland LP, Coyle JT, editors. Neurobiology of brain disorders: biological basis of neurological and psychiatric disorders. London: Academic; 2015. p. 497–520.
8. Polman CH, Reingold SC, Banwell B, Clanet M, Cohen JA, Filippi M, et al. Diagnostic criteria for multiple sclerosis: 2010 revisions to the McDonald criteria. Ann Neurol. 2011;69:292–302.
9. Lublin FD, Reingold SC, Cohen JA, Cutter GR, Sørensen PS, Thompson AJ, et al. Defining the clinical course of multiple sclerosis: the 2013 revisions. Neurology. 2014;83:278–86.
10. Ontaneda D, Fox RJ. Progressive multiple sclerosis. Curr Opin Neurol. 2015;28:237–43.
11. Ontaneda D, Fox RJ, Chataway J. Clinical trials in progressive multiple sclerosis: lessons learned and future perspectives. Lancet Neurol. 2015;14:208–23.
12. Mahad DH, Trapp BD, Lassmann H. Pathological mechanisms in progressive multiple sclerosis. Lancet Neurol. 2015;14:183–93.
13. Ciccarelli O, Barkhof F, Bodini B, De Stefano N, Golay X, Nicolay K, et al. Pathogenesis of multiple sclerosis: insights from molecular and metabolic imaging. Lancet Neurol. 2014;13:807–22.
14. Haider L, Simeonidou C, Steinberger G, Hametner S, Grigoriadis N, Deretzi G, et al. Multiple sclerosis deep grey matter: the relation between demyelination, neurodegeneration, inflammation and iron. J Neurol Neurosurg Psychiatry. 2014;85:1386–95.
15. Stys PK, Zamponi GW, van Minnen J, Geurts JJ. Will the real multiple sclerosis please stand up? Nat Rev Neurosci. 2012;13:507–14.
16. Kamm CP, Uitdehaag BM, Polman CH. Multiple sclerosis: current knowledge and future outlook. Eur Neurol. 2014;72:132–41.
17. Feinstein A, Freeman J, Lo AC. Treatment of progressive multiple sclerosis: what works, what does not, and what is needed. Lancet Neurol. 2015;14:194–207.
18. Koch MW, Cutter G, Stys PK, Yong VW, Metz LM. Treatment trials in progressive MS -current challenges and future directions. Nat Rev Neurol. 2013;9:496–503.
19. Dutta R, Trapp BD. Relapsing and progressive forms of multiple sclerosis: insights from pathology. Curr Opin Neurol. 2014;27:271–8.
20. Calabrese M, Magliozzi R, Ciccarelli O, Geurts JJ, Reynolds R, Martin R. Exploring the origins of grey matter damage in multiple sclerosis. Nat Rev Neurosci. 2015;16:147–58.
21. Lassmann H. Multiple sclerosis: Lessons from molecular neuropathology. Exp Neurol. 2014;262:2–7.
22. Dutta R, Trapp BD. Mechanisms of neuronal dysfunction and degeneration in multiple sclerosis. Prog Neurobiol. 2011;93:1–12.
23. Salvetti M, Landsman D, Schwarz-Lam P, Comi G, Thompson AJ, Fox RJ. Progressive MS: from pathophysiology to drug discovery. Mult Scler. 2015;21:1376–84.
24. Criste G, Trapp B, Dutta R. Axonal loss in multiple sclerosis: causes and mechanisms. In: Goodin DS, editor. Handbook of clinical neurology (vol 122): Multiple sclerosis and related disorders. Amsterdam: Elsevier; 2014. p. 101–13.
25. Bramow S, Frischer JM, Lassmann H, Koch-Henriksen N, Lucchinetti CF, Sørensen PS, et al. Demyelination versus remyelination in progressive multiple sclerosis. Brain. 2010;133:2983–98.
26. Lubetzki C, Stankoff B. Demyelination in multiple sclerosis. In: Goodin DS, editor. Handbook of clinical neurology (vol 122): Multiple sclerosis and related disorders. Amsterdam: Elsevier; 2014. p. 89–99.
27. Prins M, Schul E, Geurts J, van der Valk P, Drukarch B, van Dam AM. Pathological differences between white and grey matter multiple sclerosis lesions. Ann N Y Acad Sci. 2015;1351:99–113.
28. Fischer MT, Wimmer I, Höftberger R, Gerlach S, Haider L, Zrzavy T, et al. Disease-specific molecular events in cortical multiple sclerosis lesions. Brain. 2013;136:1799–815.
29. Frischer JM, Weigand SD, Guo Y, Kale N, Parisi JE, Pirko I, et al. Clinical and pathological insights into the dynamic nature of the white matter multiple sclerosis plaque. Ann Neurol. 2015;78:710–21.
30. Lassmann H. Pathology and disease mechanisms in different stages of multiple sclerosis. J Neurol Sci. 2013;333:1–4.
31. Metz I, Weigand SD, Popescu BF, Frischer JM, Parisi JE, Guo Y, et al. Pathologic heterogeneity persists in early active multiple sclerosis lesions. Ann Neurol. 2014;75:728–38.
32. Absinta M, Vuolo L, Rao A, Nair G, Sati P, Cortese IC, et al. Gadolinium-based MRI characterization of leptomeningeal inflammation in multiple sclerosis. Neurology. 2015;85:18–28.
33. Correale J. The role of microglial activation in disease progression. Mult Scler. 2014;20:1288–95.
34. Campbell GR, Worrall JT, Mahad DJ. The central role of mitochondria in axonal degeneration in multiple sclerosis. Mult Scler. 2014;20:1806–13.
35. Hametner S, Wimmer I, Haider L, Pfeifenbring S, Brück W, Lassmann H. Iron and neurodegenration in the multiple sclerosis brain. Ann Neurol. 2013;74:848–61.
36. Filippi M, Rocca MA, Barkhof F, Brück W, Chen JT, Comi G, et al. Association between pathological and MRI findings in multiple sclerosis. Lancet Neurol. 2012;11:349–60.
37. Rovira À, Wattjes MP, Tintoré M, Tur C, Yousry TA, Sormani MP, et al. Evidence-based guidelines: MAGNIMS consensus guidelines on the use of MRI in multiple sclerosis-clinical implementation in the diagnostic process. Nat Rev Neurol. 2015;11:471–82.
38. Wattjes MP, Rovira À, Miller D, Yousry TA, Sormani MP, de Stefano MP, et al. Evidence-based guidelines: MAGNIMS consensus guidelines on the use of MRI in multiple sclerosis–establishing disease prognosis and monitoring patients. Nat Rev Neurol. 2015;11:597–606.
39. Filippi M, Rocca MA, Ciccarelli O, De Stefano N, Evangelou N, Kappos L, et al. MRI criteria for the diagnosis of multiple sclerosis: MAGNIMS consensus guidelines. Lancet Neurol. 2016;15:292–303.
40. Filippi M, Rocca MA, De Stefano N, Enzinger C, Fisher E, Horsfield MA, et al. Magnetic resonance techniques in multiple sclerosis: the present and the future. Arch Neurol. 2011;68:1514–20.
41. Rocca MA, Absinta M, Filippi M. The role of advanced magnetic resonance imaging techniques in primary progressive MS. J Neurol. 2012;259:611–21.
42. Enzinger C, Barkhof F, Ciccarelli O, Filippi M, Kappos L, Rocca MA, et al. Nonconventional MRI and microstructural cerebral changes in multiple sclerosis. Nat Rev Neurol. 2015;11:676–86.
43. Butt AM, Fern RF, Matute C. Neurotransmitter signaling in white matter. Glia. 2014;62:1762–79.

44. Kanwar JR, Kanwar RK, Krissansen GW. Simultaneous neuroprotection and blockade of inflammation reverses autoimmune encephalomyelitis. Brain. 2004;127:1313–31.

45. Baranzini SE, Srinivasan R, Khankhanian P, Okuda DT, Nelson SJ, Matthews PM, et al. Genetic variation influences glutamate concentrations in brains of patients with multiple sclerosis. Brain. 2010;133:2603–11.

46. Pampliega O, Domercq M, Soria FN, Villoslada P, Rodríguez-Antigüedad A, Matute C. Increased expression of cystine/glutamate antiporter in multiple sclerosis. J Neuroinflammation. 2011;8:63.

47. Matute C, Torre I, Pérez-Cerdá F, Pérez-Samartín A, Alberdi E, Etxebarria E, et al. P2X(7) receptor blockade prevents ATP excitotoxicity in oligodendrocytes and ameliorates experimental autoimmune encephalomyelitis. J Neurosci. 2007;27:9525–33.

48. Oyanguren-Desez O, Rodríguez-Antigüedad A, Villoslada P, Domercq M, Alberdi E, Matute C. Gain-of-function of P2X7 receptor gene variants in multiple sclerosis. Cell Calcium. 2011;50:468–72.

49. Gu BJ, Field J, Dutertre S, Ou A, Kilpatrick TJ, Lechner-Scott J, et al. A rare P2X7 variant Arg307Gln with absent pore formation function protects against neuroinflammation in multiple sclerosis. Hum Mol Genet. 2015;24:5644–54.

50. Montalban X, Hemmer B, Rammohan K, Giovannoni G, de Seze J, Bar-Or A, et al. Efficacy and safety of ocrelizumab in primary progressive multiple sclerosis-results of the placebo-controlled, double-blind, Phase III ORATORIO study. Mult Scler. 2016;22(S1):17.

51. Kappos L, Li D, Calabresi PA, O'Connor P, Bar-Or A, Barkhof F, et al. Ocrelizumab in relapsing-remitting multiple sclerosis: a phase 2, randomised, placebo-controlled, multicentre trial. Lancet. 2011;378:1779–87.

52. Chataway J, Miller DH. Multiple sclerosis-quenching the flames of inflammation. Lancet. 2011;378:1759–60.

53. Sorensen PS, Blinkenberg M. The potential role for ocrelizumab in the treatment of multiple sclerosis: current evidence and future prospects. Ther Adv Neurol Disord. 2016;9:44–52.

54. Steinman L, Zamvil SS. Beginning of the end of two-stage theory purporting that inflammation then degeneration explains pathogenesis of progressive multiple sclerosis. Curr Opin Neurol. 2016;29: Epub ahead of print. doi:10.1097/WCO.0000000000000317

55. Sheridan C. Anti-CD20 antibody wows in multiple sclerosis. Nat Biotechnol. 2015;33:1215–6.

56. Milo R. Therapeutic strategies targeting B-cells in multiple sclerosis. Autoimmun Rev. 2016; doi:10.1016/j.autrev.2016.03.006.

57. Wolinsky JS, Arnold D, Bar-Or A, de Seze J, Giovannoni G, Hemmer B, et al. Efficacy of ocrelizumab in patients with PPMS with and without T1 gadolinium-enhancing lesions at baseline in a Phase III, placebo-controlled trial. Mult Scler. 2016;22(S1):67–8.

58. Shirani A, Okuda DT, Stüve O. Therapeutic advances and future prospects in progressive forms of multiple sclerosis. Neurotherapeutics. 2016;13:58–69.

59. Hutchinson M. Neurodegeneration in multiple sclerosis is a process separate from inflammation: No. Mult Scler. 2015;21:1628–31.

60. Louapre C, Lubetzki C. Neurodegeneration in multiple sclerosis is a process separate from inflammation: Yes. Mult Scler. 2015;21:1626–8.

11

Inpatient versus outpatient rehabilitation for multiple sclerosis patients: effects on disability and quality of life

Angelo Pappalardo[1,2†], Emanuele D'Amico[1†], Carmela Leone[1], Silvia Messina[1], Clara Chisari[1], L. Rampello[1], Lina Torre[3] and Francesco Patti[1*]

Abstract

Background: The most suitable setting of rehabilitation for Persons with Multiple Sclerosis (PwMS) has not been identified so far because there is a general lacking of controlled studies. Aim of this study was to evaluate the treatment efficacy in terms of functional independence between two different settings.

Methods: A randomized, wait-list controlled study was performed at the MS Center of the University of Catania, and Rehabilitation Center of the Hospital of Acireale, Italy. Inclusion criteria were: a) range of age 18–75, b) Expanded Disability Status Scale ≥4.0 and ≤8.0 c) self-reported worsening of standing or walking abilities in the last 6 months. The examining physician was blind to patient allocation program. The Functional Independence Measure (FIM), and the 36-Health Survey Questionnaire (SF-36) data were collected at T0 (baseline) and T1 (follow-up).

Results: One-hundred forty-six patients were randomly assigned to three groups. Forty-nine PwMS were allocated in the outpatient treatment group (Group A), 49 patients in the inpatients treatment group (Group B) and 48 patients in the control waiting list (Group C).
Both Group A and Group B showed a significant improvement in total FIM scores ($p = 0.03$, $p = 0.008$; respectively) at T1 compared to T0. No difference was found between Group A and B with regard to the FIM scores in the intergroup analysis. Group A showed significant improvement at T1 compared to T0 in all sub-items of SF-36 ($p < 0.05$), contrary to Group B. A significant difference in total FIM score between the three groups was found ($p = 0.0003$). The pairwise comparisons showed a significant difference between Group A vs Group C ($p = 0.003$) and Group B versus Group C ($p = 0.001$).

Conclusions: Inpatients and ouapatients rehabilitation approaches both showed efficacy in improving total FIM score. Outpatient rehabilitation setting seems to be more effective in improving patients QoL.

Keywords: Multiple sclerosis, Neurorehabilitation, Outpatient, Inpatient, FIM, QoL

Background

Physical rehabilitation is generally accepted as useful for persons with MS (pwMS). A wide range of rehabilitation approaches is employed, ranging from more traditional strategies to newer techniques emphasizing the learning and practice of functional motor skills within a "task-specific" context [1, 2]. It is also important to identify

* Correspondence: patti@unict.it
†Equal contributors
[1]GF Ingrassia Department, Neuroscience Section, First Neurology Clinic, Multiple Sclerosis Centre Sicilia Region, University Hospital Catania, Catania, Italy, Via S. Sofia 78, 90100 Catania, Italy
Full list of author information is available at the end of the article

the optimal approach for a given PwMS and to determine how long the effects last, estimating the cost-effectiveness. Studies verifying the efficacy of physical rehabilitation require reliable, valid, and practical outcome measures. Functional independence and health-related quality of life (HRQoL) are among the outcome measures more investigated. Some studies showed as rehabilitation can improve the motor parameters of functional independence measures (FIM) in PwMS [3–7].

However, the clinical trials performed so far, focusing on different rehabilitation approaches have showed some limitations. Heterogeneity of MS phenotype, concomitant treatments with either disease modifying or symptomatic drugs, quantitative and qualitative disparity of rehabilitation treatment, lacking of appropriate and sensitive outcome instruments are all limits in performing a rehabilitative clinical trials. All of these factors can strongly influence the setting, the development and the outcomes of a rehabilitation program in clinical practice.

To date, four possible options of rehabilitation's setting are described in clinical practice: home-based therapy, outpatient ambulatory therapy, inpatient hospital-based therapy and outpatient hospital-based therapy [3–5, 8–20].

However, guidelines addressing the clinicians to the rational allocation of PwMS in a specific rehabilitative program are lacking.

Aim of our study is to investigate the treatment efficacy in terms of FIM scores between inpatient and outpatient neurorehabilitation programs. Furthermore, we evaluated the effects of two different settings of rehabilitation on quality of life.

Methods

A randomized, wait-list controlled study was performed at the MS Center of the University of Catania, Italy and, at the Rehabilitation Center of the S. Marta & S. Venera Hospital in Acireale, Catania, Italy. The formal plan of the study was approved by the local Ethics Committee in September 2007. All enrolled PwMS signed a written informed consent.

A total of 260 pwMS, consecutively admitted to MS Center from 1st January to 30th June 2008, were screened for the inclusion and exclusion criteria. All the PwMS suffered by a clinically defined MS according to 2005 revisions to the McDonald diagnostic criteria [21]. The required inclusion criteria were: a) range of age between 18–75, b) disability status assessed by Expanded Disability Status Scale (EDSS) [22] ≥4.0 and ≤8.0, c) self-reported worsening of standing or walking abilities for at least 6 months.

Exclusion criteria were: a) PwMS with a diagnosis of MS less than six months; b) history of recent (<3 months) disease relapse; c) recent (<6 months) admission to MS-specific hospital-based rehabilitation; d) presence of cognitive deficits (Mini Mental State Examination-MMSE <24) [23]; presence of depressive symptoms (Beck Depression Inventory-BDI >11) [24]; e) severe heart or lung disease; drug or alcohol abuse; any other illness that could have excluded the participation in the study. PwMS were monitored along the study period for any neurological and other medical complications. Experiencing a relapse during the study period was considered criteria for dropping out.

Randomization was performed using a computer generated sequence at MS center in Catania. The randomization was stratified according to gender, age, EDSS score. The treating physician in charge of the rehabilitation project invited the PwMS to participate in the study and explained the rehabilitative intervention.

The examining physician, blind to patient allocation program, assessed each PwMS at baseline (T0) and at last day of rehabilitation period (T1). Both T0 and T1 were performed at the MS Center of the University of Catania. Both in-and-outpatient, just discharged from the rehabilitation hospital, went to MS Center to perform T1-evaluation; soon after they returned home. In Group C, T1-evaluation was carried out 40 days after T0.

EDSS, FIM [25] and 36-Health Survey Questionnaire (SF-36) [26] were administered as outcome measures.

The PwMS were randomly assigned to three different groups: Group A, outpatients rehabilitation treatment, Group B, inpatients rehabilitation treatment and Group C, no rehabilitation treatment (PwMS in waiting list of rehabilitation treatment).

In Group A, rehabilitative treatment was performed once daily, six days per week, for five consecutive weeks. Overall, PwMs received 30 sessions of treatment. Every session lasted at least 60 min, as described elsewhere (4,12). PwMS reached the Rehabilitation Center by car or public transport.

In Group B rehabilitation treatment was performed twice-daily, for six days per week. The period of treatment was 35 days. Overall, PwMS received 60 sessions of treatment. Every session lasted at least 60 min. Rehabilitation treatment for both groups was performed at the Rehabilitation Center of the S. Marta & S. Venera Hospital in Acireale. Patients were not allowed to come back home on the day without rehabilitative treatment.

Group C included PwMS in a waiting list (between 4 and 6 months for being involved in an inpatient or an outpatient setting).

The rehabilitative team was composed by 13 rehabilitation therapists. All therapists were specialized in neurological rehabilitation and had 5 to 10 years of work experience.

The study ended in June 2009.

Rehabilitation program

The aim of rehabilitation program was to address motor, sensor, balance, strength, sphincter functions whether present; specific physiotherapy sessions, languages or swallowing or pelvic rehab were administered for at least 4 days a week; pelvic or speech one day a week; finally one day a week all patients were treated with a global therapy approach consisting of five sessions. The rehabilitative treatment was tailored to the specific individual needs and was planned on volitional tasks mainly focused on motor performances. We kept into account the assertion that potential changes are specific to a given task and not a general effect of any training [27, 28]. PwMS were treated according to a protocol based on voluntary exercises for neuromuscular control, aimed to improve muscle strength of both upper and lower limbs, proprioceptive sensibility, stability and co-ordination for balance. These exercises were mainly task-oriented and aimed to ameliorate the activities of daily living. More in details, we set up a protocol of treatment, which was identical in the two treated groups. In the first thirty minutes of each daily session, every PwMS was asked setting a table, screwing a cap on a bottle, sweeping a table, binding and untying some laces, and creating objects with clay. In the subsequent fifteen minutes, PwMS performed some non-task oriented exercises including: catching wooden cubes of different sizes, building geometric shapes with cubes and grabbing moving objects. In the last fifteen minutes of each session, all pwMS underwent a specific training of locomotion and exercises facilitating the elicitation of postural adjustments for static and dynamic balance. The examining physician avoided to discuss any issue related to the rehabilitative treatment setting.

Primary outcome

The primary outcome was to evaluate the difference in FIM score between T0 and T1 in groups A and B. To detect a 20 % difference between time-point, 146 PwMS entered this parallel-design study. The probability is 99 percent that the study will detect a treatment difference at a two-sided 0.05 significance level, if the true difference between treatments is 0.842 times the standard deviation.

Statistical analysis

PwMS was defined as a responder to rehabilitation treatment if she/he showed a 20 % improvement in T1 total FIM score compared to T0.

Quantitative variables were described using mean and standard deviation, categorical variable were described by proportions. To assess the change in total FIM score, Motor FIM subitems score, Cognitive FIM subitems score between groups, we calculated the delta value by subtracting T0 pre-treatment score from T1 score.

Data were analyzed using STATA 10.0 software packages. A p value < 0.05 was considered as statistically significant. The difference between means and the difference between proportions was evaluated by the t-test and the Fisher exact test respectively. In case of not a normal distribution appropriate non-parametric tests were performed. ANOVA with a Bonferroni correction for multiple comparison was performed to assess the differences between groups. Mann–Whitney was performed to assess the difference between time-points.

Results

Out of the 260 screened PwMS, 114 were not enrolled, because 59 did not satisfy inclusion criteria, 40 refused to participate and 15 lived far away from the rehabilitation center (a long distance to the Rehabilitation Center was arbitrarily considered a disadvantage to be enrolled in the study). Thus, 146 PwMS were included and randomized using a computer generated sequence.

Forty-nine were allocated in the Rehabilitation Outpatients Treatment (Group A); 49 in the Rehabilitation Inpatient Treatment (Group B) and 48 in Control Waiting List (Group C). Baseline demographic and clinical characteristics of the 146 enrolled PwMS are summarized in Table 1. There were not significant differences among the three groups for all variables. All randomized PwMS completed the study and were analyzed. No drop-outs were observed for any of the three groups of the study.

Total FIM score improved in 22.6 % of patient in group A and 14.6 % in group B ($p = 0.5$). Motor FIM subitems improved in 32 % of patients in group A and 21.4 % in group B ($p = 0.4$) while cognitive FIM subitems showed no improvement in group A and an improvement in 3.5 % of patients in group B.

Intragroup analysis

We found a significant difference in term of total FIM score between T0 and T1 in Group A (91 ± 9.9 vs 98.6 ± 15.2, $p = 0.03$), in Group B (89.4 ± 20 vs 98.3 ± 17.3, $p = 0.008$) and Motor FIM subitems score in Group A (59 ± 9.4 vs 66 ± 13.4, $p = 0.02$) (Table 2). In Group C, was found no significant variation between T0 and T1in terms of total FIM scores and its subitems.

Variations of SF-36 domains are presented in Table 3. Significant differences were observed at T1 compared to

Table 1 Randomized patients' clinical and demographic characteristics

	Group A	Group B	Group C	p
Number-N. of pts	49	49	48	
N. Male (%)	18 (37)	17 (35)	18 (37)	No significant -ns
N. Women (%)	31 (63)	32 (65)	30 (62)	ns
Age, mean ± sd (min-max)	48.0 ± 10.0 (25–60)	46.0 ± 9.0 (32–74)	45.0 ± 5.0 (30–57)	ns
Employed patients N. (%)	13 (26)	8 (16)	14 (29)	
Disease course				
Secondary-Progressive N. (%)	31 (63)	32(65)	30 (62)	ns
Primary-Progressive N. (%)	18 (37)	17(35)	18 (37)	ns
Mean ± sd EDSS	6.5 ± 1.0	6.5 ± 1.1	6.4 ± 0.6	ns

Table 2 Comparison of FIM total score; motor and cognitive sub-items between T0 and T1 in three groups

Variables	Group A			Group B			Group C		
	T0 m ± sd	T1 m ± sd	p	T0 m ± sd	T1 m ± sd	p	T0 m ± sd	T1 m ± sd	p
Total FIM	91 ± 9.9	98.6 ± 15.2	0.03	89.4 ± 20	98.3 ± 17.3	0.008	89.5 ± 15.9	89.3 ± 15.9	ns
Motor subtotal score	59 ± 9.4	66 ± 13.4	0.02	59 ± 18.5	67 ± 16.1	0.09	58 ± 12.8	58 ± 12.9	ns
Cognitive subtotal score	32 ± 2.8	32 ± 2.4	ns	31 ± 3.8	32 ± 3.4	ns	31.5 ± 4.5	31 ± 4.5	ns

Mann–Whitney test was performed between T0 and T1

T0 only in Group A. In particular, the most significant change was found in physical role functioning (31.8 ± 34.8 vs 55 ± 42.9, $p < 0.0001$), vitality (46.7 ± 16.8 vs 58.4 ± 15.1, $p < 0.0001$), social role functioning (56.6 ± 22.1 vs 76.7 ± 18.7, $p < 0.0001$) and mental health (54.4 ± 18.5 vs 64.8 ± 17.3, $p < 0.0001$).

Intergroup analysis

Delta values of total FIM score, motor FIM subitems score and cognitive FIM subitems score were compared between the three groups (group A, group B, group C). A significant difference in total FIM score between the three groups was found ($p = 0.0003$). When the pairwise comparisons were investigated, we found a significant difference between Group A vs Group C ($p = 0.003$) and Group B versus Group C ($p = 0.001$). Motor FIM subitems score was significantly different between groups ($p = 0.0001$). The pairwise comparison showed a significant difference between Group A versus Group C ($p < 0.001$) and in Group B versus Group C ($p < 0.001$). No significant differences in cognitive FIM subitems scores were observed between the three groups (see Table 4).

Discussion

The results of this randomized study showed significant and clinically meaningful changes in term of impact on the functional independence inpatient and outpatient rehabilitation in comparison with no intervention. In particular, the subcategories of motor FIM demonstrated higher improvement compared to the other subcategories, showing as PwMS can gain benefits in their daily-living activities as well as in their mobility. The improvement of motor FIM was found in 32 and 21.4 % of patients respectively in Group A and B. These percentages, although not high, were obtained as we defined a patient as responder to rehabilitation whether he/she showed a 20 % improvement in T1 compared to T0. We choose a low cut-off in order to more spot the potential of neurorehabilitation in PwMS.

The efficacy of rehabilitation in PwMS was just described elsewhere [3, 4, 8–20, 29–34].

A Cochrane review including 260 patients showed strong evidence for exercise therapy compared to no exercise therapy in terms of muscle power function, exercise tolerance functions and mobility-related activities [30]. A recent systematic review including 54 studies, found strong evidence that exercise performed two times per week increases aerobic capacity and muscular strength, whereas the evidence was not consistent regarding the effects of exercise training on mobility, fatigue, and health-related quality of life [29].

Over the past 20 years, numerous studies have been published that for the design, number of enrolled patients, outcome measures, rehabilitative strategy and setting; that is studies performed in inpatient, outpatient and home-based rehabilitation. Inpatient setting was

Table 3 SF-36 domains. Comparison among the three groups at T0 and T1

Domains	Group A			Group B			Group C		
	Baseline m ± sd	T_1 m ± sd	p	Baseline m ± sd	T_1 m ± sd	p	Baseline m ± sd	T_1 m ± sd	p
Physical function	31.2 ± 20.7	37.8 ± 28	$p < 0.05$	25.8 ± 19.1	26.6 ± 20.2	ns	23.5 ± 15.5	24.4 ± 17.7	ns
Physical role functioning	31.8 ± 34.8	55 ± 42.9	$p < 0.0001$	30 ± 22	31.4 ± 18.5	ns	31.2 ± 37	28.4 ± 35.3	ns
Bodily pain	52.7 ± 25.8	67.2 ± 23.8	$p < 0.001$	62.9 ± 28.2	67.5 ± 26.9	ns	64.4 ± 28.6	63.1 ± 28.4	ns
General health perceptions	48.8 ± 19.6	52.5 ± 19.2	$p < 0.001$	44.6 ± 17.8	49.5 ± 20.5	ns	51 ± 20.2	50.2 ± 19.5	ns
Vitality	46.7 ± 16.8	58.4 ± 15.1	$p < 0.0001$	41.2 ± 16.7	43 ± 18.8	ns	48.5 ± 20.1	46.2 ± 18.3	ns
Social role functioning	56.6 ± 22.1	76.7 ± 18.7	$p < 0.0001$	62.9 ± 22.8	64 ± 26.2	ns	60.8 ± 25.8	59 ± 25	ns
Emotional role functioning	60.8 ± 39.6	73.1 ± 34.6	$p < 0.05$	48.8 ± 41.1	49.6 ± 38.3	ns	45.3 ± 43.6	44.3 ± 43.5	ns
Mental health	54.4 ± 18.5	64.8 ± 17.3	$p < 0.0001$	62 ± 25.5	67 ± 23.5	ns	59 ± 26.1	56.9 ± 24.9	ns

$p < 0.05$ - Wilcoxon signed rank for Group A versus both Group B and Group C

Table 4 Delta value between three groups

Variables	Group A	Group B	Group C	p
Total FIM	8 ± 12	8,9 ± 9,7	−0,2 ± 0,6	0.0003*
Motor subtotal score	8 ± 9,5	8 ± 9,2	0 ± 0,7	0.0001**
Cognitive subtotal score	0 ± 3,1	0,7 ± 1,3	0	0.3053

*Bonferroni Correction: Group A vs Group C p = 0.003; Group B vs Group C p = 0.001; Group A vs Group B ns
**Bonferroni Correction: Group A vs Group C p < 0.001; Group B vs Group C p < 0.001; Group A vs Group B ns

associated with a significant improvement in functional impairment [15], disability [10, 32], functional independence [3] and HRQoL [3, 10, 32]. Trials conducted in outpatient setting demonstrated effectiveness of rehabilitation in improvement of muscular strength (9), walking capacity [34], functional independence [4], HRQol [9, 11, 12, 34]. Home-based rehabilitation showed significant improvement in HRQoL [13, 16], balance [17, 19], leg extensor power [14], gait parameters [20], fatigue [10].

Very recently, an exercise-based patient education program conducted at home or at outpatient set, demonstrated improvements in PwMS' mobility, gait ability, endurance, fatigue, and health-related quality of life after completing the 12-week intervention [31].

As exposed in the introduction, we searched to address an unresolved question in MS clinical practice: what is the most suitable setting for PwMS? This issue is becoming crucial, considering that the majority of MS patients required rehabilitation treatment [35] and that leads to increasing health costs [36]. To the best of our knowledge, only few studies were designed considering a comparison between two different settings of rehabilitation (outpatient versus inpatient). Francabandera et al. [8] reported that inpatient rehabilitation resulted in small but significant improvements in ambulatory status and level of independence in self-care as compared with outpatient treatment. But that study enrolled PwMS with a more severe disability (EDSS score 6.0 – 9.0) than ours and the outpatient group received physical and occupational therapy not only i a clinic but also at home; therefore a comparison with our work is difficult to perform.

In a more recent randomized study [5], both in-and –outpatient PwMS showed statistically significant improvement in FIM total score and in the FIM motor domains compared to controls; whereby the rehabilitation programme for PwMS determined important reduction in disability with a large treatment effect sizes for a number of FIM domains. In that study, unlike ours, the authors also enrolled PwMS affected by the Relapsing-Remitting phenotype; beside, they did not separately provide the data of the two setting of rehabilitation, as the objectives of that study were different from those of our study.

Traditionally, rehabilitation has been targeted at maintaining and preserving patient's personal and social activities. The findings of our study, as well as those of others studies, advice us that the goals of neurorehabilitation should be renewed, targeting to the improvement of the residual capacities and so, enhancing the functional independence. To this aim, we believe that active rehabilitation, based on voluntary task-oriented exercises, could determine beneficial effects in terms of functional independence. In agreement with this assertion, Bonzano et al. demonstrated that rehabilitation treatment based on voluntary movements may contribute to preserve the white matter integrity in the corpus callosum and corticospinal tracts and to maintain the coordination ability; such benefits were not observed in control group [27]. These findings confirms the hypothesis that the sensorimotor deficits observed in PwMS over the disease course could be mainly due to the progression of white matter damage and that neurorehabilitation may attenuate this neurodegenerative process [37, 38].

In our study, just Group A showed a significant improvement social and psychological parameters in SF-36. In Group B, we found a slight but not statistically significant improvement in all domains of SF-36. Some years ago, other authors were reached to the same finding; inpatient treated group improved in functional impairment but not in HRQoL [15]. Therefore, the lack of efficacy on HRQoL in Group B might be related to the hospitalization, which could have determined a greater psychological stressful effect and we sought to screen that in the future. To the outpatients were offered the possibility to came back home after every treatment session, and therefore, they could continue their jobs and their social activities. That support the evidence of the most meaningful benefit in QoL domain social role functioning for these PwMS.

These findings may draw the conclusion that a different setting for rehabilitation treatment should be chosen taking into account many personal needs and desires of each patient. A physician dealing with a rehabilitative treatment should bear in mind the emotional aspects in PwMS to come back home at the end of each daily session. A recent study showed that PwMS had less functional improvement than other populations using the inpatient rehabilitation setting and the higher rates of depression was found within the MS population [39]. This finding must be an important consideration for rehabilitation service needs in PwMS.

The willingness and the economic possibilities of the patients to get the rehabilitative center every day have to be considered as well their wishes of improvement.

However, which is the real impact of the hospitalization on the previous habitual activities of the patient's daily life? How could the hospitalization impact patient's social and psychological profile?

Nowadays it is very important the economic costs and relative cost-effectiveness of the different rehabilitative settings [36]. There is no doubt that outpatient rehabilitation is less expensive than the inpatient rehabilitation program, independently from the comparable effectiveness. At the same time, outpatient rehabilitation seems to be more burdensome for patients in terms of economic resources and familiar commitment (travel cost, caregiver time management, etc.).

We are aware about the limitations of our study. A percentage of about 45 % of PWMS were nor enrolled and only patients with an EDSS ≥4.0 and ≤8.0 were recruited. That cannot generalize our results to a global MS population. However, the three groups had comparable baseline characteristics and adequate cognitive performing that allowed to reduce a major source of bias. Moreover, we did not perform follow-up assessment, but we aimed to set another study to ride over these limitations and to evaluate the eventual carry-on effects of both rehabilitation settings.

Despite the above limitations, we found that both rehabilitative treatment settings, inpatient and outpatient, are equally effective in diminishing the disability in PwMs. Interestingly, only the outpatient treatment was found to be effective in improving the HRQoL.

Conclusions

In conclusion, we believe that outpatient setting is usually well accepted by PwMS with minimal impact on patients habitual familiar and social life. However it should be underlined that inpatient setting could be more suitable for both patients with a more severe disability that have difficulties in terms of reaching the rehabilitative center and for those preferring to be treated without involvement of relatives or caregivers. More studies needed.

Competing interests
Dr. Patti has served on the scientific advisory board for Teva, Biogen-Idec, Bayer-Schering, Novartis and has received honoraria as a speaker for Teva, Biogen, Merck-Serono, Bayer-Schering, Genzyme/Sanofi, Novartis.
Dr. D'Amico, Dr. Messina, Dr. Pappalardo, Dr. Rampello, Lina Torre have nothing to disclose.

Authors' contributions
AP carried out the study, participated in drafting the manuscript. ED carried out the study, participated in drafting the manuscript. SM carried out the study, participated in drafting the manuscript participated in the sequence alignment. CL carried out the study, participated in drafting the manuscript. CC carried out the study, participated in drafting the manuscript. LT carried out the study. FP carried out the study, participated in drafting the manuscript, giving the final approval. All authors read and approved the final manuscript.

Acknowledgments
The authors would like to thank for the precious collaboration the physiatrist Laura Longo and Giuseppe Sicuso and the physioterapists Barchitta Rocco, Scuderi Letizia, La Spina Concetta, Buzzone Concetta, Corallo Serena, De Carlo Davide, Vinci Ornella, D'Urso Patrizia, Blanco Mario, Cuddè Agrippina, Casablanca Paolo, Pennisi Stefania, Pennisi Angela, Alfio Nicolosi, Biagio Papotto, Mario Vincenzino.

Author details
[1]GF Ingrassia Department, Neuroscience Section, First Neurology Clinic, Multiple Sclerosis Centre Sicilia Region, University Hospital Catania, Catania, Italy, Via S. Sofia 78, 90100 Catania, Italy. [2]Department of Rehabilitation, S. Marta & S.Venera Hospital, ASP Catania, Acireale, Catania, Italy. [3]Rehabilitation Unit, Opera Diocesana Assistenza, Catania, Italy.

References
1. Beer S, Khan F, Kesselring J. Rehabilitation interventions in multiple sclerosis: an overview. J Neurol. 2012;259:1994–2008.
2. Morgen K, Kadom N, Sawaki L, et al. Training-dependent plasticity in patients with multiple sclerosis. Brain. 2004;127:2506–17.
3. Solari A, Filippini G, Gasco P, et al. Physical rehabilitation has a positive effect on disability in multiple sclerosis patients. Neurology. 1999;52(1):57–62.
4. Patti F, Ciancio MR, Cacopardo M, et al. Effects of a short outpatient rehabilitation treatment on disability of multiple sclerosis patients–a randomised controlled trial. J Neurol. 2003;250(7):861–6.
5. Khan F, Pallant JF, Brand C, et al. Effectiveness of rehabilitation intervention in persons with multiple sclerosis: a randomised controlled trial. J Neurol Neurosurg Psychiatry. 2008;79(11):1230–5.
6. Schwartz I, Sajin A, Moreh E, et al. Robot-assisted gait training in multiple sclerosis patients: a randomized trial. Mult Scler. 2012;18(6):881–90.
7. Khan F, Pallant JF, Zhang N, et al. Clinical practice improvement approach in multiple sclerosis rehabilitation: a pilot study. Int J Rehabil Res. 2010;33(3):238–47.
8. Francabandera FL, Holland NJ, Wiesel-Levison P, et al. Multiple Sclerosis Rehabilitation: Inpatient vs. Outpatient Rehabil Nurs. 1988;13:251–3.
9. Petajan JH, Gappmaier E, White AT, et al. Impact of aerobic training on fitness and quality of life in multiple sclerosis. Ann Neurol. 1996;39(4):432–41.
10. Freeman JA, Langdon DW, Hobart JC, et al. The impact of inpatient rehabilitation on progressive multiple sclerosis. Ann Neurol. 1997;42(2):236–44.
11. Di Fabio RP, Choi T, Soderberg J, et al. Health-related quality of life for patients with progressive multiple sclerosis: influence of rehabilitation. Phys Ther. 1997;77(12):1704–16.
12. Patti F, Ciancio MR, Reggio E, et al. The impact of outpatient rehabilitation on quality of life in multiple sclerosis. J Neurol. 2002;249(8):1027–33.
13. Pozzilli C, Brunetti M, Amicosante AM, et al. Home based management in multiple sclerosis: results of a randomised controlled trial. J Neurol Neurosurg Psychiatry. 2002;73(3):250–5.
14. DeBolt LS, McCubbin JA. The effects of home-based resistance exercise on balance, power, and mobility in adults with multiple sclerosis. Arch Phys Med Rehabil. 2004;85(2):290–7.
15. Romberg A, Virtanen A, Ruutiainen J, et al. Long-term exercise improves functional impairment but not quality of life in multiple sclerosis. J Neurol. 2005;252(7):839–45.
16. McCullagh R, Fitzgerald AP, Murphy RP, et al. Long-term benefits of exercising on quality of life and fatigue in multiple sclerosis patients with mild disability: a pilot study. Clin Rehabil. 2008;22(3):206–14.
17. Finkelstein J, Lapshin O, Castro H, et al. Home-based physical telerehabilitation in patients with multiple sclerosis: a pilot study. Rehabil Res Dev. 2008;45(9):1361–73.
18. Vikman T, Fielding P, Lindmark B, et al. Effects of inpatient rehabilitation in multiple sclerosis patients with moderate disability. Adv Physiother. 2008; 10(2):58–65.
19. Prosperini L, Fortuna D, Giannì C, et al. Home-based balance training using the Wii balance board: a randomized, crossover pilot study in multiple sclerosis. Neurorehabil Neural Repair. 2013;27(6):516–25.
20. Conklyn D, Stough D, Novak EA, et al. Home-based walking program using rhythmic auditory stimulation improves gait performance in patients with multiple sclerosis: a pilot study. Neurorehabil Neural Repair. 2010;24(9):835–42.
21. Polmann CH, Reingold SC, Edan G, et al. Diagnostic criteria for multiple sclerosis: 2005 revisions to the "McDonald Criteria". Ann Neurol. 2005;58(6):840–6.
22. Kurtzke JF. Rating neurologic impairment in multiple sclerosis: an expanded disability status scale (EDSS). Neurology. 1983;33(11):1444–52.
23. Beatty WW, Goodkin DE. Screening for cognitive impairment in multiple sclerosis. An evaluation of the Mini-Mental State Examination. Arch Neurol. 1990;47:297–301.
24. Sullivan MJ, Weinshenker B, Mikail S, et al. Screening for major depression in the early stages of multiple sclerosis. Can J Neurol Sci. 1995;22:228–31.

25. Keith RA, Granger CV, Hamilton BB, et al. The functional independence measure: a new tool for rehabilitation. Adv Clin Rehabil. 1987;1:6–18.

26. Garratt AM, Ruta DA, Abdalla MI, et al. The SF36 health survey questionnaire: an outcome measure suitable for routine use within the NHS? BMJ. 1993;306(6890):1440–4.

27. Bonzano L, Tacchino A, Brichetto G, et al. Upper limb motor rehabilitation impacts white matter microstructure in multiple sclerosis. Neuroimage. 2014;90:107–16.

28. Thomas C, Baker CI. Teaching an adult brain new tricks: a critical review of evidence for training-dependent structural plasticity in humans. Neuroimage. 2013;73:225–36.

29. Latimer-Cheung AE, Pilutti LA, Hicks AL, et al. The effects of exercise training on fitness, mobility, fatigue, and health related quality of life among adults with multiple sclerosis: a systematic review to inform guideline development. Arch Phys Med Rehabil. 2013;94(9):1800–28.

30. Rietberg MB, Brooks D, Uitdehaag BM, Kwakkel G. Exercise therapy for multiple sclerosis. Cochrane Database Syst Rev. 2005;1, CD003980.

31. Kersten S, Mahli M, Drosselmeyer J et al. A Pilot Study of an Exercise-Based Patient Education Program in People with Multiple Sclerosis. Mult Scler Int. 2014;Epub 2014 Dec 21.

32. Gaber TA, Oo WW, Gautam V, et al. Outcomes of inpatient rehabilitation of patients with multiple sclerosis. NeuroRehabilitation. 2012;30(2):97–100.

33. Romberg A, Virtanen A, Ruutiainen J, et al. Effects of a 6-month exercise program on patients with multiple sclerosis: a randomized study. Neurology. 2004;63(11):2034–8.

34. Rampello A, Franceschini M, Piepoli M, et al. Effect of aerobic training on walking capacity and maximal exercise tolerance in patients with multiple sclerosis: a randomized crossover controlled study. Phys Ther. 2007;87(5):545–55.

35. Khan F, Turner-Stokes L, Ng L, Kilpatrick T. Multidisciplinary rehabilitation for adults with multiple sclerosis. Cochrane Database Syst Rev. 2007;2, CD006036. Review.

36. Patti F, Amato MP, Trojano M, et al. Multiple sclerosis in Italy: cost-of-illness study. Neurol Sci. 2011;32(5):787–94.

37. Ge Y, Law M, Grossman RI. Applications of diffusion tensor MR imaging in multiple sclerosis. Ann N Y Acad Sci. 2005;1064:202–19.

38. Evangelou N, Esiri MM, Smith S, et al. Auantitative pathological evidence for axonal loss in normal appearing white matter in multiple sclerosis. Ann Neurol. 2000;47:391–5.

39. Morley MA, Coots LA, Forgues AL, et al. Inpatient rehabilitation utilization for Medicare beneficiaries with multiple sclerosis. Arch Phys Med Rehabil. 2012;93(8):1377–83.

12

Alemtuzumab for multiple sclerosis: the new concept of immunomodulation

Paolo Gallo[1*], Diego Centonze[2] and Maria Giovanna Marrosu[3]

Abstract

Alemtuzumab (Lemtrada®) is a humanized anti-CD52 IgG1 monoclonal antibody that depletes CD52-expressing cells from the circulation. Robust clinical and radiologic data, derived from clinical trials and long-term observational studies, indicate that alemtuzumab induces a marked immunosuppression related to the depletion of circulating T and B lymphocytes. However, recent advances suggest that the long-term clinical effects of alemtuzumab are probably due to unique *qualitative* changes in the process of lymphocyte repopulation of the immune system. This leads to a particular rebalancing of the immune system. In this paper we review the immunomodulatory mechanisms underlying the therapeutic effect of alemtuzumab in pre-clinical models and in patients with relapsing remitting multiple sclerosis (RRMS), and stress the importance of a monoclonal antibody-based immunosuppression for treating the severe forms of RRMS. Alemtuzumab has many features of the ideal immunomodulatory drug: rapid biological and clinical actions and and long-lasting benefit. Alemtuzumab can be used as rescue therapy or as first line drug in severe-onset MS. Thus, the availability of alemtuzumab constitutes a significant step forward in the therapy of MS.

Keywords: Alemtuzumab, Multiple sclerosis, Immunomodulation

Background

Alemtuzumab, previously known as Campath-1H, is a recombinant, humanised, monoclonal immunoglobulin IgG1 kappa, that targets the cell-surface glycoprotein CD52 [22, 23]. Alemtuzumab induces antibody-dependent cellular cytotoxicity (ADCC) and complement-dependent cytotoxicity (CDC), and activates pro-apoptotic pathways on CD52-expressing cells. One phase-2 trial (CAMMS-223) and two phase-3 studies (CARE-MS1 and CARE-MS2) have clearly demonstrated the efficacy of alemtuzumab in the treatment of naive patients and have established its superiority over high-dose high-frequency interferon beta-1a (IFNb-1a) in patients who continue to experience relapses despite of first-line therapy [9–11]. Alemtuzumab primary safety concern is the development of secondary autoimmunity, that occurs up to five years after the first cycle of infusions and peaks at two years. Indeed, about 30% of patients develop thyroid autoimmunity and 1% idiopathic thrombocytopenic purpura (ITP). In addition, 4 out of

1486 patients (<0.3%) enrolled in phase II and II trials developed autoimmune glomerulonephritis.

In September 2013, the European Medicine Agency (EMA) approved alemtuzumab as a first-line therapy for adults with active relapsing remitting multiple sclerosis, under the trade name Lemtrada. Lemtrada is now also approved as a treatment of multiple sclerosis in US, Canada, Australia, Switzerland, Israel, and many countries in South America. This review focuses on the mechanisms of action of alemtuzumab on the immune system (Table 1) and tries to explain the long lasting biological and clinical effects of this monoclonal antibody on multiple sclerosis (MS).

CD52, the target

CD52 is a short peptide of 12 amino acids highly expressed on T and B lymphocytes, and at very low levels on natural killer cells, monocytes and macrophages (Fig. 1), while neutrophils, dentritic cells and bone marrow stem cells don't express this molecule (Buggings et al., 2002). Further, CD52 is found within the male genital tract and is present on the surface of mature sperm cells. Since it is highly negatively charged it has been supposed that its

* Correspondence: paolo.gallo@unipd.it
[1]Department of Neuroscience DNS, Multiple Sclerosis Centre, University Hospital, Via Giustiniani, 5, 35129 Padova, Italy
Full list of author information is available at the end of the article

Table 1 Biological effects of Alemtuzumab

Effects	Mechanisms	References
Fast and long-lasting immune suppression	Rapid and complete depletion of circulating T and B lymphocytes; limited effect on lymphoid organs. Differentiated CD20, CD4 and CD8 lymphocyte repopulation (B before T, T4 before T8) Long-lasting re-modelling of the lymphocyte network: earlier appearance of regulatory B and T cells, later appearance of Th1 and Th17. Anti-inflammatory changes in the cytochine network. More tolerogenic immune network during reconstitution.	Hu et al., 2009 [29] Thompson et al., 2010 [38] Jones et al., 2009 [30] Zhang et al., 2013 [42] Turner et al., 2013 [40] Havari et al., 2015 [25] Wang et al., 2015 [43] Wang et al., 2015 [43] Watanabe et al., 2006 [44]
Decrease in brain inflammation and neurodegeneration	Almost complete suppression of brain inflammation. Increased production of neurotrophic/growth factors by antigen-specific T cells.	Jones et al., 2010 [31] Turner et al., 2015 [41]
No impact on immune competence	Immunocompetent cells in the lymphoid organs are largely preserved. B and T cell response against bacterial and viral antigens are maintained during therapy. Innate immunity is not affected.	Hu et al., 2009 [29] Buggins et al., 2002 [6] McCarthy et al., 2013 [34] Clark et al., 2012 [7] Turner et al., 2013 [40]
Cytokine release syndrome	Transient, cytolysis-related release of pro-inflammatory acute-phase cytokines (TNF, IL-1, IL-6).	Breslin et al., 2007 [4] Wing et al., 1996 [45] Bugelski et al., 2009 [5]

function consisted in hampering cell adhesion, thus allowing cells to freely move around (see the review of [23]). Although a recent study has found that activated CD4 T cells expressing high levels of CD52 may have regulatory activities on T effector lymphocytes [2] the function of CD52 remains partially unknown.

Human and mouse antigen-activated T cells with high CD52 expression were demonstrated to suppress other T cells. CD4 + CD25 + CD52^{high} T cells are distinct from CD4 + CD25^{high}Foxp3+ regulatory T cells inasmuch as they suppress auto-reactive T cell subsets by releasing soluble CD52 (CD52s). CD52s binds to the inhibitory receptor sialic acid-binding immunoglobulin-like lectins-

10 (Siglec-10) thus impairing the phosphorylation of the T cell receptor (TCR)–associated kinases Lck and Zap70 (Fig. 2). The final result is a down regulation of TCR assembly and, consequently, T cell activation. Humans with autoimmune diabetes were found to have a lower frequency and diminished function of CD4 + CD25 + CD52^{high} T cells responsive to the autoantigen GAD65. In diabetes-prone mice of the non-obese diabetic (NOD) strain, transfer of lymphocyte populations depleted of CD4 + CD25 + CD52^{high} cells results in a more severe disease [2].

Beside the CD52-Siglec-10 ligand-receptor mechanism, the CD52 molecule may down-regulate T cell activation

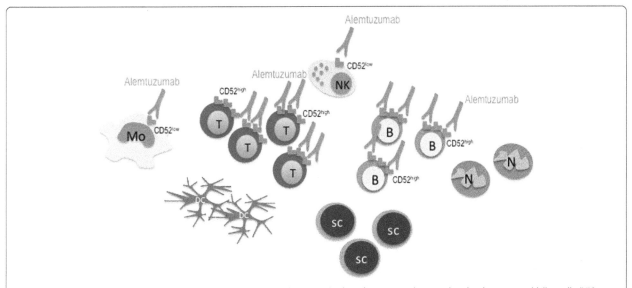

Fig. 1 CD52 is a short peptide of 12 amino acids highly expressed on T and B lymphocytes, and at very low levels on natural killer cells (NK), monocytes and macrophages (Mo), while neutrophils (N), dendritic cells (DC) and bone marrow stem cells (SC) do not express this molecule

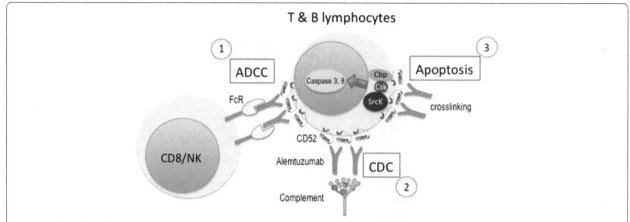

Fig. 2 On T and B cells expressing high concentrations of CD52, alemtuzumab (IgG1k) activates: 1) antibody-dependent cell-mediated (CD8 and NK) cytotoxicity (ADCC), 2) complement-dependent cytotoxicity (CDC), 3) caspase-dependent apoptosis

by molecular cross-linkage mediated by an as yet unidentified endogenous ligand that, in vitro, might be mimicked by a bivalent anti-CD52 antibody [3]. These two (cytolitic and pro-apoptotic) mechanisms may operate in a synergistic manner.

Since one third of alemtuzumab-treated patients develop autoimmune diseases, in particular autoimmune thyroiditis [17, 18], it might be possible that the long-lasting deletion of CD4 + CD25 + CD52^{high} T cells following therapy needs may account for these adverse events.

However, the impairment of the CD4 + CD25 + CD52^{high}–mediated T-cell regulation following alemtuzumab administration does not constitute a concern

with regard of MS since alemtuzumab exerts a strong immunosuppressive activity by activating (see below) the ACDC and CDC mediated lysis of T and B lymphocytes and inducing caspase-dependent cell apoptosis, leading to a marked global lymphocyte depletion that includes autoreactive pathogenic lymphocytes. The density of CD52 on cell surface is believed to influence the susceptibility of lymphoid cells to alemtuzumab-induced ACDC and CDC [37], but other factors, e.g. the level of expression of complement-inhibitory proteins, were also suggested to play a role especially in protecting cell lysis in the lymphoid organs [Genzyme, EU summary of product characteristics, 2013; [36] (Fig. 3).

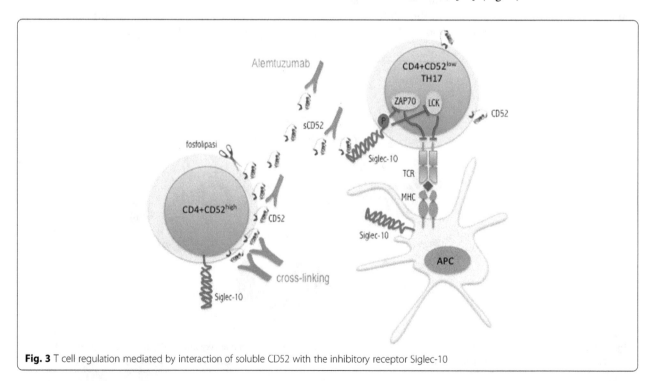

Fig. 3 T cell regulation mediated by interaction of soluble CD52 with the inhibitory receptor Siglec-10

Pre-clinical studies

Transgenic hu-CD52 mice

Since alemtuzumab does not cross-react with mouse CD52, a transgenic mouse model expressing the human CD52 molecule (huCD52) was created to assess, in pre-clinical experimental/animal settings, the effects of alemtuzumab on lymphocyte subsets in lymphoid organs [29]. The administration of a single 10 mg/kg dose of alemtuzumab to huCD52-transgenic mice replicated the depletion of B and T lymphocyte circulating populations observed in human studies, with little effect on cells of the innate immune system (neutrophils and NK cells). Lymphocyte depletion in lymphoid organs (spleen, thymus, lymph nodes) was less profound than in the blood and was mediated primarily through ADCC exerted by neutrophils and NK cells, and largely independent of CDC [29]. At higher alemtuzumab doses, the degree of lymphopenia in the lymphoid organs (especially in spleen and lymph nodes) was definitely less profound compared to that observed in the peripheral circulation. This can be explained by the fact that, at the therapeutic dosage, alemtuzumab is largely absorbed by circulating lymphocytes, thus making its penetration in the lymphoid organs very limited. Moreover, it might be possible that the effector mechanisms responsible for cell depletion are less abundant or effective in lymphoid organs compared with peripheral blood. Interestingly, a relative sparing of T cells with a regulatory phenotype (CD4 + CD25^{high}FoxP3+) compared to total CD4+ T cell population was observed in both the blood and spleen even though both populations express equivalent levels of CD52 on their surface. The mechanism and significance of this apparent sparing of T cells with a regulatory phenotype remain unclear but could be a relevant factor in determining the long term suppression of inflammation obtained by alemtuzumab therapy.

In hu52 mice, lymphocyte repopulation was also very similar to that observed in humans. Namely, B lymphocytes returned to baseline levels by 7–10 weeks post-treatment while CD4+ and CD8+ T cells recovered more slowly and were still below the baseline levels at weeks 25. One possible explanation for the differential timing of T and B cell repopulation in the blood might be that alemtuzumab did not significantly affect the bone marrow thus allowing for the rapid recovery of B lymphocytes, while the effect on thymus determined a partial depletion of thymocytes, which could account, at least partly, for the slower recovery of T lymphocytes. Indeed, examination of the thymus of the transgenic mouse disclosed a partial depletion of single-positive and double-positive thymocytes (reaching 50% at the dose of 10 mg/kg of alemtuzumab). However, while the partial loss of thymocytes may, at least partly, explain the delay in T-cell recovery, the

explanation for the long-lasting duration of T-cell lymphopenia is still missing.

In the huCD52-transgenic mice it was also possible to replicate the transient increase in serum cytokine levels observed in humans, and responsible for the so-called 'cytokine released syndrome' and mainly related to the acute liberation of pro-inflammatory cytokines, such as TNFalpha, IL-1 beta, IL-6.

The functional properties of immune cells that remained following alemtuzumab treatment in huCD52 mice were also evaluated [29]. T lymphocytes showed in vitro proliferation rates and cytokine production in response to anti-CD3 Mab stimulation very similar to that observed in vehicle-treated mice. The T-cell receptor repertoire and the efficiency of T-cell response against a viral challenge were also maintained after alemtuzumab treatment. The primary T-cell response against viruses was explored by challenging the huCD52 transgenic mice with the adenovirus vector Ad2 at 7, 21, or 35 days after alemtuzumab treatment. T-cell responses were reduced at 7 and 21 days post alemtuzumab treatment, but comparable to that observed in control animals after five weeks later, before T-cell counts returned to pre-treatment levels. The primary B-cell response was also modestly affected. The antibody response to a T-dependent antigen was attenuated 3 days after alemtuzumab treatment (the nadir of lymphocyte depletion), but was similar to vehicle-treated controls at 21 days [29]. Preserved immune responses in alemtuzumab-treated animals may be due, in part, to the activity of residual B and T lymphocytes within peripheral lymphoid organs.

These observations were further confirmed in a study aimed at evaluating the impact of alemtuzumab treatment on number and function of innate immune cells in the same murine [40]. Following alemtuzumab administration, a transient decrease in primary adaptive immune responses was observed, but there was little effect on memory responses. Namely, the antibody response to a T-independent antigen was not significantly affected by the treatment suggesting that the remaining B lymphocytes were still capable to mount a normal antibody response. On the contrary, the antibody response to a T-dependent antigen was impaired when immunization was performed few days after alemtuzumab treatment, but returned to control levels by day 21 post-therapy. A mild, transient decline on primary T cell responses was also observed in mice immunized with adenovirus Ad2, but the difference with not treated mice did not reach statistical significance. Interestingly, T cell response to Ad2 returned to control levels by despite peripheral T lymphocyte counts were still suppressed.

Data in hu-CD52 transgenic mice and in experimental autoimmune encephalomyelitis (EAE) suggest that the effect of alemtuzumab on the immune network is multifaceted, and probably includes a disequilibrium in the lymphocyte numbers, alterations in the functional properties of some lymphocyte subsets, and a transient effects on components of innate immunity. Particular intriguing is the observation that, after alemtuzumab treatment, naïve CD4+ and CD8+ T cells in the spleen were the most susceptible to depletion, whereas central and effector memory T cells, as well as Tregs, were depleted to a lesser extent, despite equivalent levels of CD52 expression on their surfaces.

All together, the observations done in Hu-CD52 transgenic mice suggest that protective levels of T cell immunity against infection can still be present despite the marked T and B cell lymphopenia. Animal data agree with the clinical data in humans showing that the highest risk of infection occurs in the first month post-alemtuzumab treatment and declines thereafter even though blood T cell counts remain below the normal range [12]. This may be partly explained by the recovery of sufficient numbers of lymphocytes in the lymphoid organs that can participate in the development of immune responses.

Experimental autoimmune encephalomyelitis

The effect of anti-CD52 therapy was tested in three murine models of the brain autoimmune inflammation, the EAE, that reproduces some of the histological features of MS: EAE induced by MOG35–55 (myelin oligodendrocyte glycoprotein) in C57BL/6 mice, which represents a standard acute model of disease primarily driven by peptide-specific CD4+ lymphocytes; chronic EAE induced by MOG1–121, that is believed to involve the contribution of both T and B lymphocytes in the pathogenesis; and relapsing remitting EAE induced by PLP139–151 (proteolipid protein) in SJL mice [40]. Treatment with a single course of anti-muCD52 in mice with early symptoms (day 12–16 from immunization) achieved long term control of disease in all 3 models demonstrating efficacy against the different aspects of disease pathogenesis. In the MOG$_{35-55}$ model, the delayed administration of anti-muCD52 at the time the mice attained more significant disability, with a disease score of 2 that corresponds to a full tail paralysis and hind limb paresis, was still efficacious and resulted in the almost complete reversal of disease symptoms. Interestingly, the control of disease was maintained up to ~ day 90 without further retreatment in spite of complete lymphocyte repopulation in the blood and lymphoid organs.

Histological examination disclosed a significant reduction of immune cell infiltration in all regions of the spinal cord in anti-muCD52-treated mice vs control mice. This was accompanied by a significant reduction in the degree of spinal cord demyelination and axonal damage. Administration of anti-muCD52 not only reduces the number of circulating T lymphocytes, but also reduces the number of infiltrating T lymphocytes in the CNS of EAE mice, decreases the number of MOG-reactive CD4 T cells and overall cytokine production and strongly inhibited the development of CNS inflammation and concomitant demyelination and axonal damage. Electrophysiological assessment showed preservation of axonal conductance in the spinal cord suggesting that anti-CD52 therapy may help to preserve CNS integrity [41]. Taken all together, these results demonstrate the robust general and local immunosuppressive action of anti-muCD52 treatment in several models of EAE and parallel the long term control of disease observed in the majority of RRMS patients treated with alemtuzumab.

Thus, experimental studies in vitro and in animal models have 1) confirmed the mechanism of action of alemtuzumab, 2) reproduced the kinetics of lymphocyte depletion and repopulation observed in humans and 3) correlated the strong, rapid and long-lasting immunosuppression to a significant reversion/amelioration of autoimmune-mediated brain inflammation.

Studies in humans

Alemtuzumab-treated patients exhibited a nearly complete depletion of circulating CD4(+) lymphocytes within few hours after administration with a nadir between day 3 and 7. The reconstitution of the circulating lymphocyte repertoire was found to follow peculiar kinetics. In the CARE-MS-I and -II studies, alemtuzumab was associated with a decrease in circulating lymphocyte counts after each treatment course, but had few or transient effects on other leukocytes (neutrophils, monocytes, eosinophils, basophils and natural killer cells) [8, 11, 12]. The total lymphocyte count returned to the lower limit of the normal values by month 6 in about 40% of patients and by month 12 in about 80% of patients. In one study, however, CD4+ lymphocytes remained significantly decreased for up to 24 months [42], while in another study both CD4+ and CD8+ lymphocyte counts remained below baseline levels for a median of 61 and 30 months, respectively [13]. B cell numbers returned to baseline by 3 months, and in some cases their number increased beyond baseline levels at 27 months (but rarely exceeded the upper limit of normal values) [13, 19].

In a follow-up study in 36 MS patients (384 person years), aimed at analysing the long term effects of a single course of alemtuzumab (100 mg over 5 infusion days, a dose higher than that currently use in MS) on lymphocyte reconstitution, the geometric mean recovery time of total lymphocyte counts to the lower limit of the normal range (≥1.0X10^9 cells/L) was 12.7 months. For B cells the recovery time was 7.1 months, while CD8+ and CD4+ lymphocytes returned within the normal ranges in

20 and 35 months, respectively, but only in a minority of the patients they returned within the baseline values (30% and 21%, respectively). In spite of prolonged lymphocyte depletion, no infective safety concerns were observed [28].

The lymphocyte reconstitution profile that follows alemtuzumab-induced lymphocyte depletion appear very similar to that observed after marked immunosuppression obtained with other therapies, for instance haematopoietic stem cell transplantation, and suggests that it might be driven by common homeostatic mechanisms, such as proliferation of mature lymphocytes that escaped depletion, or by ex-novo lymphocyte production from precursors in the thymus [19, 32].

During the reconstitution phase of the circulating lymphocyte repertoire, CD4(+)CD25(+)CD127(low) regulatory T cells preferentially expanded within the CD4(+) lymphocyte population, reaching peak expansion at month 1. The increase in the percentage of TGF-β1, IL-10, and IL-4 producing CD4(+) cells (Th2 phenotype) reached the higher level at month 3, whereas Th1 and Th17 Th cells increased much slowly and returned within the normal values at months 12. However, a significant decrease in the percentages of Th1 and Th17 cells was still detected at months 12 and 24 in comparison with the baseline values. A gradual increase in serum IL-7 and IL-4 and a decrease in IL-17A, IL-17 F, IL-21, IL-22, and IFN-γ levels were also demonstrated following treatment. These observations are in line with in vitro studies that disclosed that IL-7 induced an expansion of CD4(+)CD25(+)CD127(low) regulatory T cells and a decrease in the percentages of Th17 and Th1 cells, and further indicates that the differential reconstitution of T cell subsets and selectively delayed CD4(+) T cell repopulation following alemtuzumab-induced lymphopenia may partly contribute to its long-lasting suppression of disease activity [42] (Fig. 4).

In a recent 24-month multicentre study aimed at evaluating Th and Treg repopulation and function during alemtuzumab therapy in 29 MS patients, CD4+ cell percentage remained significantly lower compared to baseline, while a significant increase in Treg percentage was observed at month 24 and was accompanied by an increase in Treg suppressive activity against myelin basic protein-specific Th1 and Th17 cells [20]. Although the meaning of the increase in percentage and function of Treg in the late phase of alemtuzumab therapy is unclear and need to be investigated in larger numbers of patients, these findings further suggest that CD52 depletion induces a transient re-arrangement of the T cell network.

With regard to the analysis of lymphocyte subsets, data coming from CARE-MS-I and II showed that the relative proportion of CD4+ naive T cells decreased (from 36 to 5% [CARE-MS-I] and from 37 to 2% [CARE-MS-II]) and the relative proportion of CD4+ memory T cells increased (from 63 to 94% and from 63 to 97%, respectively) by month 1 and returned to near-baseline levels by month 12, while the relative proportions of CD4 + CD25+ regulatory T cells increased by month 1 (from 3 to 14% and from 4 to 13%, respectively) and remained elevated at month 12 [24]. A similar pattern was observed for CD8 + T cells. Moreover, the relative proportion of mature naïve B cells decreased and the relative proportion of immature B cells increased by month 1 and approached baseline levels by month 6. It has been suggested that early T-cell reconstitution occurs via the expansion of existing cells which have escaped depletion, rather than via generation of new T cells in the thymus [32]. This may, at least partly, contribute to the development of secondary autoimmunity following alemtuzumab treatment, as peripheral expansion favours immune populations that respond to self-antigens [32]. However, as above mentioned, human and

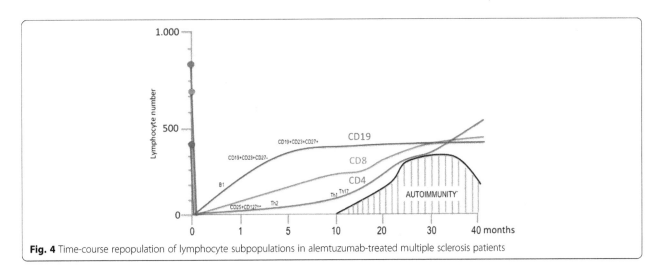

Fig. 4 Time-course repopulation of lymphocyte subpopulations in alemtuzumab-treated multiple sclerosis patients

mouse antigen-activated CD4+ T cells with high expression of CD52 on their surface (CD4 + CD52^{high}) were demonstrated to exert a suppressive action on other T cells by releasing CD52s. The demonstration that humans with autoimmune diabetes have a lower frequency and diminished function of CD52^{hi}CD4+ T cells responsive to the autoantigen GAD65 is particularly worth of interest, since it suggests a role of this T cell subpopulation in human autoimmunity. While these findings identify a CD52-mediated T cell regulatory mechanism that may protect from autoimmune diseases, they suggest that the impairment of this mechanism may contribute, at least partly, to the appearance of auto-immune disorders in alemtuzumab-treated individuals [2].

Alemtuzumab administration is associated with the acute induction of several pro-inflammatory cytokines, such as tumour necrosis factor-alpha (TNFa), interleukin-6 (IL-6) and interferon gamma (IFNg). This is due to the cross-linking of natural killer cells and to the lysis of lymphocytes and cells of the monocyte/macrophage lineage with subsequent release of pro-inflammatory cytokines that peaks 2-6 h after infusions and causes the so-called "cytokine-release syndrome).

However, the long-lasting effect of alemtuzumab on the cytokine network consists in the down-regulation of pro-inflammatory interleukins that may also be considered a major mechanism underlying the therapeutic effect of the drug. Indeed, in a study investigating cytokine production by ex vivo stimulated T cells obtained from MS patients treated for 12 months with alemtuzumab a long-lasting decrease in the secretion of IL-17 and IL-22 (produced by Th17 cells) was observed [27].

The immune-competence following alemtuzumab therapy was assessed in a pilot case-control study involving 24 patients [34]. The antibody responses to 3 vaccines (1. diphtheria, tetanus, and poliomyelitis vaccine, 2. Haemophilus influenzae type b and meningococcal group C conjugate vaccine, and 3. pneumococcal polysaccharide vaccine). The antibody titres against common viruses (mumps, rubella, varicella-zoster, and Epstein-Barr virus) were measured before alemtuzumab treatment and 1 and 9–11 months after treatment. Serum antibodies against common viruses remained detectable after treatment, and vaccine responses were normal to T-cell–dependent recall antigens (tetanus, diphtheria, and polio), to T-cell–dependent novel antigen (meningococcus C), and to T-cell–independent antigens (pneumococcal). No evidence for a diminished response to vaccinations in 5 patients studied within 6 months of alemtuzumab treatment was observed. Thus, alemtuzumab treated individuals retain 1) humoral immunologic memory (in the form of antibodies against common viruses and response to recall antigens), and 2) the ability to mount a humoral immune response against a novel

antigen. These data indicate that patients with relapsing remitting multiple sclerosis appear immunocompetent after treatment with alemtuzumab.

Alemtuzumab treatment was found to significantly reduce the risk of relapse and accumulation of disability compared with high-dose, high-frequency interferon beta 1a. The post hoc subgroup analyses of the CAMMS223 trial disclosed that among patients with no clinical disease activity immediately before treatment, or any clinical or radiological disease activity on-trial, disability improved after alemtuzumab but not following interferon beta. These observations led to the hypothesis that disability improvement after alemtuzumab was not only the result of the anti-inflammatory activity of the drug, but could in part be due to a sort of 'protective' effect mediated by neurotrophic factors possibly produced by lymphocytes. Indeed, after alemtuzumab, and only when specifically stimulated with myelin basic protein, peripheral blood mononuclear cell (PBMC) cultures produced increased concentrations of brain-derived neurotrophic factor, platelet-derived growth factor and ciliary neurotrophic factor [31]. Analysis by reverse transcriptase polymerase chain reaction of cell separations showed that the increased production of ciliary neurotrophic factor and brain-derived neurotrophic factor after alemtuzumab was attributable to increased production by T lymphocytes. Media from these post-alemtuzumab PBMC cultures promoted survival of rat neurones and increased axonal length in vitro, effects that were partially reversed by neutralizing antibodies against brain-derived nerve growth factor and ciliary neurotrophic factor. This conditioned media also enhanced oligodendrocyte precursor cell survival, maturation and myelination. The hypothesis that alemtuzumab-induced lymphocyte-derived neurotrophins mat play a neuro-protective role in vivo in MS patients needs further investigations.

Pharmacokinetic data

The pharmacokinetics of alemtuzumab were investigated in a study involving 216 patients with RRMS who received a first treatment course of intravenous infusions of alemtuzumab 12 or 24 mg/day on 5 consecutive days, followed by a second course with the same dosage on 3 consecutive days one year later. The highest serum concentration of alemtuzumab was observed following the last infusion of each treatment course; serum concentration increased with each consecutive dose within the course. The mean maximum serum concentration (Cmax) was 3014 ng/mL on day five of the initial treatment course, in recipients of alemtuzumab 12 mg; the mean Cmax was 2,276 ng/mL on day three of the second treatment course.

Classical biotransformation studies have not been conducted for alemtuzumab, as yet. The alpha elimination half-life was & 4–5 days in both treatment courses, and low or undetectable serum concentrations occurred within & 30 days of the end of each treatment course. No sufficient data are available to draw conclusion on the effect of race or sex on alemtuzumab pharmacokinetics and no formal drug interaction studies have been conducted for alemtuzumab at the recommended dosage in patients with MS (Genzyme Therapeutics Ltd. LemtradaTM, EU summary of productcharacteristics. 2013. [21] http://www.ema.europa.eu/docs).

Clinical trials and extension data

The effects of alemtuzumab on clinical and magnetic resonance parameters in patients with active RRMS have been investigated in one Phase II (Campath-1H in Multiple Sclerosis, CAMMS223) and two Phase III (Comparison of Alemtuzumab and Rebif efficacy in Multiple Sclerosis, CARE-MS-I and CARE-MS-II) randomized, rater-blinded, active comparator-controlled, multinational trials. Five years extension data have been made recently available from all these studies ([8, 10–12], Coles et al., 2013).

In CAMMS223 (enrolment period: December 2002-July 2004), 334 treatment naïve RRMS patients with a disease duration <3 years were randomized to receive 1) treatment with i.v. infusion of alemtuzumab 12 ($n = 113$) or 24 ($n = 110$) mg/day on 5 consecutive days, followed by a second treatment course at the same dosage on 3 consecutive days at months 12 and 24, or 2) subcutaneous interferon beta-1a 44 mcg tiw ($n = 111$). On September 2005, the trial was suspended for the appearance of three cases (one death) of alemtuzumab-related immune thrombocytopenic purpura (ITP). Interferon beta-1a treatment continued as planned. In 2008, the dosing suspension was lifted, an option redosing was given to the patients and a safety monitoring programme (ended in January 2010) was planned and carried on. Compared to IFNb-1a, alemtuzumab 12 mg/day was significantly more effective in reducing the relapse rate (-67% $p <0.0001$), in increasing the number of relapse-free patients (76% vs. 50%, $p <0.0001$) and in decreasing the sustained accumulation of disability (SAD) (8%vs. 27%, $p = 0.0006$). The MRI finding were also impressive: compared to IFNb, alemtuzumab-treated patients had a lower increase in T2WM lesion volume ($p = 0.005$) and a lower reduction in brain volume on T1 images ($p = 0.05$).

In CARE-MS-I naïve RRMS patients were randomized 2:1 to treatment with i.v. alemtuzumab 12 mg (on days 1–5 at baseline and on days 1–3 in a second course 12 months later) or s.c. IFNb-1a 44 mcg tiw.

In CARE-MS II, RRMS considered not responder to DMD were randomized 2 : 2 : 1 to alemtuzumab 12 or 24 mg (on days 1–5 at baseline and on days 1–3 in a second course 12 months later) or IFNb-1a 44 mcg tiw. Alemtuzumab 12 mg/day was more effective than IFNb-1a in the reduction of relapse rate (co-primary endpoint) in patients with treatment-naive (54.9%) or previously treated (49.4%) RRMS ($p <0.0001$ in both studies). Alemtuzumab 12 mg/day was also significantly ($p <0.0001$) more effective than IFNb-1a with regard to time to first relapse in both treatment-naive (HR 0.45 [95% CI 0.33–0.61]) and previously treated patients (HR 0.53 [95% CI 0.41–0.69]).

The number of patients who were relapse-free at 2 years was significantly ($p <0.0001$) higher in the alemtuzumab 12 mg/day group than in the IFN-1a group in both studies.. Similarly, alemtuzumab 12 mg/day was more effective than IFNb-1a in the reduction of 6-month confirmed sustained accumulation of disability rate (coprimary endpoint) in patients previously treated RRMS, but there was no significant between-group difference in patients with treatment-naive RRMS. Alemtuzumab was associated with a risk reduction of 30% (not significant) in treatment-naive and 42% ($p = 0.0084$) in previously treated patients for this endpoint. In previously treated patients (CARE-MS-II), significantly ($p = 0.0002$) more alemtuzumab 12 mg/day than interferon beta-1a recipients had a sustained reduction in disability score from baseline, confirmed over 6 months, in patients with baseline EDSS scores of >2.0) [HR 2.57 (95% CI 1.57–4.20]). Between-group differences in the change in EDSS score were significant ($p <0.0001$) in previously treated patients, but not in treatment-naive patients.

Alemtuzumab 12 mg/day was significantly ($p <0.05$) more effective than IFNb-1a with regard to the proportion of patients with Gadolinium-enhancing lesions at 24 months or new or enlarging T2 lesions, and the median change in brain parenchymal fraction in patients with treatment-naïve or previously treated RRMS. No significant between-group difference was observed in the median change in volume of hyperintense lesions in either study. Significantly more recipients of IFNb-1a had new T1 hypointense lesions than recipients of alemtuzumab in previously treated patients; the difference was not significant in treatment-naive patients. Alemtuzumab was associated with a significantly ($p <0.01$) greater proportion of patients who were clinically disease free (absence of both relapses and sustained accumulation of disability) and those who were both clinically disease free and MRI disease free (absence of both Gadolinium- enhancing lesions and new or enlarging T2 lesions) than IFNb-1a in both treatment-naive and previously treated patients with RRMS. In a sub-analysis of patients with highly-active RRMS in CARE-MS II (101 alemtuzumab and 42 IFNb-1a recipients), 33.3 and 0%, respectively, were disease activity-free at 1 year (p <0.0001) and 24.2% of the alemtuzumab recipients remained disease activity-free at 24 months. At 24 months, 35.8 and 60.0%, respectively, had relapses, 7.4 and 17.5% had sustained accumulation of disability, 22.1 and 52.5% had gadolinium-enhancing lesion activity, and 60.0 and 92.5% had T2 -lesion activity.

Supportive analyses demonstrated that significantly fewer alemtuzumab 12 mg/day than interferon beta-1a recipients had severe relapses (reduction of 61 and 48%; both p <0.05) or relapses leading to steroid treatment (reduction of 58 and 56%; both p <0.0001) in both treatment-naïve and previously treated patients, respectively, and relapses that led to hospitalization in previously treated patients (reduction of 55%; p = 0.0045).

Data of the five-years extension study of Phase III Clinical Trials have been recently presented at ECTRIMS 2015 [1, 14, 16, 25, 33, 39] The proportion of patients having no evidence of 6-months confirmed disability progression remained high through year 5: 80% in CARE-MS-I and 76% in CARE-MS-II compared to respectively 92 and 87% observed at the end of the trials (2 years). More than 50% of the patients of both studies maintained the NEDA (non evidence of disease activity) at the end of the follow-up. Interestingly, alemtuzumab continued to slow-down the loss of brain volume over the five years: the mean annual rate of brain volume loss ranged between 0.07% (CARE-MS-II) and 0.2% (CARE-MS-I), a rate similar to that observed in normal individuals (0.1–0.3%). Furthermore, the proportion of patients with sustained improvement in pre-existing disability (defined as ≥1-point EDSS decrease over 6 month for patients with EDSS ≥2.0 at core study baseline) increased progressively through 5 years, and was respectively 33% in CARE-MS-I and 43% in CARE-MS-II. Finally, the cytokine-release syndrome became progressively milder with repeated administration and the rate of antibody-mediated autoimmunity (thyroid) decreased from 20% to 10% from year 3 to year 5.

Recently, data of 10-year follow-up of patients enrolled in the CAMMS-223 study have been presented at the American Academy Neurology annual congress [15]. Of the 60 patients who enrolled in the long-term follow-up, 20 (33%) received only the initial 2 courses over 10 years. Of the 39 (65%) patients receiving >2 alemtuzumab courses, 26 (67%) only received 3 courses, 7 (12%) received 4 courses, and 6 (10%) received a total of 5 courses.

Through 10 years of follow-up, a low ARR (0.08) was maintained, while the mean EDSS score change from baseline (SD) was +0.12 over 10 years. Interestingly, EDSS remained stable or improved over 10 years

in the majority of patients, and most patients (76%) showed no evidence of 6-month confirmed disability worsening. These observations indicate that alemtuzumab may provide a unique treatment approach with durable efficacy in the absence of continuous treatment for RRMS patients through 10 years.

Safety profile of alemtuzumab
The adverse events (AE) complained by up to 90% of patients during or within 24 h after alemtuzumab infusion constitute the so-called 'cytokine release syndrome', and appear more frequently on the first day of infusion. The majority of these AE are mild to moderate in severity and are managed by premedication with steroids, anti-pyretics, and anti-histamines. The proportion of patients with AE is higher during the first course of alemtuzumab than the second.

In the RCT CAMMS223, CARE-MS-I and CARE-MS-II, infections were slightly more common with alemtuzumab than with sc IFNb-1a, but most were mild or moderate in severity. Serious infections were reported rarely (2–4% alemtuzumab versus 1% IFNb-1a). The most common infections were those of the respiratory and urinary tracts. Herpetic infections occurred in 16% of patients in the CARE-MS I and CARE-MS II studies. The risk of herpetic infection was greatest in the first month post-treatment, and could be reduced by prophylactic oral aciclovir (only 0.5% of patients receiving aciclovir developed a herpetic infection after the first course of alemtuzumab). Despite the marked immune-depression, no case of progressive multifocal leukoencephalopathy has been reported in alemtuzumab-treated MS patients up to date.

No statistically difference in the risk of cancers was observed after alemtuzumab compared to IFNb-1a in any of the trials (that, however, were not powered to pick up differences in low-frequency events).

Autoimmune AE constitute the most relevant risk of alemtuzumab therapy and have been associated with the characteristic time-course lymphocyte repopulation above described. Three major types of autoimmune disorders have been reported: thyroid diseases in about 30% of patients (Graves' hyperthyroidism, 65.8%, hypothyroidism, 20.5%, and subacute thyroiditis (12.3%), idiopatic throbocytopenic purpura (ITP) in 1% and nephropathy due to anti-glomerular basement membrane antibodies in 0.3% [8, 12]. In addition, single case of autoimmune neutropenia, pancytopenia and haemolytic anaemia, have been reported in less than 0.5% of treated patients.

The monitoring schedule recommended in the Lemtrada's Summary of Product Characteristics should be rigorously applied to identify rapidly the first symptoms of autoimmune disease so as to institute appropriate therapy.

Table 2 Alemtuzumab meets almost all the criteria that are expected from the ideal disease-modifying immunosuppressive/immunomodulatory drug for multiple sclerosis

Criteria of the ideal immunosuppressive drug	YES	Partially	NO
Rapid biological action	X		
Rapid clinical effects	X		
Long-lasting effects	X		
Low frequency of injections/administrations	X		
Respect the patient's quality of life	X		
Acceptable costs		X	
No non-specific toxicity	X		
Low risk of opportunistic infections	X		
No increase risk in cancer	X		
No increase in antibody-mediated autoimmunity			X
No increase in severe antibody-mediated autoimmunity		X	
No increase in mortality	X		
Manageable cytokine-release syndrome	X		
Immune system re-modelling/re-shaping	X		

Reviews with more detailed information on safety profile of alemtuzumab are available in the literature (Havrdova et al., 2015; [24, 26, 35]).

Conclusions

Alemtuzumab can be considered an immunosuppressive drug having complex, yet unexplored, immunomodulatory activities (Table 2). Its biological and clinical actions are fast and, in a large proportion of patients, long-lasting. This allows a low frequency of administration, thus making acceptable the infusion-related side effects (the cytokine release syndrome) and the costs of the therapy. In front of an increased in antibody-related autoimmune disorders (mainly autoimmune thyroiditis), it has to be pointed out that the risk of severe, life-threatening adverse events is extremely low and actually manageable. Moreover, Alemtuzumab seems not to expose the patients to an increased risk of cancer, no-specific toxicity and mortality, and the risk of infectious diseases appears very low. All these features make alemtuzumab a significant step forward in the therapy of MS.

Acknowledgements
NA.

Funding
NA since the paper is a review.

Authors' contributions
All authors have equally contributed to the manuscript.

Competing interests
All authors have no competing interest.

Author details
[1]Department of Neuroscience DNS, Multiple Sclerosis Centre, University Hospital, Via Giustiniani, 5, 35129 Padova, Italy. [2]Neurology and Neuroriabilitation Unit, IRCCS Neuromed, Pozzilli, and Univerity of Tor Vergata, Rome, Italy. [3]Multiple Sclerosis Centre, Ospedale Binaghi, University of Cagliari, Cagliari, Italy.

References

1. Arnold DL, Traboulsee A, Coles AJ, Cohen JA, Fox EJ, Hartung H, Havrdova E, Selmaj KW, Margolin DH, Zhao Y, et al. Durable effect of alemtuzumab on MRI activity in treatment-naive active relapsing-remitting multiple sclerosis patients: 4-year follow-up of CARE-MS I. In: Proceedings of the AAN meeting, Washington, DC, USA. 2015.
2. Bandala-Sanchez E, Zhang Y, Reinwald S, Dromey JA, Lee BH, Qian J, Bohmer RM, Harrison LC. T cell regulation mediated by interaction of soluble CD52 with the inhibitory receptor Siglec-10. Nat Immunol. 2013;14:741–8.
3. Ban-Hock T, Tin K, Peter T, Alex B. Immune regulation by CD52-expressing CD4 T cells. Cell Mole Immunol. 2013;10:379–82.
4. Breslin S. Cytokine-release syndrome: overview and nursing implications. Clin J Oncol Nurs. 2007;11(1 Suppl):37–42.
5. Bugelski PJ, Achuthanandam R, Capocasale RJ, Treacy G, Bouman-Thio E. Monoclonal antibody-induced cytokine-release syndrome. Expert Rev Clin Immunol. 2009;5(5):499–521.
6. Buggins AG, Mufti GJ, Salisbury J, et al. Peripheral blood but not tissue dendritic cells express CD52 and are depleted by treatment with alemtuzumab. Blood. 2002;100:1715–20.
7. Clark RA, Watanabe R, Teague JE, Schlapbach C, Tawa MC, Adams N, Dorosario AA, Chaney KS, Cutler CS, Leboeuf NR, Carter JB, Fisher DC, Kupper TS. Skin effector memory T cells do not recirculate and provide immune protection in alemtuzumab-treated CTCL patients. Sci Transl Med. 2012;4(117):117ra7. doi: 10.1126.
8. Cohen JA, Coles AJ, Arnold DL, Confavreux C, Fox EJ, Hartung HP, Havrdova E, Selmaj KW, Weiner HL, Fisher E, et al. Alemtuzumab versus interferon β 1a as first-line treatment for patients with relapsing-remitting multiple sclerosis: a randomised controlled phase 3 trial. CARE-MS I. Lancet. 2012;380:1819–28.
9. Coles AJ, Compston DA, Selmaj KW, Lake SL, Moran S, Margolin DH, Norris K, Tandon PK. Alemtuzumab vs. Interferon β-1a in early multiple sclerosis. N Engl J Med. 2008;359:1786–801.
10. Coles AJ, Fox E, Vladic A, Gazda SK, Brinar V, Selmaj KW, Bass AD, Wynn DR, Margolin DH, Lake SL, et al. Alemtuzumab versus interferon β-1a in early relapsing-remitting multiple sclerosis: Post-hoc and subset analyses of clinical efficacy outcomes. Lancet Neurol. 2011;10:338–48.
11. Coles AJ, Fox E, Vladic A, Gazda S.K, Brinar V, Selmaj K.W, Skoromets A, Stolyarov I, Bass A, Sullivan H, et al. Alemtuzumab more effective than interferon β-1a at 5-year follow-up of CAMMS223 clinical trial. Neurology. 2012a;78:1069–1078
12. Coles AJ, Twyman C.L, Arnold D.L, Cohen J.A, Confavreux C, Fox EJ, Hartung, H.P, Havrdova E, Selmaj K.W, Weiner H.L, et al. Alemtuzumab for patients with relapsing multiple sclerosis after disease-modifying therapy: A randomised controlled phase 3 trial. CARE-MS II. Lancet 2012b, 380, 1829–1839
13. Coles AJ. Alemtuzumab treatment of multiple sclerosis. Semin Neurol. 2013; 33(1):66–73.
14. Coles AJ, Arnold DL, Cohen JA, Fox EJ, Hartung H, Havrdova E, Selmaj KW, Margolin DH, Kasten L, Panzara M, et al. Alemtuzumab slows brain volume loss over 4 years despite most relapsing-remitting multiple sclerosis patients not receiving treatment for 3 years. In: Proceedings of the AAN meeting, Washington, DC, USA. 2015.
15. Coles AJ, Habek M, Bass AN, Brinar V, Vladic A, Margolin DH, Fox EJ, on behalf of the CAMMS223 Investigators. Durable efficacy of alemtuzumab over 10 years: long-term follow-up of patients With RRMS from the CAMMS223 study. In: Poster P3.053, 68th American academy of neurology (AAN) annual meeting, Vancouver, BC, Canada. 2016.

16. Compston DAS, Giovannoni G, Arnold DL, Fox EJ, Hartung H, Havrdova E, Selmaj KW, Margolin DH, Palmer J, Panzara M, et al. Durable effect of alemtuzumab on clinical outcomes in treatment-naïve relapsing-remitting multiple sclerosis patients: 4-year follow-up of CARE-MS I. In: Proceedings of the AAN meeting, Philadelphia, PA, USA. 2015.

17. Cossburn M, Pace AA, Jones J, Ali R, Ingram G, Baker K, Hirst C, Zajicek J, Scolding N, Boggild M, Pickersgill T, Ben-Shlomo Y, Coles A, Robertson NP. Autoimmune disease after alemtuzumab treatment for multiple sclerosis in a multicenter cohort. Neurology. 2011;77(6):573–9.

18. Costelloe L, Jones J, Coles A. Secondary autoimmune diseases following alemtuzumab therapy for multiple sclerosis. Expert Rev Neurother. 2012; 12(3):335–41.

19. Cox AL, Thompson SA, Jones JL, Robertson VH, Hale G, Waldmann H, Compston DA, Coles AJ. Lymphocyte homeostasis following therapeutic lymphocyte depletion in multiple sclerosis. Eur J Immunol. 2005;35:3332–42.

20. De Mercanti S, Rolla S, Cucci A, Bardina V, Cocco E, et al. Alemtuzumab long-term immunologic effect. Neurol Neuroimmunol Neuroinflamm. 2016;3:e194.

21. Genzyme Therapeutics Ltd. LemtradaTM (alemtuzumab 12 mg concentrate for solution for infusion): EU summary of productcharacteristics. 2013. http://www.ema.europa.eu/docs/en_GB/document_library/EPAR_-_Product_Information/human/003718/WC500150521.pdf. Accessed 16 Oct 2013.

22. Hale G, Bright S, Chumbley G, Hoang T, Metcalf D, Munro AJ, Waldmann H. Removal of T cells from bone marrow for transplantation: a monoclonal anti-lymphocyte antibody that fixes human complement. Blood. 1983;62:873–82.

23. Hale G, Waldmann H. From laboratory to clinic : the story of CAMPATH-1. Methods Mol Med. 2000;40:243–66.

24. Hartung H-P, Aktas O, Boyko AN. Alemtuzumab: a new therapy for active relapsing–remitting multiple sclerosis. Mult Scler. 2015;21(1):22–34.

25. Havari E, Turner M, Dodge J, Treleaven C, Shihabuddin L, et al. Anti-murine CD52 antibody treatment does not adversely affect the migratory ability of immune cells. In: Proceedings of the AAN Meeting, Philadelphia, PA, USA. 2015.

26. Havrdova E, Horakova D, Kovarova I. Alemtuzumab in the treatment of multiple sclerosis: key clinical trial results and considerations for use. Ther Adv Neurol Disord. 2015;8(1):31–45.

27. Helliwell CL, Coles AJ. Monoclonal antibodies in multiple sclerosis treatment: current and future steps. Ther Adv Neurol Disord. 2009;2(4):195–203.

28. Hill-Cawthorne GA, Button T, Tuohy O, Jones JL, May K, Somerfield J, Green A, Giovannoni G, Compston DA, Fahey MT, Coles AJ. Long term lymphocyte reconstitution after alemtuzumab treatment of multiple sclerosis. J Neurol Neurosurg Psychiatry. 2012;83(3):298–304.

29. Hu Y, Turner MJ, Shields J, Gale MS, Hutto E, et al. Investigation of the mechanism of action of alemtuzumab in a human CD52 transgenic mouse model. Immunology. 2009;128:260–70.

30. Jones JL, Phuah CL, Cox AL, Thompson SA, Ban M, Shawcross J, Walton A, Sawcer SJ, Compston A, Coles AJ. IL-21 drives secondary autoimmunity in patients with multiple sclerosis, following therapeutic lymphocyte depletion with alemtuzumab (Campath-1H). J Clin Invest. 2009;119(7):2052–61.

31. Jones JL, Anderson JM, Phuah CL, Fox EJ, Selmaj K, Margolin D, Lake SL, Palmer J, Thompson SJ, Wilkins A, et al. Improvement in disability after alemtuzumab treatment of multiple sclerosis is associated with neuroprotective autoimmunity. Brain. 2010;133:2232–47.

32. Jones JL, Thompson SA, Loh P, et al. Human autoimmunity after lymphocyte depletion is causedby homeostatic T-cell proliferation. Proc Natl Acad Sci U S A. 2013;110:20200–5.

33. LaGanke C, Hughes B, Berkovich R, Cohen JA, Giovannoni G, Kasten L, Margolin DH, Havrdova E. Durable effect of alemtuzumab on disability improvement in patients with relapsing-remitting multiple sclerosis who relapsed on a prior therapy. In: Proceedings of the AAN meeting, Washington, DC, USA. 2015.

34. McCarthy CL, Tuohy O, Compston DA, Kumararatne DS, Coles AJ, Jones JL. Immune competence after alemtuzumab treatment of multiple sclerosis. Neurology. 2013;81(10):872–6.

35. Menge T, Stuve O, Kieseier BC, Hartung H-P. Alemtuzumab. The advantages and challenges ofa novel therapy in MS. Neurology. 2014;83:87–97.

36. Rao SP, Campos-Rivera J, Sancho J, et al. Differential sensitivity of human PBMC subsets to alemtuzumab mediated cytotoxicity. Mult Scler. 2010;16: S139–40.

37. Rao SP, Sancho J, Campos-Rivera J, Boutin PM, Severy PB, et al. Human peripheral blood mononuclear cells exhibit heterogeneous CD52 expression levels and show differential sensitivity to alemtuzumab mediated cytolysis. PLoS One. 2012;7:e39416.

38. Thompson SA, Jones JL, Cox AL, Compston DA, Coles AJ. B-cell reconstitution and BAFF after alemtuzumab (Campath-1H) treatment of multiple sclerosis. J Clin Immunol 2010;30(1):99–105.

39. Traboulsee A, Coles AJ, Cohen JA, Compston DAS, Fox EJ, Hartung H, Havrdova E, Selmaj KW, Margolin DH, Zhao Y, et al. Durable effect of alemtuzumab on MRI outcomes in patients with relapsing-remitting multiple sclerosis who relapsed on prior therapy: 4-year follow-up of CARE-MS II. In: Proceedings of the AAN meeting, Washington, DC, USA. 2015.

40. Turner MJ, Lamorte MJ, Chretien N, Havari E, Roberts BL, et al. Immune status following alemtuzumab treatment in human CD52 transgenic mice. J Neuroimmunol. 2013;261:29–36.

41. Turner MJ, Pang PT, Chretien N, Havari E, LaMorte MJ, et al. Reduction of inflammation and preservation of neurological function by anti-CD52 therapy in murine experimental autoimmune encephalomyelitis. J Neuroimmunol. 2015;285:4–12.

42. Zhang X, Tao Y, Chopra M, Ahn M, Marcus KL, et al. Differential reconstitution of T cell subsets following immunodepleting treatment with alemtuzumab (anti-CD52 monoclonal antibody) in patients with relapsing-remitting multiple sclerosis. J Immunol. 2013;191:5867–74.

43. Wang H, Dong J, Shi P, et al. Anti-mouse CD52 monoclonal antibody ameliorates intestinal epithelial barrier functionin interleukin-10 knockout mice with spontaneous chronic colitis. Immunology 2015;144(2):254–262.

44. Watanabe T, Masuyama J, Sohma Y, Inazawa H, Horie K, et al. CD52 is a novel costimulatory molecule for induction of CD4+ regulatory T cells. Clin Immunol. 2006;120(3):247–59.

45. Wing MG, Moreau T, Greenwood J, Smith RM, Hale G, et al. Mechanism of first-dose cytokine-release syndrome by CAMPATH 1-H: involvement of CD16 (FcgammaRIII) and CD11a/CD18 (LFA-1) on NK cells. J Clin Invest. 1996;98(12):2819–26.

13

Longitudinal change in Paced Auditory Serial Addition Test (PASAT) performance following immunoablative therapy and haematopoietic stem cell transplant in multiple sclerosis

Lisa A. S. Walker[1,2,3,4], Jason A. Berard[2,4,6*], Marjorie Bowman[2], Harold L. Atkins[2,3], Hyunwoo Lee[5], Douglas Arnold[5] and Mark S. Freedman[2,3]

Abstract

Background: Immediately following immunoablation and hematopoietic stem cell transplantation (IA-HSCT) for MS a median decrease in brain volume of 3.2 % over 2.4 months occurs. After 2 years, rates of atrophy are comparable to normal volunteers. Potential impact of atrophy on cognition was evaluated by examining performance on the Paced Auditory Serial Addition Test (PASAT) pre- and post-IA-HSCT.

Methods: Twenty-three individuals with rapidly progressing/poor prognosis MS underwent high dose IA-HSCT. Individuals completed the 3" PASAT at baseline and 6/12/18/24/30/36 months post-procedure.

Results: Mean decline in performance between baseline and 6-months occurred, though it was not statistically significant. Minor declines were offset by an overall trend for improvement over time. The largest (non-significant) cognitive gains were between months 30 and 36. Neither level of impairment at baseline, nor demographic variables, influenced likelihood of improvement. No relationship between changes in cognition and changes in volumes was detected, likely secondary to small sample size.

Conclusions: While an initial decline in cognition was noted 6 months post-IA-HSCT, there were no lasting negative effects of treatment given the overall trend for improvement. Initial cognitive decline and marked volume loss are likely secondary to acute toxic effects of chemotherapy. Gains in cognition noted over 36 months suggest long-term follow-up is essential.

Keywords: Multiple sclerosis, Cognition, Stem cell, Immunoablation, MRI

Background

Although advances in the therapeutic treatment of MS have improved remarkably over the last several years, current therapies are not curative. Rather, pharmacological treatments simply slow the progression of the disease. Given that MS is an autoimmune disease treatments aim to address the immunological aspects of the illness. Immunoablation and hematopoietic stem cell

transplantation (IA-HSCT) has been postulated as a potential tool to treat a number of autoimmune diseases [1, 2]. A few groups of researchers across the globe have initiated the use of IA-HSCT procedures in individuals with MS in hopes of halting disease progression [3, 4]. The treatment is quite aggressive and thus the selection criteria for inclusion in these trials have been restricted to those with rapidly progressing MS and poor prognosis.

The Ottawa Hospital MS Clinic has completed a study evaluating the impact of IA-HSCT on MS. Of the 23 individuals to undergo the procedure, no new attacks or

* Correspondence: jberard@toh.on.ca; jberard@ottawahospital.on.ca
[2]The Ottawa Hospital Research Institute, Ottawa, Canada
[4]School of Psychology, University of Ottawa, Ottawa, Canada
Full list of author information is available at the end of the article

MRI lesions have been reported [5, 6]. These individuals have been followed extensively and their progress has been monitored in multiple ways, including neuroimaging studies. This data has revealed that the IA-HSCT procedure results in brain atrophy occurring at a significantly greater rate than is expected on the basis of natural disease progression. For a more detailed discussion on the atrophy observed, please see Lee et al. 2016 [7].

Atrophy has also been noted by other research groups [8–10] and various explanations have been postulated to explain the volume loss including: a selection bias for patients with aggressive disease and potentially faster rates of atrophy; long-term consequences of previous disease activity on tissue integrity; "pseudoatrophy" from reductions in edema (at least during the first year); and finally, neurotoxicity of the chemotherapy conditioning regimen [10]. In an attempt to address this issue our group examined atrophy in 9 secondary progressive MS patients compared to a patient with non-CNS non-Hodgkin's lymphoma (NHL) who underwent a comparable IA-HSCT procedure [11]. Volume loss exceeded change in T2 lesion volume by 2- to 20-fold. Acute atrophy was not explained by resolution of edema. Both the MS group and the NHL patient showed a median 3.2 % volume loss over a median of 2.4 months. The comparable rates of atrophy suggest that volume loss was not related to edema resolution, but rather to the toxicity of therapy (which among other agents consisted of cyclophosphamide, busulfan, and steroids); a known consequence of such treatment.

The impact of this decrease in brain volume on cognition has been evaluated by our group in 7 of the 23 individuals who underwent the IA-HSCT procedure [12]. Results from a large battery of neuropsychological tests (apart from the PASAT results reviewed here) revealed a decline in executive functioning at 2 months post-procedure. However, in those four individuals who completed 24-month follow-up, performance returned to baseline levels. Thus, despite a decline in cognition in the early period following treatment, with temporal distance from the HSCT procedure, cognition returned to baseline levels in those who completed the follow-up. No significant correlations were found between cognitive decline and change in imaging variables or stem cell dosage; although the small sample size may have masked any such relationships. Results from this study, though quite preliminary, are promising and suggest that immunoablation and HSCT may have no lasting deleterious effects on cognition.

The current study aims to further examine patterns of cognitive change in all 23 individuals from the Ottawa Hospital MS Clinic who underwent the IA-HSCT procedure. Whereas only the small subset of 7 individuals completed full neuropsychological batteries,

all 23 participants underwent serial evaluation with the Paced Auditory Serial Addition Test (PASAT). As such, we were able to evaluate the impact of IA-HSCT on information processing speed (IPS) and working memory (WM) using the PASAT. Testing took place at baseline (i.e. before the IA-HSCT procedure) and every 6 months for a period of 3 years.

The PASAT is the only cognitive measure in the Multiple Sclerosis Functional Composite (MSFC) [13]. Although there are clear limitations to the PASAT [14] and alternative measures such as the Symbol Digit Modalities Test have been discussed, [15, 16] the PASAT remains a measure that is highly sensitive to cognitive impairment and has become widely used in MS research. It has become a common outcome measure in clinical trials and, in particular, has become a useful tool to monitor cognitive change over time. Longitudinal change in PASAT scores do not correlate with change in EDSS scores, [17] but PASAT performance does correlate with imaging parameters such as DTI measures, [18] MTR in normal appearing white matter, [19, 20] brain activation using fMRI, [21, 22] atrophy, [23] and gadolinium enhancement (a marker of active inflammatory activity), [24] as well as electrophysiological measures such as P3 ERP [25]. Thus, this measure is an easily administered clinical tool that can be a marker for underlying disease progression. Higher scores on the PASAT are associated with better quality of life outcomes, demonstrating that it also has relevance to outcomes important to people suffering from MS [26, 27]. Rosti and colleagues (2007) [28] found that the PASAT was able to detect deterioration in cognition after only 1 year, but this phenomenon was found only in those individuals with MS who were already cognitively impaired at baseline (i.e., cognitively intact individuals with MS did not change over that time interval). One of the complications when using the PASAT in serial testing is its susceptibility to practice effects [13, 28]. Nonetheless, this can be controlled statistically (see below).

Given our previous work which documented cognitive decline immediately post-IA-HSCT in some individuals, [12] it was hypothesized that a similar decline in PASAT scores would be found at the 6 month mark with improvement expected at all other time points. MRI scans were obtained in conjunction with the cognitive testing to examine the potential correlation between volume loss and cognition. Our past preliminary work has shown little relationship between volume and cognitive variables early after transplant, but the current study evaluated this potential relationship over a longer follow-up interval [12].

Methods
Participants
This study was approved by the Ottawa Hospital Research Ethics Board and informed consent was obtained.

Twenty-three individuals with rapidly progressing MS who failed to respond to routine therapy (i.e. progression or continued relapses or worsening MRI after at least 1 year of therapy with interferon-β1, glatiramer acetate, mitoxantrone, or other conventional dose immunosuppressive drug therapy) were enrolled. High risk of progression was defined as ≥5 relapses in the first 2 years of disease or attainment of a Functional System (FS) Score of at least 3 (or findings consistent with a FS of 3) affecting pyramidal/cerebellar subscores within 5 years of onset. If a patient had previously received a cytotoxic agent (mitoxantrone, cyclophosphamide, etc.) they must have had normal bone marrow morphology and cytogenetics before being considered eligible for this study. MRI brain scans satisfied the MRI criteria of Paty or Fazekas for the diagnosis of MS. None of the subjects had evidence of hepatic inflammation or fibrosis. In the 23 subjects enrolled baseline EDSS ranged from 1.5 to 6.5 (mean = 4.87 (1.40)). Education ranged from high school to graduate school with the median value being equivalent to college level. Age ranged from 23 to 44 years (mean = 32.65 (5.82) years). Of the 23 subjects, 12 were diagnosed with relapsing-remitting MS and 11 with secondary progressive MS. Those with primary progressive MS were excluded.

Procedure and measures

The study was a tri-center phase II efficacy study of the role of intensive immunosupression and autologous HSCT on the natural history of MS. Participants underwent stem cell mobilization with IV cyclophosphamide (4.5 g/m^2) and 10 days of granulocyte colony-stimulating factor (10 µg/kg/day) followed by stem cell collection using peripheral vein leukopheresis. All stem cell grafts were CD34 selected and cryopreserved until transplantation. Immunoablation was accomplished using cyclophosphamide (200 mg/kg), dose-adjusted IV busulfan (maximum 16 mg/kg) and IV rabbit antithymocyte globulin (5 mg/kgSolumedrol was administered concurrently with ATG to reduce the risk of hypersensitivity reactions. Participants did not receive further MS-disease modifying drugs or experimental therapy after IA-HSCT.

Participants underwent MRI scans with pre- and post-gadolinium enhanced T1-weighted and dual spin-echo (Proton Density/T2-weighted) sequences at baseline and then serially every 6 months until 36 months post-IA-HSCT. T1-weighted pre-contrast scans were used to calculate volumes of GM, WM, and regional structures. At the same time points as the MRI, subjects completed the 3" PASAT. Note that a run-in procedure was not used for the PASAT. However, see below for the manner in which this was controlled statistically. Two participants did not complete the follow-up interval past 18 months as they underwent an unproven therapy for disease progression against the advice of their treating neurologist, and

inclusion of their data would have made it more challenging to interpret findings in the context of the treatment of interest.

Data analysis

The GM and WM volumes, normalized for subject head size, were calculated with FSL-SIENAX (cross-sectional variation of Structural Image Evaluation, using Normalisation, of Atrophy) [29]. Subcortical gray matter structures were segmented and their volumes were calculated with FSL-FIRST (FMRIB's Integrated Registration and Segmentation Tool: http://www.fmrib.ox.ac.uk/fsl/first) [30]. Volumes of cortical and other subcortical structures were calculated with Freesurfer v5.1 (http://surfer.nrm.mgh.harvard.edu/) [31, 32].

Because group comparisons of tests scores can mask significant individual differences (as can practice effects due to prior task exposure), the reliable change index (RCI) (corrected for practice) was calculated for the PASAT in order to assess an individual's change over time. A variation of the RCI was used that included an adjustment for practice effects that result from serial testing [33]. Note that practice effects were accounted for up to 12 months given that research has shown stability in practice after the third PASAT retest session [14, 34].

$$RCI = \left(\frac{(time\ 2 - time\ 1) - practice}{SE_{Diff}} \right)$$

SEdiff is the standard error of the difference which represents the spread of distribution of change scores expected had no change occurred. Given that, to the best of our knowledge, there is no published data for the 3" PASAT which provides means and standard deviations for multiple administrations, the *practice effect* was calculated by taking the mean difference between the second and first administration of the 3" PASAT (as well as between the third and second administration) for a group of healthy controls (from a different study in our lab) who received multiple administrations up to a week apart. For a more specific examination of the demographics of this control sample, please see Walker et al. 2012 [35]. The RCI scores were considered to be statistically significant and reliable at 90 % confidence intervals if the degree of change fell outside ±1.64.

Chi-square analysis was conducted to determine if those who were impaired at baseline were more or less likely to show improvement over time compared to those who were not impaired at baseline.

Analysis of variance (ANOVA) was performed to determine if demographic variables (such as age, gender, and education) explained the differences noted between those who show improvement in their performance from baseline to 36 months post-IA-HSCT and those who do not.

Finally, Pearson bivariate correlational analyses were performed to determine if PASAT RCI values (e.g. baseline to 6 months, 6 to 12 months, etc.) correlated with change in brain volume (i.e. difference scores) of the cortical and subcortical structures.

Results

Reliable Change Index (RCI) analyses

Please see Table 1 for RCI values per subject.

On average, there was a decline in RCI values between performance at baseline and performance at 6-month follow-up (mean RCI =−0.13) (see Fig. 1).

This value, although reflective of decline, does not reach statistical significance. An RCI value must exceed +/- 1.64 in order to be considered significant.

Following the 6-month mark, a trend for improvement was noted until 24 months, although this trend did not reach statistical significance. There was a decline noted at 30-months but examination of the raw scores revealed a trend for stability, with the mean decline being driven by one outlier who declined significantly. The largest cognitive gains took place between months 30 and 36, but again not to a statistically significant degree.

Chi-square analyses

Subjects' impairment status at baseline (cognitively impaired vs. cognitively intact) did not impact whether they declined, remained stable, or improved over time.

Table 1 RCI values per subject

Subject	Baseline - 6m	6m - 12m	12m - 18m	18m - 24m	24m - 30m	30m - 36m	Baseline - 36m
1	2.23	-1.26	1.53	0.31	0.35	-0.16	3.76
2	0.12	-0.94	-0.35	0.94	-1.76	2.35	0.23
3	-0.7	-1.26	0	1.57	0.12	1.26	1.06
4	-0.47	0	-1.17	1.73	0	0.16	1.17
5	-0.94	0.16	-0.47	1.1	-0.47	1.1	0.35
6	-0.12	0.78	0.23	-0.47	1.29	-1.57	0.94
7	-0.82	-1.41	0.82	-1.26	*	*	-1.76
8	-0.47	*	*	*	*	-0.31	-0.35
9	-0.59	0.16	-0.47	0.94	-0.23	0.94	0.7
10	*	*	0.12	0.94	0.47	-0.12	0.47
11	-0.23	0.63	0	-0.63	0.59	1.41	0.47
12	0	0	0.35	0.31	*	0.94	1.42
13	-2.47	1.1	0.82	-0.16	*	*	*
14	-0.23	0.78	0	-0.16	0.12	-0.16	0.7
15	0.47	1.1	-0.12	-1.26	-0.12	1.41	1.64
16	1.41	-1.26	0.82	0.47	-0.47	1.1	2.47
17	0.12	0.16	0.12	0.63	0.23	-0.16	1.41
18	-1.29	0.16	0.47	*	*	*	*
19	-0.35	0.16	0	-0.16	0.12	*	*
20	-0.12	0.94	-0.23	-0.16	*	*	*
21	0.47	0.16	-0.12	0.16	-0.12	*	*
22	2.11	0.94	-0.23	0.63	-0.59	*	*
23	-0.70	0.47	0.59	*	*	*	*

* missing data

RCI significant improvement

RCI significant decline

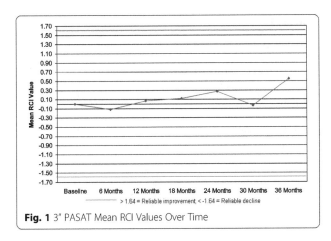

Fig. 1 3″ PASAT Mean RCI Values Over Time

Analysis of variance

There were no differences in demographics (age, gender, education) between those who showed reliable improvement and those who did not.

Correlational analyses

Change in PASAT performance did not correlate significantly with the change in percent normalized brain volume (PNBV), percent cortical grey matter volume (PGMV), or percent white matter volume (PWMV) at any time point (see Table 2 for mean percent normalized brain volumes over time).

Similarly, there was no relationship between change in PASAT performance and change in any of the cortical and subcortical structure volumes at any time point. For a more comprehensive examination of the observed MRI changes please see Lee et al. 2016 [7].

Discussion

Consistent with the hypothesis, we were able to document a slight trend toward the expected decline in PASAT performance in the initial period post-IA-HSCT given that there was a mean RCI decline between baseline and 6 months. Similarly, there was a much more encouraging trend for improvement over the longer follow-up interval. It is important to note however, that these findings did not reach statistical significance when group means were considered. The lack of significance cannot be attributed to changes associated with practice effects given that the RCI analyses take this into account; nor are these findings likely to be attributed to small sample size given that these analyses were at the level of

the individual. Six individuals demonstrated significant improvement during at least one of the time periods evaluated but several more exhibited more subtle improvements. The lack of statistical significance overall suggests that the changes in WM and IPS experienced post-IA-HSCT are subtle. This is consistent with others who describe only subtle changes in cognition associated with chemotoxicity and the resolution of initial declines as time progresses post-treatment [36, 37]. In our previous report, we outline why we believe that chemotoxicity played a significant role in the increased rate of atrophy [11]. The neurotoxic effects of chemotherapy have been well documented in the literature [36, 38] and thus, in addition to the atrophic changes, this is also likely the reason for the initial transient decline in cognition noted here. Current findings mirror what was documented by our group when examining performance on a subset of participants on a full neuropsychological evaluation [12]. Indeed, it was found that cognition declined briefly in the initial period post-procedure and returned to baseline levels by the 24-month follow-up. The current study evaluated cognition at more frequent time intervals, and examination of the mean RCI values (see Fig. 1) suggests that cognition returns to baseline levels by 12 months. Thus, the latter half of the first year post-IA-HSCT appears to be a critical period with regard to cognitive gains. The IA-HSCT procedure did not differentially impact cognition based upon cognitive status before the procedure, nor did demographic variables influence outcome.

After 12 months, there is a trend for ongoing subtle cognitive gains (with the exception of the outlier influencing performance at 30 months). Does the fact that PASAT values at 36 months follow-up exceed initial baseline levels (after accounting for practice) argue for neuronal repair? Clearly, it is too soon to make a claim like this, but results are promising and warrant further study. If cognition is improved over baseline levels then perhaps the IA-HSCT procedure does not simply halt disease progression, but fosters repair (i.e. the cognitive findings may be a marker for this potential improved pathology). Certainly past research has confirmed that PASAT performance correlates with imaging markers of pathology [18, 19, 21, 22, 24]. Nine of the 23 individuals undergoing this study have demonstrated improvement in neurological function (i.e. EDSS improvement of 1 or more) compared to baseline levels, [6] so this would

Table 2 Mean percent normalized brain volumes over time

	Baseline	6 m	12 m	18 m	24 m	30 m	36 m
Percent Normalized Brain Volume	100.00	97.68 (1.58)	97.44 (1.90)	97.31 (1.72)	97.25 (1.75)	96.26 (2.20)	96.45 (2.57)
Percent Grey Matter Volume	100.00	94.12 (2.59)	94.89 (2.98)	95.28 (2.79)	94.09 (2.71)	93.78 (4.20)	93.50 (5.18)
Percent White Matter Volume	100.00	100.66 (1.90)	99.29 (3.12)	98.97 (2.60)	99.83 (3.62)	98.60 (3.37)	98.59 (3.36)

appear to provide converging evidence for this possibility. Further investigations must occur in order to test this notion and draw any firm conclusions.

The lack of association between PASAT performance and atrophy measures is consistent with our past preliminary findings, [12] but inconsistent with the research literature that typically demonstrates a correlation between PASAT performance and neuroimaging [18, 19, 21, 22, 24]. The primary reason for the lack of relationship is likely that the sample size was insufficient. A larger sample size would garnermore statistical power to detect such a relationship. The small sample size is a function of the nature of this particular study. Enrollment criteria was quite restrictive and was limited to those with rapidly progressive disease who had not responded well to established therapies. Although the current IA-HSCT procedure appears quite promising with regard to halting disease progression and with regard to these preliminary cognitive findings, it remains a procedure that should be considered only after other options have been exhausted given the risks with which it is associated. A multi-centre trial holds the most promise with regard to enrollment of larger numbers, and indeed, discussions are underway. In such a circumstance, greater statistical power may allow us to detect the expected relationship between change in cognition and changes in brain volumes.

An additional limitation of this study is the lack of a control group. Attempts were made to obtain an appropriate control; however, we were unsuccessful. We attempted to approach individuals undergoing bone marrow transplant for other indications besides MS (i.e. haematological cancers). However, recruitment proved to be extremely difficult due to the fact that individuals undergoing such procedures are typically extremely ill. Their motivation to participate in research is low and those who are more motivated are more likely to volunteer for research targeting their own health condition (i.e. they have no impetus to contribute to MS research given that it does not relate to them directly).

Conclusions

The results of this study are clearly preliminary, but hold some promise. Initial subtle declines in cognition post-IA-HSCT are presumably due to chemotoxic effects, but these subtle declines are reversible with scores improving over time and eventually exceeding initial baseline levels. Thus, any negative impact on cognition of the IA-HSCT procedure appears to be only minor and temporary and does not appear to cause any lasting damage to the CNS. Results at 36 months highlight the necessity of long-term follow-up. Future research should attempt to replicate these findings in larger sample sizes via multi-centre initiatives. The question of possible neural repair should also be evaluated.

Abbreviations

ANOVA, analysis of variance; FS, functional system score; IA-HSCT, immunoablation and hematopoietic stem cell transplantation; IPS, information processing speed; MSFC, Multiple Sclerosis Functional Composite; NHL, non-Hodgkin's lymphoma; PASAT, Paced Auditory Serial Addition Test; PGMV, percent cortical grey matter volume; PMWV, percent white matter volume; PNBV, percent normalized brain volume; RCI, reliable change index; WM, working memory

Acknowledgments

We would like to thank the participants of this study for their time and effort.

Funding

This research was supported by a grant from the Research Foundation of the Multiple Sclerosis Society of Canada. The funding body had no role in the study design, manuscript preparation, nor the collection/analysis of the data or its interpretation.

Authors' contributions

LASW and JAB—data acquisition, analysis and interpretation of data, manuscript preparation and revision, final publication approval. MB—data acquisition, analysis and interpretation of data, manuscript revision, final publication approval. HLA and MSF—study design, data acquisition, interpretation of data, manuscript revision, final publication approval. HL and DA—MRI data acquisition, interpretation of data, manuscript revision, final publication approval.

Competing interests

The authors declare that they have no competing interests. Dr. Mark Freedman is a member of the Editorial Board for the Multiple Sclerosis and Demyelinating Disorders Journal.

Author details

[1]Neuropsychology Service, The Ottawa Hospital, Ottawa, Canada. [2]The Ottawa Hospital Research Institute, Ottawa, Canada. [3]Faculty of Medicine, University of Ottawa, Ottawa, Canada. [4]School of Psychology, University of Ottawa, Ottawa, Canada. [5]Montreal Neurological Institute and Hospital, Montreal, Canada. [6]The Ottawa Hospital—General Campus, Suite 7300, 501 Smyth Road, Ottawa, Ontario K1H 8 L6, Canada.

References

1. Gratwohl A, Passweg J, Gerber I, et al. Stem cell transplantation for autoimmune diseases. Best Pract Res Clin Haematol. 2001;14(4):755–76.
2. Tyndall A, Farge D. Progress in hematopoietic stem cell transplantation for autoimmune diseases. Expert Rev Clin Immunol. 2005;1(1):159–67.
3. Pasquini MC, Griffith LM, Arnold DL, et al. Hematopoietic stem cell transplantation for multiple sclerosis: Collaboration of the CIBMTR and EBMT to facilitate international clinical studies. Biol Blood Marrow Transplant. 2010;16:1076–83.
4. Rogojan C, Frederiksen JL. Hematopoietic stem cell transplantation in multiple sclerosis. Acta Neurol Scand. 2009;120:371–82.
5. Atkins HL, Bowman M, Allan D, et al. Immunoablation and autologous haemopoietic stem-cell transplantation for aggressive multiple sclerosis: a multicentre single-group phase 2 trial. Lancet:2016 http://dx.doi.org/10.1016/S0140-6736(16)30169-6
6. Freedman MS. Bone marrow transplantation: Does it stop MS progression? J Neurol Sci. 2007;259:85–9.
7. Lee H, Narayanan RAB, Chen JT, et al. Brain atrophy after bone marrow transplantation for treatment of multiple sclerosis. Mult Scler:2016 http://dx.doi.org/10.1016/10.1177/1352458516650992.
8. Rocca MA, Mondria T, Valsasina P, et al. A three-year study of brain atrophy after autologous hematopoietic stem cell transplantation in rapidly evolving secondary progressive multiple sclerosis. Am J Neuroradiol. 2007;28:1659–61.
9. Frischer JM, Bramow S, Dal-Bianco A, et al. The relation between inflammation and neurodegeneration in multiple sclerosis brains. Brain. 2009;132:1175–89.

10. Inglese M, Mancardi GL, Pagani E, et al. Brain tissue loss occurs after suppression of enhancement in patients with multiple sclerosis treated with autologous r. J Neurol Neurosurg Psychiatry. 2004;75:643–4.

11. Chen JT, Collins DL, Atkins HL, et al. Brain atrophy after immunoablation and stem cell transplantation in multiple sclerosis. Neurology. 2006;66:1935–7.

12. Walker LAS, Berard JA, Atkins HL, et al. Cognitive change and neuroimaging following immunoablative therapy and hematopoietic stem cell transplantation in multiple sclerosis: A pilot study. Mult Scler Relat Disord. (2014), http://dx.doi.org/10.1016/j.msard.2013.05.001.

13. Fischer JS, Jak AJ, Kniker JE, et al. Administration and Scoring Manual for the Multiple Sclerosis Functional Composite Measure (MSFC). New York: National Multiple Sclerosis Society; 2001.

14. Tombaugh TN. A comprehensive review of the Paced Auditory Serial Addition Test (PASAT). Arch Clin Neuropsychol. 2006;21:53–76.

15. Drake AS, Weinstock-Guttman B, Morrow SA, et al. Psychometrics and normative data for the Multiple Sclerosis Funcational Composite: replacing the PASAT with the Symbol Digit Modalities Test. Mult Scler. 2010;16(2):228–37.

16. Brochet B, Deloire MSA, Bonnet M, et al. Should SDMT substitute for PASAT in MSFC? A 5-year longitudinal study. Mult Scler. 2008;14:1242–9.

17. Hoogervorst ELJ, Kalkers NF, Uitdehaag MJ, et al. A study validating changes in the Multiple Sclerosis Functional Composite. Arch Neurol. 2002;59:113–6.

18. Van Hecke W, Nagels G, Leemans A, et al. Correlation of cognitive dysfunction and diffusion tensor MRI measures in patients with mild and moderate multiple sclerosis. J Magn Reson Imaging. 2010;31:1492–8.

19. Audoin B, Van Au Duong M, Ranjeva JP, et al. Magnetic resonance study of the influence of tissue damage and cortical reorganization on PASAT performance at the earliest stage of multiple sclerosis. Hum Brain Mapp. 2005;24:216–28.

20. Lin X, Tench CR, Morgan PS, et al. Use of combined conventional and quantitative MRI to quantify pathology related to cognitive impairment in multiple sclerosis. J Neurol Neurosurg Psychiatry. 2008;79:437–41.

21. Audoin B, Reuter F, Duong MVA, et al. Efficiency of cognitive control recruitment in the very early stage of multiple sclerosis: a one-year fMRI follow-up study. Mult Scler. 2008;14:786–92.

22. Cardinal KS, Wilson SM, Giesser BS, et al. A longitudinal fMRI study of the paced auditory serial addition test. Mult Scler. 2008;14:465–71.

23. Morgen K, Sammer G, Courtney SM, et al. Evidence for a direct association between cortical atrophy and cognitive impairment in relapsing-remitting MS. Neuroimage. 2006;30:891–8.

24. Bellmann-Strobl J, Wuerfel J, Aktas O, et al. Poor PASAT performance correlates with MRI contrast enhancement in multiple sclerosis. Neurology. 2009;73:1624–7.

25. Kiiski H, Reilly RB, Lonergan R, et al. Change in PASAT performance correlates with change in P3 ERP amplitude over a 12-month period in multiple sclerosis patients. J Neurol Sci. 2011;305:45–52.

26. Jongen PJ, Sindic C, Carton H, et al. Improvement of health-related quality of life in relapsing remitting multiple sclerosis patients after 2 years of treatment with intramuscular interferon-beta-1a. J Neurol. 2010;257:584–9.

27. Hayton T, Furby J, Smith KJ, et al. Clinical and imaging correlates of the multiple sclerosis impact scale in secondary progressive multiple sclerosis. J Neurol. 2012;259:237–45.

28. Rosti E, Hämäläinen P, Koivisto K, et al. One-year follow-up study of relapsing-remitting MS patients' cognitive performances: Paced Auditory Serial Addition Test's susceptibility to change. J Int Neuropsychol Soc. 2007;13:791–8.

29. Smith SM, Zhang Y, Jenkinson M, et al. Accurate, robust and automated longitudinal and cross-sectional brain change analysis. Neuroimage. 2002;17:479–89.

30. Patenaude B, Smith SM, Kennedy D, Jenkinson M. A Bayesian model of shape and appearance for subcortical brain. Neuroimage. 2011;56(3):907–22.

31. Fischl B, Salat DH, Busa E, et al. Whole brain segmentation: automated labeling of neuroanatomical structures in the human brain. Neuron. 2002;33:341–55.

32. Fischl B, van der Kouwe A, Destrieux C, et al. Automatically parcellating the human cerebral cortex. Cereb Cortex. 2004;14:11–22.

33. Shilling V, Jenkins V, Morris R, et al. The effects of adjuvant chemotherapy on cognition in women with breast cancer - preliminary results of an observational longitudinal study. Breast. 2005;14:142–50.

34. Solari A, Radice D, Manneschi L, et al. The multiple sclerosis functional composite: different practice effects in the three test components. J Neurol Sci. 2005;228:71–4.

35. Walker LA, Berard JA, Berrigan LI, et al. Detecting cognitive fatigue in multiple sclerosis: method matters. J Neurol Sci. 2012;316(1-2):86–92.

36. Stewart A, Bielajew C, Collins B, et al. A meta-analysis of the neuropsychological effects of adjuvant chemotherapy treatment in women treated for breast cancer. Clin Neuropsychol. 2006;20:76–89.

37. Collins B, Mackenzie J, Stewart A, et al. Cognitive effects of chemotherapy in post-menopausal breast cancer patients 1 year after treatment. Psychooncology. 2009;18:134–43.

38. Schagen SB, Muller MJ, Boogerd W, et al. Late effects of adjuvant chemotherapy on cognitive function: a followup study in breast cancer patients. Ann Oncol. 2002;132:1387–97.

14

Increased expression of dedicator-cytokinesis-10, caspase-2 and Synaptotagmin-like 2 is associated with clinical disease activity in multiple sclerosis

Ion Agirrezabal[1], Ricardo Palacios[1], Beatriz Moreno[1], Jorge Sepulcre[2], Alice Abernathy[1], Albert Saiz[1], Sara Llufriu[1], Manuel Comabella[3], Xavier Montalban[3], Antonio Martinez[4], David Arteta[4] and Pablo Villoslada[1,5*]

Abstract

Background: We aim to identify differentially expressed genes (DEGs) and its pathways associated with clinical activity of relapsing–remitting Multiple Sclerosis (RRMS).

Methods: We screened DEG in blood samples from patients with clinically stable or active RRMS (≥ 2 relapses or increase in ≥ 1 point in the EDSS (due to relapses) in 2 years follow-up), and healthy controls using DNA arrays. The DEGs identified were validated by RT-PCR in a prospective cohort of MS patients. We used Gene Ontology (GO) analysis for identifying the associated pathways and Jaspar database for identifying the associated transcriptions factors.

Results: We identified 45 DEG between the three groups (stable RRMS, active RRMS and control), being 14 of them significantly different between stable and active RRMS. We validated 14 out of the 45 DEG in the second cohort, eight out of the 14 being differentially expressed between active and stable patients (ARHGEF7, CASP2, DOCK10, DSP, ITPR1, KLDHC5, RBBP4, SYTL2). We found an overrepresentation of several pathways associated with lymphocyte activation. The analysis of regulatory networks identified the gene triplet of Dedicator of Cytokinesis-10 (DOCK10) – Caspase-2 (CASP2) - Synaptotagmin-like 2 (SYTL2) as being co-regulated by common transcription factors, pointing to lymphocyte activation pathways associated with disease activity.

Conclusions: We describe the triplet DOCK10 - CASP2 - SYTL2 as associated with the clinical activity of RRMS that suggest the role of lymphocyte activation, type 1 interferon and MAPkinase pathways in driving the presence of new relapses and disability accumulation.

Keywords: Multiple sclerosis, Biomarker, Disease activity, EDSS, Relapse rate, Gene expression pattern, Differentially expressed gene, DOCK10, CASP2, SYTL2, T cell activation, B cell activation

* Correspondence: pvilloslada@clinic.ub.es
[1]Center of Neuroimmunology, Institut d'Investigacions Biomèdiques August Pi i Sunyer (IDIBAPS) - Hospital Clinic of Barcelona, Barcelona, Spain
[5]University of California, San Francisco, USA
Full list of author information is available at the end of the article

Background

Multiple sclerosis (MS) is a clinically heterogeneous disease with a largely unpredictable course in individual patients. Clinical management of MS is hampered by the difficulty in obtaining an accurate prognosis. To achieve an accurate prognosis during the early or mid-stages of the disease, and to monitor both disease course and the response to therapy, it is essential to identify clinical or biological markers that can serve as surrogate end-points of the phenotype [1–4]. Such biomarkers would also greatly facilitate the design and monitoring of clinical trials to test new disease-modifying drugs by identifying the most appropriate patient subgroups for a specific therapy of interest.

The activity of relapsing-remitting MS (RRMS) is defined by the presence of new clinical relapses, presence of new lesions in the MRI, or increase in disability due to such relapses. The underlying pathogenesis of RRMS activity is therefore dependent on the presence of new inflammatory plaques within the brain parenchyma, as a result of the activation of the immune system. At present, it is not well known which pathways are activated during relapses and which ones are critical for defining a more active disease activity [5]. Previous gene expression studies have identified several genes such as GPR3, NFKB, SOCS3, STAT3, STAT1, CX3CR1, IDO, SLC9A9, HO-1 among others, associated with a more active disease [6–16]. However, at present none of such genes have been validated as a known biomarker of disease activity in MS and also, the pathways driving a more active disease are not well known [2, 5].

In the present study, we sought to identify gene signature patterns and pathways associated with RRMS and associated with clinical activity (relapses and disability worsening). Although clinical activity was defined prospectively, our study did not included MRI assessment, limiting the definition of disease activity and the opportunity to relate findings with imaging markers. We first screened gene expression from blood using DNA arrays to identify gene expression patterns that distinguish between clinically stable and active disease. Then, we validated these genes by RT-PCR in an independent prospective cohort of RRMS patients. Finally, we analyzed the regulatory network of validated genes, identifying a gene triplet composed by DOCK10, CASP2 and SYTL2 that pointed to interferon and T and B cell activation pathways as associated with disease activity in MS.

Methods

Subjects

We recruited two cohorts of patients with RRMS defined using the 2005 criteria [17]. Patients were classified as having clinically stable or active disease using following definitions: 1) stable disease - no relapses and no changes in the EDSS score during 2 years of follow-up; 2) active

disease - 2 or more relapses or a 1-point increase in the EDSS score due to relapses during 2 years of follow-up. The screening cohort contained RRMS patients in the early to mid phase of the disease: stable MS patients (n = 3; sex: 1 M/2 F; age: 38 ± 6 years; disease duration: 7 ± 0.8 years; relapse rate during the 2 years follow-up: 0; EDSS: 0 [range: 0–1]); active MS patients (n = 3; sex: 1 M/2 F; age: 33 ± 7 years; disease duration: 3 ± 0.5 years; relapse rate over the 2 years follow-up: 2.5 ± 0.5, EDSS: 3 [range: 2–4]); and healthy controls (n = 3; sex: 1 M/2 F; age: 36). None of the patients in the screening cohort were treated with disease modifying therapies at the time of the study or in the previous month. The validation cohort was a longitudinal prospective cohort of RRMS, including stable MS patients (n = 20; sex: 5 M/15 F; age: 34.0 ± 5.3 years; disease duration: 2.6 ± 2.3; relapses follow-up: 0; EDSS: 0.6 ± 0.7), active MS patients (n = 20; sex: 10 M/10 F; age: 30.5 ± 4.5; disease duration: 9.7 ± 6.6; relapse rate 2 years follow-up: 2.0 ± 0.5; EDSS: 3.8 ± 1.4) and sex and age matched healthy controls (n = 20; sex: 8 M/12 F; age: 32.5 ± 9.6 years). Use of DMTs (Interferon-beta or Glatiramer acetate) were allowed in the validation cohort, and 33 % of patients were receiving either therapy. Definition of clinical disease activity in this validation cohort was based in longitudinal prospective data and disability worsening was confirmed 6 months apart.

Ethics, consent and permissions

This study was approved by the Ethics committee of the Hospital Clinic of Barcelona. Patients were invited to participate by their neurologist after signing informed consent.

RNA extraction and DNA arrays

RNA was obtained from whole blood in the screening cohort using the PAXgene™ Blood RNA Kit (Quiagen). For the validation cohort, RNA was obtained from PBMCs purified using the Ficoll-Paque gradient system (Pharmacia Biotech). PBMCs were stored in RNAlater stabilization solution (Applied Biosystems) at – 80 °C until RNA extraction was performed. RNA was purified using the RNeasy Mini Kit and digested with the RNase Free DNase Set (both from Qiagen). The quality and quantity of the RNA was determined using a NanoDrop 2000 spectrophotometer and its integrity assessed using a 2100 bioanalyzer (Agilent Technologies). For DNA array analysis, RNA (6 μg) was transcribed to cDNA using the SuperScript Choice System (Life Technologies) according to the Affymetrix Expression Analysis Technical Manual. Subsequently, cRNA was synthesized using the BioArray HighYield RNA Transcript Labeling kit (Enzo), purified with the Kit Clean-up module (Affymetrix) and finally hybridized to the HG-U133 Plus 2.0 DNA array (Affymetrix). For the validation and treatment cohorts, cDNA synthesis was performed from total RNA using the High-Capacity cDNA Archive Kit

(Applied Biosystems). Raw DNA array data was uploaded to the ArrayExpress database (accession code E-GEOD-2012082010000219) (Additional file 1).

Real time PCR
RT-PCR was performed using Low Density Arrays (LDA: Applied Biosystems) that were designed selecting TaqMan assays provided by Applied Biosystems for 45 genes plus five housekeeping genes using the following criteria: 1) minimal distance between the Affymetrix probe set and the Applied Biosystems probe set; 2) no genomic DNA detection (Additional file 2). All samples were analyzed in duplicate (384 wells) and the arrays were analyzed in

triplicate. RT-PCR was carried out in the 7900 Fast Real-Time PCR system using TaqMan Gene Expression Master Mix kit (both from Applied Biosystems) as follows: 2 min at 50 °C; 10 min at 94.5 °C; 40 cycles of 30 s at 97 °C, 1 min at 59.7 °C and 4 °C indefinitely [18]. SDS 2.2.1 software was used to analyze migration on microfluid plates.

Western blot analysis
Protein levels of DOCK10, CASP2 and SYTL2 were measured by Western blots from brain tissue as previously described [6]. Antibodies used for Western blot were as follows: mouse anti-DOCK10 (Novus Biologicals), mouse

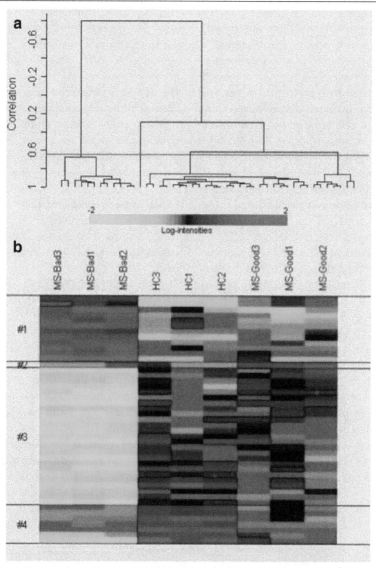

Fig. 1 Screening for differentially expressed genes in controls and in patients with clinically stable or active RRMS. 45 genes differentially expressed between all 3 conditions in patients with stable MS (MS-good), active MS (MS-bad) and controls (HC) were found. **a** Cluster analysis identified 4 clusters of genes using as a cut-off a correlation of 0.65; **b** shows the heat map of the 45 DEG grouped in the 4 clusters indentified (F-test after FDR correction)

Table 1 Differentially expressed genes between clinically stable MS, active MS and controls by DNA array analysis (Additional file 1)

Cluster	Gene symbol	p-value	Description
Cluster #1	TNPO1	2.00E-07	Transportin 1
	CXCR3	0.0009282	Chemokine (C-X-C motif) receptor 3
	ATP9A	0.0007041	ATPase, Class II, type 9A
	CASP2	0.0003848	Caspase 2
	PRX	0.0009587	Periaxin
	DSP	0.0006427	Desmoplakin
	MALAT1	0.0009593	Metastasis associated lung adenocarcinoma transcript 1; PRO1073
	CXorf56	0.0001169	chromosome X open reading frame 56, hypothetical protein FLJ22965
	SSBP4	2.07E-05	single stranded DNA binding protein 4
	CCT8	2.13E-05	Chaperonin containing TCP1, subunit 8 (theta)
		9.61E-05	Homo sapiens cDNA clone IMAGE:4824925
	ELSPBP1	0.0006039	Epididymal sperm binding protein 1
Cluster #2	**DOCK10**	0.0003135	Dedicator of cytokinesis 10
Cluster #3	**ZNF75**	0.0005587	Zinc finger protein 75 (D8C6)
	MRS2L	0.0007168	MRS2-like, magnesium homeostasis factor (S. cerevisiae)
	TTC10	0.0006527	Tetratricopeptide repeat domain 10, IFT88: intraflagellar transport 88
		0.0002011	Homo sapiens cDNA clone IMAGE:2348094 3
	MIA3	0.0004529	Melanoma inhibitory activity family, member 3, C219-reactive peptide
	KMO	7.40E-06	Kynurenine 3-monooxygenase (kynurenine 3-hydroxylase)
	FREB	1.19E-05	Fc receptor homolog expressed in B cells; FCRLA
	MRPL16	0.0005844	Mitochondrial ribosomal protein L16
	RNFT1	0.0004832	ring finger protein, transmembrane 1; PTD016 protein
	PRO1693	0.0002505	Homo sapiens PRO1693 protein
	ANXA4	0.0002741	Annexin A4
	MTM1	0.0004095	Myotubularin 1
	KLHDC5	0.0004232	Kelch domain containing 5; KIAA1340 protein
	METTL21A	2.0004554	Methyltransferase like 21A
	RBBP4	0.0003732	Retinoblastoma binding protein 4
	PPP2CB	0.0008942	Protein phosphatase 2, catalytic subunit, beta isoform
	TRAPPC11	0.0003224	Trafficking protein particle complex subunit 11 isoform a
	SLC7A7	0.0008726	Solute carrier family 7 (cationic amino acid transporter, y + system)
	ALG13	0.0005845	Asparagine-linked glycosylation 13 homolog; chromosome X ORF45
	PDIA3	0.000489	Protein disulfide isomerase family A; glucose regulated protein, 58 kDa
	INPP4A	0.0007406	Inositol polyphosphate-4-phosphatase, type I, 107 kDa
	TFEC	0.0002318	Transcription factor EC
	DDX23	0.0006295	DEAD (Asp-Glu-Ala-Asp) box polypeptide 23

Table 1 Differentially expressed genes between clinically stable MS, active MS and controls by DNA array analysis (Additional file 1) *(Continued)*

	KIFAP3	0.0003059	Kinesin-associated protein 3
	NEK4	0.0002713	NIMA (never in mitosis gene a)-related kinase 4
Cluster #4	ZNF24	0.0009911	Zinc finger protein 24 (KOX 17)
	BTBD7	6.14E-05	BTB (POZ) domain containing 7
	ITPR1	0.0003003	Inositol 1,4,5-triphosphate receptor, type 1
	WDR20	1.07E-05	WD repeat domain 20
	LOC100507376	3.00E-07	CDNA FLJ90295 fis, clone NT2RP2000240.
	SYTL2	0.0002614	Synaptotagmin-like 2
	ARHGEF7	0.0003018	Rho guanine nucleotide exchange factor (GEF) 7

We identified 45 DEGs between stable MS, active MS and healthy controls (F-test, FDR corrected *p*-value). Cluster analysis grouped the DEG in 4 clusters. Genes validated in the second cohort are highlighted in bold

anti-CASP2 and mouse anti-SYTL2 (both from Santa Cruz).

Bioinformatics analysis

In order to estimate the power of our analysis, we assumed that 95 % of the evaluated probes were not differentially expressed. We aimed to detect an isolated mean difference of 1 in log-expression between groups, and set to control the rate of false positives at 10 %. Assuming a standard deviation of 0.5 in the difference in log-expression between groups, the power of our analysis was 0.65. Therefore, it could be expected that 65 % of genes that showed a two-fold differential expression between any of the groups would be identified.

DNA array results were normalized using Micro-array Suite 5.0 (MAS 5.0; Affymetrix®) and analyzed using the Biometric Research Branch (BRB) Array Tools 3.2.3 (Dr Richard Simon and Amy Peng Lam). To filter the genes with the BRB software we used the following

criteria: 1) genes with an intensity >10 were assigned a value of 10; 2) genes were deleted if in the < 20 % of cases the change gene expression was < 1.5 with respect to the median, if the percentage of missing values was > 50 %, or if the percentage of absents was > 70 %. For group comparison we used the F-test and for pair group comparison we used *T*-test, with a significance threshold set to $p < 0.001$. Multiple comparisons were adjusted using the false discovery method with the significance threshold was set to $p < 0.05$. For LDA analysis, we first discarded samples with an SD > 0.38. The normalization factor was calculated using geNorm software (https://gen-orm.cmgg.be) and normalized values were transformed to a logarithmic scale. For group comparison we used the Kruskal-Wallis and for pair group comparison we used Mann–Whitney U non-parametric tests, with a significance threshold set to $p < 0.01$. Multiple comparisons were performed using the Bonferroni method with the significance threshold was set to $p < 0.05$. Statistical

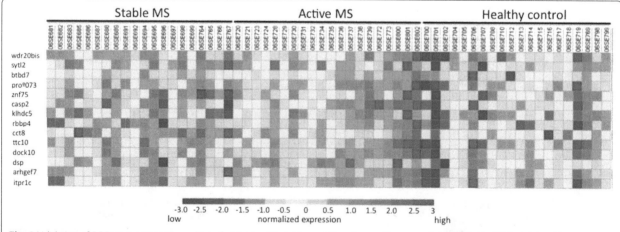

Fig. 2 Validation of DEGs in a prospective cohort of patients with stable or active disease. Heat map showing the 14 DEGs validated by RT-PCR in the validation cohort: ARHGEF7, BTBD7, CASP2, CCT8, DOCK10, DSP, ITPR1, KLDHC5, PRO1073, RBBP4, SYTL2, TTC10, WDR20, ZNF75. The normalization factor was calculated using geNorm software and normalized values were transformed to a logarithmic scale. Group comparison were performed using the Kruskal-Wallis test with a significance threshold set to $p < 0.01$ after correction for multiple testing (Bonferoni)

analyses were performed using SPSS 11.0 (SPSS Inc., Chicago, USA) and R software (R Core Development Team, 2011). Correlation between DEG in the array and RT-PCR study was 0.379. Gene Ontology was analyzed using Genecodis software (http://www.cnb.csic.es). To identify transcription factors (TF) that act as common regulators of the genes of interest, we searched for common TF binding sites based on frequency matrices obtained from the Jaspar database [19], using the position specific weight matrix (PSWM) method with both PSCAN [20] and R software.

Results

Patients with either clinically active or stable RRMS were screened, along with healthy sex- and age-matched controls. RNA extracted from whole blood was analyzed using the HG-U133 Plus 2.0 DNA array (Affymetrix), obtaining 14,705 of the 54,675 available probes which fulfilled the criteria for analysis. We performed group analysis and pairwise comparisons between each of the three groups. The group analysis identified 45 differentially expressed genes (DEGs) grouped in four clusters between the three groups (F-test, $p < 0.001$, FDR correction) (Fig. 1; Table 1; Additional file 3). Genes GABPA; FREB; ZNF146; GATA3; KMO; MSH2; GP1BA; DSP; GIPC2; HAK; SSBP4; SP192; MGC35130; KIAA0826; C6orf115 significantly discriminate between patients with clinically stable and active disease (T-test, $p < 0.001$, FDR correction). To validate the DEGs associated with clinical activity in RRMS, we analyzed the expression of the DEGs by RT-PCR in a second independent cohort of MS patients. We determined which genes differed significantly between the three conditions, validating 14 out of the

previously identified 45 DEGs that differed significantly (Kruskal-Wallis test, $p < 0.01$ after Bonferroni correction for multiple testing): ARHGEF7, BTBD7, CASP2, CCT8, DOCK10, DSP, ITPR1, KLDHC5, MALAT-1 (PRO1073), RBBP4, SYTL2, IFT88 (TTC10), WDR20, ZNF75 (Fig. 2). Eight out these 14 genes, ARHGEF7, CASP2, DOCK10, DSP, ITPR1, KLDHC5, RBBP4, SYTL2, were expressed significantly different between MS patients with clinically stable or active disease (Mann–Whitney U test, $p < 0.01$ after Bonferroni correction for multiple testing).

In order to obtain insights about the biological role of the validated DEGs we performed Gene Ontology (GO) analysis and regulatory network analysis. The GO analysis of the DEGs revealed an overrepresentation of several pathways associated with lymphocyte activation as follows: a) GO biological process: B cell receptor signaling pathway, and positive regulation of apoptosis; b) GO molecular functions: Rho GTPase binding, Rab GTPase binding and GTPase binding; c) Enrichment analysis of KEGG pathways: cell adhesion molecules and T cell receptor signaling. In order to analyze the regulatory networks associated with the validated DEGs associated with disease activity, we searched for high correlation in gene expression as indication or co-regulated expression.

Among the 14 DEGs, we found only one triplet with high degree of correlation between their expression levels (by pairwise correlation). The expression of the triplet DOCK10, CASP2 and SYTL2 was highly correlated (DOCK10/CASP2: $r = 0.799$; $p = 1.637e\text{-}11$; DOCK10/SYTL2: $r = 0.591$; $p = 1.218e\text{-}05$; and CASP2/SYTL: $r = 0.613$; $p = 4.506e\text{-}06$; Fig. 3), which would suggest the existence of master regulators for these gene triplet. The gene expression levels of the gene triplet DOCK10, CASP2

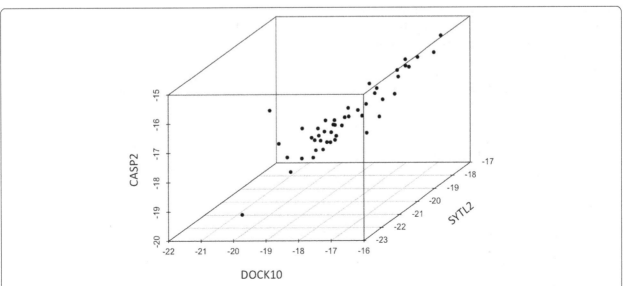

Fig. 3 Correlation of DOCK10, SYTL and CASP2 gene expression. The correlation of the gene expression levels of DOCK10, SYTL and CASP2 obtained by RT-PCR were performed using the Spearman correlation ($R^2 = 0.65$)

and SYTL2 were found to be increased in patients with MS (both clinically stable and active disease) compared to controls both in the DNA array as well as in the RT-PCR assays. Also, we analyzed protein levels of the triplet DOCK10, CASP2 and SYTL2 in PBMCs from MS patients and healthy controls. We observed higher levels of Dock10 and Sytl2 protein in MS patients compared with controls, and we observed a decrease in Caspase-2 in patients at protein level (Fig. 4). In order to search for common regulators of the expression of the gene triplet we performed a TF binding site prediction for DOCK10, CASP2 and SYTL2 genes. We identified 8 TF as potential master regulators: MAFB, STAT1, MYF5, FOXQ1, TCF3, SOX9, SRY and INSM1 (Table 2). A subsequent search of the Reactome and KEGG databases revealed that the top two TF MAFB and STAT1 are the downstream TF of the type I IFN and MAP kinase pathways.

Discussion

We found a gene expression signature associated with higher clinically disease activity in patients with RRMS. To identify pathways associated with such increased clinically disease activity, a bioinformatics search revealed the gene triplet DOCK10, CASP2 and SYTL2, which are activated in concert by the MAFB, STAT1 and MYF transcription factors. This pattern suggests the activation of type I IFN and MAPkinase pathways in response to immune cell receptor activation, which is in agreement with previous studies showing dysregulation of type I interferon pathway in MS [21, 22]. In addition, GO analysis revealed the involvement of several pathways related with lymphocyte activation (Fig. 5).

Several gene expression patterns associated with disease activity in MS have been identified previously, implicating T-cell activation and expansion, inflammation and apoptosis/cell cycle regulation in disease activity [7–9, 13, 23–26]. Biological processes that involve DEGs include the immune response, cell adhesion, cell differentiation, cellular component movement, signal transduction, blood coagulation, axon guidance, DNA and RNA transcription regulation, and the regulation of cell proliferation. Several of the TFs identified in the present study have previously been implicated in MS disease activity by the ANZ consortium [27], including TCF, MYB and the SOX family. Our findings strongly support the involvement of T and B cell activation, immune cell signaling, such as type I interferon signaling, and the regulation of cell proliferation in the pathogenesis and severity of MS. Further validation of these biomarkers in multicenter clinical studies will be required to assess its robustness in different platforms and centers.

The DOCK10/CASP2/SYTL2 gene triplet has been implicated in lymphocyte activation and function (Fig. 5). DOCK10 is a member of the dedicator of cytokinesis family, which acts as activator of the Rho family of small

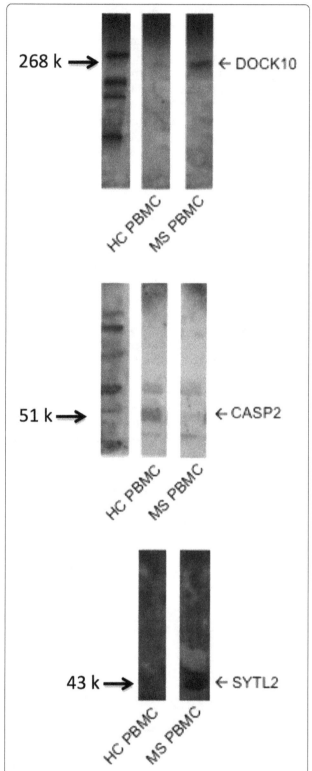

Fig. 4 Dock10, SYTL and CASP2 protein levels in PBMCs from MS patients. Representative Western blots probed to assess the Dock10, SYTL and CASP2 protein levels in PBMCs from patients and controls

Table 2 Transcription factors associated with the MS gene expression pattern

TF	Function	p
MAFB	Transcription factor MafB	0.000198
STAT1	Signal transducer and activator of transcription 1	0.001521
MYF5	Myogenic factor 5	0.005987
TCF3	Transcription factor E2-alpha	0.019014
SOX9	Transcription factor SOX-9	0.024095
SRY	Sex-determining region Y protein	0.029105
FOXQ1	Forkhead box protein Q1	0.037121
INSM1	Insulinoma-associated protein 1	0.047677

Identification of the transcription factors (TF) associated with DOCK10, CASP2 and SYTL2 triplet, using the Jaspar database. Results are presented using the name of the TF in the Jaspar database and the p value of the position-specific weight matrix analysis, ranked by the p value

GTPases and mediates signaling by G-protein receptors, cytokine receptors (protein-kinases), integrins and cadherins [28]. Dock10 is mainly expressed in lymphocytes, and it is activated by the IL-4 and Rho pathways [28], exhibiting differential splicing between T and B cells [29]. Statins modulate the activity of Rho GTPases, which contributes to the induction of the Th2 phenotype and ameliorates disease severity in an animal model of MS [30]. Finally, DOCK10 is also involved in dendrite spine morphogenesis [31]. Taken together with the present results, these findings implicate DOCK-10 in increased MS disease activity through its effects on lymphocyte migration and their differentiation to the Th2 phenotype, and B cell activation.

Caspase 2 (CASP2) is a protease that is activated in response to stress (DNA damage) and it appears to participate more in the regulation of the cell cycle than in apoptosis [32]. Moreover, CASP2 acts as a tumor suppressor by inducing cell cycle arrest. CASP2 is highly

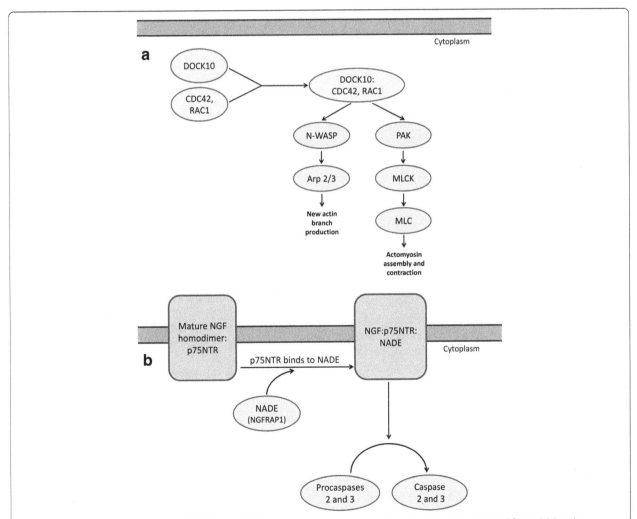

Fig. 5 Biological pathways involved in DOCK10 and CASP2 function. Pathways related with both genes were obtained from KEGG and Reactome databases

expressed in B cells during the plasmablast stage of differentiation [33], and is overexpressed in MS patients during relapses and in response to interferon-beta or intravenous immunoglobulin therapy [34–36]. In addition, CASP2 is involved specifically in apoptosis in neuronal cells [36, 37]. Together with its modulation of the immune response, this observation strongly suggests that CASP2 contributes to the dampening of lymphocyte proliferation. We believe differences in CASP2 RNA and protein levels in our study should be related with functional regulation of this protein. One hypothesis is that the increase in protein levels may be due to higher stability or lower degradation of this protein in immune cells from MS patients. Such higher levels may suppress the levels of RNA expression as a negative feedback. Alternatively, regulation of CASP2 gene expression and efficiency to translation to protein may differ in MS patients compared to controls, probably due to pro-inflammatory state, leading to higher protein levels even with lower RNA synthesis.

Synaptotagmin-like 2 (SYTL2 or SLP2) is a member of a C2 domain-containing protein family and it is involved in RAB27A-dependent vesicular trafficking. Among other functions, SYTL2 participates in the maturation of immune synapses in cytotoxic T cells in order to promote the exocytoxis of cytotoxic granules containing perforin [38]. Interestingly, SYTL2 is required for mitochondrial fusion in response to cellular stress [39], which is critical for the restoration of mitochondrial function after stress damage [40]. Its mode of action suggests that SYTL2 participates in the stress response during inflammation.

There are several limitations of the present study that should be noted. The definitions of "active" and "stable" disease are based on the clinical expression of the disease and thus, they do not account for sub-clinical activity revealed by MRI. For this reason, our findings only apply to clinically active disease and we were not able to correlate our findings with imaging markers of disease activity. Nevertheless, misclassification of patients due to lack of MRI would increase the number of false negatives more than the number of false positives, suggesting that validated biomarkers of the proposed phenotype will persist even in the presence of the noise generated due to inaccurate clinical descriptions [3]. Although our datasets were small, we followed a sequential analysis in independent cohorts for reducing number of genes and test performed. Overall, this strategy decreased the risk of false positives, which is the main limitation in gene expression studies.

Conclusion

In summary, we describe a gene expression pattern composed by DOCK10, CASP2 and SYTL2, which is associated with a more active course of disease in patients with RRMS. The biological function of the genes and pathways identified suggest that clinical disease activity in the early to medium phase of MS is associated with increased activation of the adaptive immune system, involving both T and B cells. Additional studies will be required to further validate this molecular biomarker as well as for validating such therapeutic targets for MS and other autoimmune diseases.

Competing interest
PV has received consultancy honoraria from Roche, Novartis,, Digna Biotech; contract grants from Roche and Novartis and is shareholder in Bionure Farma SL. All other authors have no conflict of interest with this work.

Authors' contribution
IA, BM, RP, AA and JS carried out the RT-PCR and western-blot studies. AM and DA performed the array studies. JS, AS, SL, MC and XM contributed with samples and clinical data and classified individuals based in disease activity. IA, RP and DA performed the bioinformatic analysis. PV conceived of the study, and participated in its design and coordination and drafted the manuscript. All authors read and approved the final manuscript.

Acknowledgements
This study was supported by grants from the Spanish Ministry of Science (PSE-010000-2008-5) and Fundacion Cellex to PV, the Instituto de Salud Carlos III - Red Española de Esclerosis Multiple (RED07-0060) to PV, AS and XM, and the 7th EU Framework Programme (Marie Curie initial training network UEPHA*MS; grant agreement n° 212877) to PV and MC.

Disclosure
PV has received consultancy honoraria from Roche, Novartis, MedImmune, Heidelberg Engineering, Neurotec Farma, Digna Biotech; contract grants from Roche and Novartis and is shareholder in Bionure Farma SL.

Author details
[1]Center of Neuroimmunology, Institut d'Investigacions Biomèdiques August Pi i Sunyer (IDIBAPS) - Hospital Clinic of Barcelona, Barcelona, Spain. [2]Division of Nuclear Medicine and Molecular Imaging, Department of Radiology, Harvard Medical School, Boston, USA. [3]Department of Neurology-Neuroimmunology, Centre d'Esclerosi Múltiple de Catalunya, Cemcat, Hospital Universitari Vall d'Hebron (HUVH), Barcelona, Spain. [4]Progenica SL, Zamudio, Spain. [5]University of California, San Francisco, USA.

References
1. Martin R, Bielekova B, Hohlfeld R, Utz U. Biomarkers in multiple sclerosis. Dis Markers. 2006;22(4):183–5.
2. Villoslada P. Biomarkers for multiple sclerosis. Drug News Perspect. 2010;23(9):585–95.
3. Graber JJ, Dhib-Jalbut S. Biomarkers of disease activity in multiple sclerosis. J Neurol Sci. 2011;305(1–2):1–10.
4. Villoslada P, Baranzini S. Data integration and systems biology approaches for biomarker discovery: challenges and opportunities for multiple sclerosis. J Neuroimmunol. 2012;248(1–2):58–65.
5. Kotelnikova E, Bernardo-Faura M, Silberberg G, Kiani NA, Messinis D, Melas IN, et al. Signaling networks in MS: a systems-based approach to developing new pharmacological therapies. Mult Scler. 2015;21(2):138–46.
6. Moreno B, Hevia H, Santamaria M, Sepulcre J, Munoz J, Garcia-Trevijano ER, et al. Methylthioadenosine reverses brain autoimmune disease. Ann Neurol. 2006;60:323–34.

7. Hecker M, Paap BK, Goertsches RH, Kandulski O, Fatum C, Koczan D, et al. Reassessment of blood gene expression markers for the prognosis of relapsing-remitting multiple sclerosis. PLoS One. 2011;6(12):e29648.

8. Gurevich M, Tuller T, Rubinstein U, Or-Bach R, Achiron A. Prediction of acute multiple sclerosis relapses by transcription levels of peripheral blood cells. BMC Med Genomics. 2009;2:46.

9. Satoh J, Misawa T, Tabunoki H, Yamamura T. Molecular network analysis of T-cell transcriptome suggests aberrant regulation of gene expression by NF-kappaB as a biomarker for relapse of multiple sclerosis. Dis Markers. 2008; 25(1):27–35.

10. Frisullo G, Mirabella M, Angelucci F, Caggiula M, Morosetti R, Sancricca C, et al. The effect of disease activity on leptin, leptin receptor and suppressor of cytokine signalling-3 expression in relapsing-remitting multiple sclerosis. J Neuroimmunol. 2007;192(1–2):174–83.

11. Frisullo G, Angelucci F, Caggiula M, Nociti V, Iorio R, Patanella AK, et al. pSTAT1, pSTAT3, and T-bet expression in peripheral blood mononuclear cells from relapsing-remitting multiple sclerosis patients correlates with disease activity. J Neurosci Res. 2006;84(5):1027–36.

12. Infante-Duarte C, Weber A, Kratzschmar J, Prozorovski T, Pikol S, Hamann I, et al. Frequency of blood CX3CR1-positive natural killer cells correlates with disease activity in multiple sclerosis patients. FASEB J. 2005;19(13):1902–4.

13. Achiron A, Gurevich M, Friedman N, Kaminski N, Mandel M. Blood transcriptional signatures of multiple sclerosis: unique gene expression of disease activity. Ann Neurol. 2004;55(3):410–7.

14. Mancuso R, Hernis A, Agostini S, Rovaris M, Caputo D, Fuchs D, et al. Indoleamine 2,3 dioxygenase (IDO) expression and activity in relapsing-remitting multiple sclerosis. PLoS One. 2015;10(6):e0130715.

15. Esposito F, Sorosina M, Ottoboni L, Lim ET, Replogle JM, Raj T, et al. A pharmacogenetic study implicates SLC9a9 in multiple sclerosis disease activity. Ann Neurol. 2015;78(1):115–27.

16. Fagone P, Patti F, Mangano K, Mammana S, Coco M, Touil-Boukoffa C, et al. Heme oxygenase-1 expression in peripheral blood mononuclear cells correlates with disease activity in multiple sclerosis. J Neuroimmunol. 2013; 261(1–2):82–6.

17. Polman CH, Reingold SC, Edan G, Filippi M, Hartung HP, Kappos L, et al. Diagnostic criteria for multiple sclerosis: 2005 revisions to the "McDonald Criteria". Ann Neurol. 2005;58(6):840–6.

18. Di Penta A, Moreno B, Reix S, Fernandez-Diez B, Villanueva M, Errea O, et al. Oxidative stress and proinflammatory cytokines contribute to demyelination and axonal damage in a cerebellar culture model of neuroinflammation. PloSONE. 2013;8(2):e54722.

19. Bryne JC, Valen E, Tang MH, Marstrand T, Winther O, da Piedade I, et al. JASPAR, the open access database of transcription factor-binding profiles: new content and tools in the 2008 update. Nucleic Acids Res. 2008; 36(Database issue):D102–6.

20. Zambelli F, Pesole G, Pavesi G. Pscan: finding over-represented transcription factor binding site motifs in sequences from co-regulated or co-expressed genes. Nucleic Acids Res. 2009;37(Web Server issue):W247–52.

21. Comabella M, Lunemann JD, Rio J, Sanchez A, Lopez C, Julia E, et al. A type I interferon signature in monocytes is associated with poor response to interferon-beta in multiple sclerosis. Brain. 2009;132(Pt 12):3353–65.

22. Baranzini SE, Mousavi P, Rio J, Caillier SJ, Stillman A, Villoslada P, et al. Transcription-based prediction of response to IFNbeta using supervised computational methods. PLoSBiol. 2005;3(1):e2.

23. Satoh J, Nakanishi M, Koike F, Onoue H, Aranami T, Yamamoto T, et al. T cell gene expression profiling identifies distinct subgroups of Japanese multiple sclerosis patients. J Neuroimmunol. 2006;174(1–2):108–18.

24. Achiron A, Gurevich M, Snir Y, Segal E, Mandel M. Zinc-ion binding and cytokine activity regulation pathways predicts outcome in relapsing-remitting multiple sclerosis. Clin Exp Immunol. 2007;149(2):235–42.

25. Corvol JC, Pelletier D, Henry RG, Caillier SJ, Wang J, Pappas D, et al. Abrogation of T cell quiescence characterizes patients at high risk for multiple sclerosis after the initial neurological event. Proc Natl Acad Sci U S A. 2008;105(33):11839–44.

26. Ottoboni L, Keenan BT, Tamayo P, Kuchroo M, Mesirov JP, Buckle GJ, et al. An RNA profile identifies two subsets of multiple sclerosis patients differing in disease activity. Sci Transl Med. 2012;4(153):153ra31.

27. Riveros C, Mellor D, Gandhi KS, McKay FC, Cox MB, Berretta R, et al. A transcription factor map as revealed by a genome-wide gene expression analysis of whole-blood mRNA transcriptome in multiple sclerosis. PLoS One. 2010;5(12):e14176.

28. Yelo E, Bernardo MV, Gimeno L, Alcaraz-Garcia MJ, Majado MJ, Parrado A. Dock10, a novel CZH protein selectively induced by interleukin-4 in human B lymphocytes. Mol Immunol. 2008;45(12):3411–8.

29. Alcaraz-Garcia MJ, Ruiz-Lafuente N, Sebastian-Ruiz S, Majado MJ, Gonzalez-Garcia C, Bernardo MV, et al. Human and mouse DOCK10 splicing isoforms with alternative first coding exon usage are differentially expressed in T and B lymphocytes. Hum Immunol. 2011;72(7):531–7.

30. Paintlia AS, Paintlia MK, Singh AK, Singh I. Inhibition of rho family functions by lovastatin promotes myelin repair in ameliorating experimental autoimmune encephalomyelitis. Mol Pharmacol. 2008;73(5):1381–93.

31. Jaudon F, Raynaud F, Wehrle R, Bellanger JM, Doulazmi M, Vodjdani G, et al. The RhoGEF DOCK10 is essential for dendritic spine morphogenesis. Mol Biol Cell. 2015;26(11):2112–27.

32. Bouchier-Hayes L, Green DR. Caspase-2: the orphan caspase. Cell Death Differ. 2012;19(1):51–7.

33. Jourdan M, Reme T, Goldschmidt H, Fiol G, Pantesco V, De Vos J, et al. Gene expression of anti- and pro-apoptotic proteins in malignant and normal plasma cells. Br J Haematol. 2009;145(1):45–58.

34. Baranzini SE, Madireddy LR, Cromer A, D'Antonio M, Lehr L, Beelke M, et al. Prognostic biomarkers of IFNb therapy in multiple sclerosis patients. Mult Scler. 2015;21(7):894–904.

35. Pigard N, Elovaara I, Kuusisto H, Paalavuo R, Dastidar P, Zimmermann K, et al. Therapeutic activities of intravenous immunoglobulins in multiple sclerosis involve modulation of chemokine expression. J Neuroimmunol. 2009;209(1–2):114–20.

36. Hu HI, Chang HH, Sun DS. Differential regulation of caspase-2 in MPP(+)-induced apoptosis in primary cortical neurons. Exp Cell Res. 2015;332(1):60–6.

37. Vigneswara V, Akpan N, Berry M, Logan A, Troy CM, Ahmed Z. Combined suppression of CASP2 and CASP6 protects retinal ganglion cells from apoptosis and promotes axon regeneration through CNTF-mediated JAK/STAT signalling. Brain. 2014;137(Pt 6):1656–75.

38. Menasche G, Menager MM, Lefebvre JM, Deutsch E, Athman R, Lambert N, et al. A newly identified isoform of Slp2a associates with Rab27a in cytotoxic T cells and participates to cytotoxic granule secretion. Blood. 2008; 112(13):5052–62.

39. Tondera D, Grandemange S, Jourdain A, Karbowski M, Mattenberger Y, Herzig S, et al. SLP-2 is required for stress-induced mitochondrial hyperfusion. EMBO J. 2009;28(11):1589–600.

40. Court FA, Coleman MP. Mitochondria as a central sensor for axonal degenerative stimuli. Trends Neurosci. 2012;35(6):364–72.

15

Hippocampal neuroplasticity and inflammation: relevance for multiple sclerosis

Andrea Mancini[1], Lorenzo Gaetani[1], Maria Di Gregorio[1], Alessandro Tozzi[2,3], Veronica Ghiglieri[2,4], Paolo Calabresi[1,2] and Massimiliano Di Filippo[1*]

Abstract

Cognitive impairment is very frequent during multiple sclerosis (MS), involving approximately 40–70% of the patients, with a profound impact on patient's life. It is now established that among the various central nervous system (CNS) structures involved during the course of MS, the hippocampus is particularly sensitive to the detrimental effects of neuroinflammation. Different studies demonstrated hippocampal involvement during MS, in association with depression and cognitive impairment, such as verbal and visuo-spatial memory deficits, even during the earlier phases of the disease. These cognitive alterations could represent the visible consequences of a hidden synaptic impairment. Indeed, neuronal and immune functions are intertwined and the immune system is able to modulate the efficacy of synaptic transmission and the induction of the main forms of synaptic plasticity, such as long term potentiation (LTP). Hippocampal synaptic plasticity has been studied during the last decades as the physiological basis of human learning and memory and its disruption can be associated with behavioral and cognitive abnormalities. The aim of the present work is to review the available evidence about the presence of hippocampal synaptic plasticity alterations in experimental models of MS, specifically during the course of experimental autoimmune encephalomyelitis (EAE) and to discuss their relevance with regard to human MS. Indeed, the failure of synapses to express plasticity during neuroinflammation could potentially lead to a progressive failure of the brain plastic reserve, possibly contributing to disability progression and cognitive impairment during MS.

Keywords: Hippocampus, Multiple sclerosis, Synaptic plasticity, Neuroinflammation, Experimental autoimmune encephalomyelitis, Cognitive impairment

Background

Neurons and synapses are located behind the blood–brain barrier and the anatomical and functional characteristics of cerebral perfusion led to the erroneous believing that the physiology of neuronal communication could not be influenced by immune responses. Conversely, it is now well established that neuronal function is strongly influenced by both central and peripheral inflammation [1]. In particular, it has been shown that the immune system is able to modulate the efficacy of synaptic transmission and the induction of the main forms of synaptic plasticity [1]. Glial and microglial cells are now recognized as active elements of synapses, playing a central role in neuro-inflammatory processes [2–4]. Moreover, several soluble products that were thought to exclusively exert immunological functions, such as cytokines, are known to influence synaptic transmission during both physiological and pathological conditions [1, 5]. In particular, the inflammatory demyelinating process taking place during multiple sclerosis (MS), as well as systemic inflammatory triggers, could lead to the anomalous production of inflammatory mediators at synaptic sites with the subsequent disruption of synaptic homeostasis.

---
* Correspondence: massimiliano.difilippo@unipg.it
[1]Clinica Neurologica, Dipartimento di Medicina, Università degli Studi di Perugia, Ospedale Santa Maria della Misericordia, S. Andrea delle Fratte, Perugia 06132, Italy
Full list of author information is available at the end of the article

Systemic infections and chronic inflammatory processes are associated with behavioral and cognitive changes consisting in fatigue, depression, impaired learning and memory. These symptoms, all very frequent during MS, were collectively named as "sickness behavior" [6–8]. Specifically, during MS, cognitive impairment is very common with an important impact on patient's daily activities and quality of life [9] and it is detectable even during the earlier phases of the disease [9, 10]. Behavioral and cognitive alterations during MS could represent the clinical consequences of a subtle synaptic impairment, derived from an abnormal production of pro-inflammatory molecules by activated microglia during central inflammation [1, 11, 12]. Altered synaptic plasticity could shape the course of MS. Indeed, the plastic potential of the central nervous system (CNS) is fundamental to recover from brain injuries, and the disruption of the main forms of synaptic plasticity may exert a negative impact on disease progression and accumulation of disability [13, 14]. Among the various CNS sites involved in MS, the hippocampus is particularly vulnerable to the detrimental effects of neuroinflammation [15, 16]. Several studies demonstrated that hippocampal impairment is associated with depression and cognitive decline, such as verbal and visuo-spatial memory deficits [17–20]. The aim of the present work is to review the available evidence about the alteration of hippocampal synaptic plasticity in experimental models of MS and to discuss their relevance with regard to human MS.

The hippocampus: structure and function

"The findings reported herein led us to attribute a special importance to the anterior hippocampus and hippocampal gyrus in the retention of new experience." (Scoville and Milner, 1957) [21].

This sentence was the conclusion reached by Scoville and Milner during their neurosurgical study in 1957 [21]. In order to treat patients with psychiatric disorders or untreatable forms of epilepsy, they performed extensive bilateral medial temporal-lobe resections. One of their patient, H.M., after a bilateral medial temporal lobe resection, showed a partial retrograde and anterograde amnesia [21]. Interestingly, his perceptual abilities were spared, together with his working memory and motor skill learning. This observation contributed to a large research field about memory and its anatomical and biological background. During the last decades, many neuropsychological, behavioral and neuroimaging studies pointed to the medial temporal lobe, in particular to the hippocampus, as the critical cerebral structure for declarative and spatial memory [22, 23]. In particular,

the integrity of human hippocampus is considered fundamental for the formation of episodic memory, the ability to recall personal experiences and semantic knowledge, that could be considered the basis of personal learning and culture [22, 23]. This may explain why an impairment of these cognitive functions appears early together with a bilateral atrophy of medial temporal lobes during Alzheimer's disease [22] and why during transient global amnesia a bilateral hippocampal dysfunction occurs [24]. Moreover, the hippocampus seems to be the core structure encoding visuo-spatial information, as explained by the cognitive map theory proposed by O'Keefe and Nadel [25, 26]. This theory tries to explore the functional organization of hippocampus in rats and other animals, describing a cognitive map located in this cerebral structure, with neurons acting as *place cells* [25]. *Place cells* represent the functional units of this map, selectively increasing their firing rate when animals explore a determined and unique spatial region, helping the rodent to orientate itself and leading to the formation of an allocentric spatial memory [25, 27]. The importance of the hippocampus in spatial learning is also confirmed by the evidence that hippocampal volume is linked to spatial ability in different species of birds and small mammals [28, 29]. In humans, neuroimaging studies with structural magnetic resonance imaging (MRI) scans showed that the posterior hippocampal volume was increased bilaterally in licensed London taxi drivers, compared to age-matched controls [30]. This increased volume can be explained by the extensive training in spatial navigation made by these workers, as it correlates positively with time spent driving through the chaotic traffic in the British capital [30]. In conclusion, the hippocampus appears to be fundamental to answer questions about what, when and where something takes place and hippocampal involvement has been correlated to deficits in verbal and visuo-spatial memory during MS [17, 20, 31].

The hippocampal structure and synaptic plasticity were studied to assess their relationship with memory and human behavior. Declarative and episodic memory can be deconstructed in sequentially organized associative representations, in which each single event or variable is specifically settled in a unique flow, ultimately leading to a coherent experience or meaning [23]. Memory could be seen as a relational network in which each event correlates with others in a negative or positive way. Hippocampal structure and synaptic properties seem to fit perfectly with this functional activity, owing to its ability to create associations, intensifying some of them while lowering others [27, 32, 33]. This structure is well organized to process and associate different kinds of information, working as a C-shaped computational loop with extensive recurrent fibers (Fig. 1). A lot of

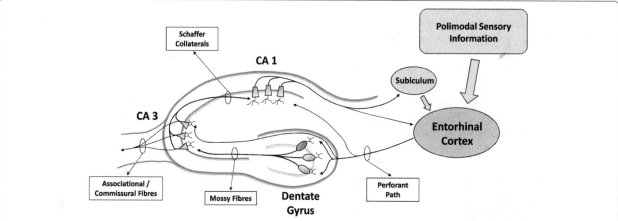

Fig. 1 Simplified functional anatomy of the hippocampus. Hippocampal circuitry is usually described as a trisynaptic loop, with a C-shaped organization. Perforant Path (PP) carries the major hippocampal input, consisting in polimodal sensory information collected by the Entorhinal Cortex (EC) from higher sensory cortices. PP contacts dendritic spines of granule cells in hippocampal Dentate Gyrus (DG), and a smaller part contacts directly neurons of the CA1 and CA3 hippocampal areas. Axons from DG granule cells are collectively named Mossy Fibres (MF) and project to hippocampal CA3 pyramidal cells. These cells represent an important computational node, since they are connected to contralateral CA3 and CA1 pyramidal cells through associational/commissural fibres. Moreover, they receive recurrent connections from ipsilateral CA3 cells, representing "internal" inputs, and they receive "external" inputs from DG and EC. CA3 pyramidal cells then project to ipsilateral CA1 pyramidal neurons, with connection fibres named Schaffer Collaterals (SC). Synapses between SC and CA1 neurons, and their plastic modulation, seem to be crucial for hippocampal computational ability and memory encoding. Lastly, CA1 axons contact directly and indirectly, through Subiculum, the EC

information from virtually all cortical associative areas converge towards the hippocampus through *entorhinal cortex* (EC) and *perforant path* (PP). PP axons make excitatory synaptic contact with all the three major areas of the hippocampus, the *dentate gyrus* (DG), *cornus ammonis* (CA)3 and CA1 areas. In particular, they contact granule cells located within the DG. These cells project through the *mossy fibres* (MF) to CA3 pyramidal neurons, which in turn send recurrent connections to other CA3 pyramidal neurons creating a kind of reverberant signaling. Thus, CA3 hippocampal area receives two kinds of information: "external" information from EC, PP and CA1 area through the MF; "internal" information from CA3 pyramidal recurrent connections [34]. Axons from CA3 neurons finally converge into *Schaffer Collaterals* (SC) and contact dendrites of CA1 pyramidal cells, whose projections ultimately contact the *subiculum* (SUB) and the EC [23, 33, 34]. This circuitry is extensively modulated by associational and commissural fibers and by inhibitory neurons distributed in all of the described hippocampal areas, creating a complex net of connections.

The plastic modulation of hippocampal synaptic activity could represent the functional basis of its computational ability. The simultaneous and repetitive stimulation of connected sub-components of this assembly, each one representing a specific external or internal stimulus, could lead to a strengthened connection between them [23, 33, 34]. Cortico-hippocampal connections act as an individual guidance to modulate behavior

in relation to the spatial, temporal and semantic context [27]. Such computational activity could predict upcoming stimuli and events in the environment, expanding its role from a static representation of reality to a probabilistic computational unit, useful to orientate human behavior towards a mutating and unexpected reality [27].

Synaptic plasticity, memory and learning in the hippocampus

"Our experiments show that there exists at least one group of synapses in the hippocampus whose efficiency is influenced by activity which may have occurred several hours previously - a time scale long enough to be potentially useful for information storage." (Bliss and Lomo, 1973) [35]

The way through which a neuronal network can storage and recall information always attracted neuroscientist's attention. Since the histological structure of the nervous system was described, several researchers tried to hypothesize how neural activity can modulate and influence neuronal connections [36]. In 1949, Donald Hebb in his book "The organization of behavior" postulated that a connection between two neuronal cells is strengthened by the simultaneously activation of both of them [37]. This Hebbian principle is a coincidence-detection rule, which reflected the long-standing idea, dating back to Cajal, that repeated stimulation of a synaptic connection could induce structural synaptic changes, as a way to form sustained memory traces from episodic experiences during learning [38]. Few decades later, an experimental support to this principle was provided. Bliss and Lomo demonstrated that repetitive high frequency stimulation (HFS) of the PP fibers to the DG of the hippocampus leads to a persistent average increase in the amplitude of the population excitatory post-synaptic potential (EPSP), meaning a powerful response of hippocampal granule cells [35]. This effect was firstly named long-lasting potentiation, successively best known as *long-term potentiation* (LTP). To date, hippocampal LTP is surely the best known activity-dependent form of synaptic plasticity [39], it is expressed by excitatory synapses throughout the brain and it appears to be dependent both on post-synaptic and pre-synaptic processes [40] (Fig. 2). LTP, together with *long-term depression* (LTD) [40, 41] and other forms of synaptic

plasticity, represent the most probable physiological basis of human learning and memory [23, 27, 33, 34], and several studies showed their occurrence *in vivo* at synaptic sites [40, 42].

Long-term forms of synaptic plasticity, such as LTP, are considered the physiological basis of human memory, since they are induced rapidly after synaptic stimulation, they are stable over time and can associate different stimuli in a functional network facilitating the encoding and recalling of information [42]. To prove these features of LTP many studies tried to demonstrate with electrophysiological techniques that it plays an important functional role in learning and memory. In 1983, Collingridge and colleagues showed that the selective blockage of *N-methyl-D-aspartate* (NMDA) glutamate receptors with the drug *amino-phosphonovaleric acid* (AP5) at excitatory hippocampal synapses, was able to

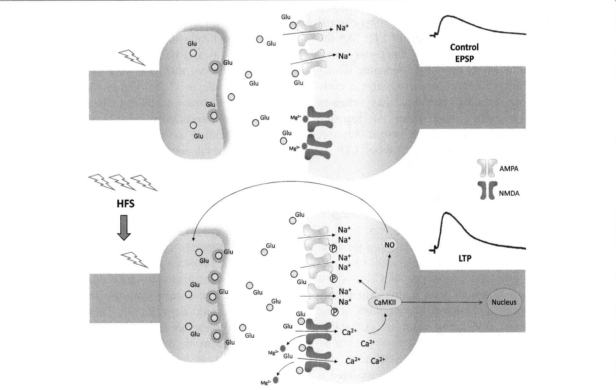

Fig. 2 Long-term potentiation (LTP) induction. In basal "control" condition, glutamate (Glu) released by the pre-synaptic terminal after an electric stimulation interacts with *a-amino-3-hydroxy-5-methyl-4-isoxazolepropionic acid* (AMPA) glutamate receptor, resulting in sodium (Na$^+$) influx and an excitatory post-synaptic potential (control EPSP). In this condition, glutamate interaction with *N-methyl-D-aspartate* (NMDA) glutamate receptors has no consequence because of the voltage-dependent blockage by magnesium (Mg^{2+}) of these receptors. During repetitive synaptic stimulation, which is mimicked in experimental conditions by the *high frequency stimulation* (HFS) protocol, the voltage-dependent NMDA blockage by Mg^{2+} is removed, allowing a Ca^{2+} influx into the post-synaptic element. This influx leads to the activation of *calcium/calmodulin-dependent protein kinase II* (CaMKII) and other several kinases, not shown in the figure, such as *protein kinase A* (PKA), *atypical protein kinase C isoforms* and *mitogen-activated protein kinases* (MAPK), which induce molecular changes in the post-synaptic dendritic spine [1, 40]. AMPA receptors are phosphorylated with an increase in Na$^+$ conductance, and more AMPA receptors are delivered to the plasma membrane from the sub-synaptic compartments. Moreover, neuronal gene expression is modulated in order to modify the morphology and the molecular structure of the dendritic spine. Finally, retrograde messengers like nitric oxide (NO), seem to play a role in LTP induction and maintenance, enhancing Glu release from the pre-synaptic element. All these synaptic modifications ultimately result in a sustained long-term increase of the EPSP (LTP), enhancing excitatory transmission between the two neurons

block the induction of LTP [43]. The role of NMDA glutamate receptor in synaptic plasticity was later supported by the studies of Morris and colleagues, who studied the behavioral effects of chronic, *in vivo*, intraventricular infusion of D,L-AP5 in rats [44]. During their experiments, rats were located into a large pool of water with a hidden platform located at a corner, and they measured the mean time needed to find the hidden platform and escape from water, a test known as Morris water maze [44]. The authors showed that the infusion of a selective NMDA antagonist, capable to block LTP induction in vitro, caused a significant impairment in learning and spatial navigation, suggesting a key role for hippocampal LTP in memory and spatial learning [44]. Whitlock and colleagues studied hippocampal synaptic alterations induced by inhibitory avoidance test (IAT), a test capable to induce a rapidly acquired and stable spatial memory, with associated changes in gene expression in the CA1 area of hippocampus [42]. They showed that the molecular changes occurring at hippocampal synapses during the *in vitro* induction of LTP, like the phosphorylation of *α-amino-3hydroxy-5methyl-4-isoxazolepropionic acid* (AMPA) glutamate receptor GluR1 subunit, where similar to those occurred after a cycle of active avoidance training, meaning that synapses responsible of controlling that form of learning probably expressed LTP [42]. These results support the hypothesis that spatial learning induces LTP in the CA1 area of the hippocampus.

In the last years, many studies explored new physiological pathways and cellular types implicated in the modulation of activity-dependent synaptic plasticity. Resident glial cells in the CNS, like astrocytes, seem to be key partners of neurons, actively regulating synaptic transmission [45]. Interestingly, also microglial cells, the resident immune cells and phagocytes of CNS, which rapidly activate in response to brain injury, dynamically interact with synapses in physiological conditions, acting like synaptic sensors modulating neuronal excitability and transmission [3, 46]. To date, synapses appear to be a more complex anatomical structure than it was believed before. Synapses are indeed now considered a "tri-partite" or even a "quad-partite" connection, in which pre- and post- synaptic neurons interact with glial cells such as astrocytes or microglia in order to modulate the efficacy of synaptic transmission [2, 3, 45–48]. Interestingly, the functional role of glial cells in synaptic plasticity could be crucial in particular during pathological conditions. For example, the regulation of water balance in CNS has been reported to be relevant in synaptic plasticity [49]. Aquaporin-4 (AQP4) is a water channel expressed by astrocytes in CNS and its abnormal modulation during pathologic conditions such as cerebral edema, epilepsy and ischemia could lead to a

defective LTP and LTD at hippocampal synapses [50]. Increasing attention is now oriented towards the functional and structural role of astrocytes in synaptogenesis and the regulation of synaptic activity [5, 51, 52]. Astrocytes are able to modulate the extracellular concentration of neurotransmitters, but they can also influence the expression and functional activity of postsynaptic receptors [53], helping in the maintenance of advantageous connections and removal of superfluous ones. Moreover, neuronal homeostasis, energy metabolism and defense against oxidative stress appear to be dependent on several astrocytic processes such as glutamate uptake and recycling, K^+ buffering, lactate release, glycogen mobilization, glutathione (GSH) synthesis and the production of neuroprotective trophic factors (for example nerve growth factor, NGF, ciliary neurotrophic factor, CNTF, glial cell-line derived neurotrophic factor, GDNF, and fibroblast growth factor 2, FGF-2) [54]. During neuroinflammatory processes, glial activation could lead to the release of a wide repertoire of immune mediators and cytokines, potentially affecting neuronal viability and synaptic transmission [54]. Indeed, an astrocyte-derived mediator, such as lactosylceramide, could play a role in CNS inflammation and neuronal degeneration in experimental models of MS, interfering with glutamate transmission [55–57]. Similarly, microglia is gaining attention as a central regulator of synaptic transmission during neuroinflammation and other neurodegenerative disorders [2, 3, 48, 58].

Microglia, neuroinflammation and synaptic plasticity: a deep impact

In the CNS, approximately 10% of the total cellular elements are represented by microglia, with variations between 0.5 to 16.6% for each human brain area [3, 59]. Microglia is constituted by mesodermal cells which migrate in the neural tube from the yolk-sac during the first ten embryonic days [2, 48]. They share the same lineage with monocytes and macrophages and represent the main resident immune innate defense within the CNS, contributing to inflammatory response against different kind of injuries [3]. Microglia is normally resting in the mature nervous system, with a phenotype characterized by long ramified processes extending from a small cell body [2]. During nervous tissue injury or inflammatory processes, microglial cells become activated, shaping into a globular "amoeboid" form with the ability to move towards the site of damage [3]. Even when in their "quiescent" or "resting" state, the thin microglial processes are highly dynamic and continuously scan neighboring neurons transiently contacting synapses near them with fast movements [60, 61]. Interestingly, microglial thin processes express several classes of neurotransmitter receptors and ion channels, normally found in neurons [3]. It has been demonstrated that NMDA receptors expressed by microglia can modulate the neuroinflammatory process, influencing reactive oxygen species (ROS) and cytokines production [62]. This rich equipment in neurotransmitter receptors and ion channels could be useful in physiological conditions to sample the extracellular matrix, monitoring neuronal activity near microglial cells. This function could lead microglia to play the role of active supervisor of neuronal firing activity and synaptic function [2, 48]. The monitoring activity of microglia seems to be crucial in the CNS development and refinement during the post-natal period [47, 63]. Microglia is indeed able to phagocytize inappropriate exuberant synapses, a process known as synaptic pruning, and apoptotic neurons, even by directly inducing programmed cell death through apoptotic signals [2, 47, 48, 63]. In fact, mice lacking the receptor for fractalkine (CX3CR1), a molecule which promotes microglia migration into CNS, show a reduced microglia brain concentration during CNS development, in association to an impaired synaptic pruning and synaptic transmission [63]. Parkhurst and colleagues studied the role of microglia in synaptic plasticity in an animal model lacking CNS microglia [64]. They generated CX3CR1(CreER) mice expressing *tamoxifen-inducible Cre recombinase* that allows for specific gene function manipulation in microglia [64]. They induced the expression of diphtheria toxin receptor in microglia, so they could later specifically remove microglia from the brain upon diphtheria toxin administration [64]. They found that microglia-depleted mice show behavioral abnormalities associated with hippocampal-dependent learning impairment. Interestingly, these abnormalities were associated with abnormal turnover of dendritic spines, and could be mimicked by the lack of brain-derived neurotrophic factor (BDNF) [64]. These results obtained by Parkhurst strongly support the crucial role played by microglia in neuroplasticity and learning. Thus, emerging evidence is converging toward a regulating role for microglia on synaptic transmission and synaptic plasticity in the adult brain. Microglia can act as modulator by several mechanisms, for example producing molecules such as interleukin-1β (IL-1β) and tumor necrosis factor α (TNF-α), which have an active influence on the main forms of synaptic plasticity, learning and memory, both during physiological and pathological condition [1, 3, 65, 66].

In particular, the effect of IL-1β on synaptic plasticity was studied by Katsuki and colleagues, who showed that recombinant human IL-1β is able to block the induction of hippocampal LTP in mouse brain slices [67]. Other research groups confirmed this evidence, suggesting a key role for this cytokine in synaptic plasticity defects observed during

neuroinflammatory processes [58, 66, 68–70]. However, endogenous IL-1β is normally expressed at low levels in control conditions, and it has been proposed to be essential for the physiological induction of hippocampal LTP and consolidation of memory [65, 71]. Accordingly, the analysis of a genetic murine model lacking IL-1β receptor showed impaired hippocampal neuro-plasticity [72]. The molecular pathway activated by IL-1β, which involves mitogen activated protein kinases (MAPKs) and nuclear factor-kappa β (NF-κβ), could indeed influence neuronal gene expression and regulate plastic processes at synaptic sites [1]. In particular, the assembly, expression and phosphorylation of glutamate receptor, glutamate secretion, intracellular calcium concentration, ROS production and cholinergic neurotransmission are influenced and regulated by IL-1β [1]. Thus, IL-1β could exert a fundamental role in modulating and favoring synaptic plasticity when expressed at physiological low levels, while an increased expression of this cytokine, such as during neuroinflammatory processes, could exert detrimental effects on neuroplasticity in the hippocampus. Interestingly, a recent study assessed the cerebro-spinal fluid (CSF) levels of this cytokine in 170 patients with relapsing-remitting MS, during clinical and radiological remission [73]. As result, higher CSF levels of IL-1β were found to be associated with mid-term disease progression [73]. This work could support the hypothesis that an inflammatory environment in the CNS, potentially leading to the failure of brain plastic capacities, could play a pathogenic role during disease progression in patients with MS.

The same observation seems to be true for microglial cells. Indeed, although their physiological activity is necessary for neuronal circuit development and function, when microglia becomes activated by inflammatory stimuli it is able to disrupt the ability of CNS synapses to express plasticity. In particular, inflammatory processes, like those occurring during EAE and MS, alter the fine balance existing between microglia and synapses/neurons, leading to excessive secretion of inflammatory products, such as cytokines and ROS, which could be harmful for neurons and neuroplastic processes [1, 3, 74].

Hippocampal synaptic plasticity in experimental models of MS

The possibility to mimic the complex pathogenic mechanism occurring during human MS still remains very difficult. The experimental model most frequently utilized to study human MS is represented by experimental auto-immune encephalomyelitis (EAE), since it mimics some of the clinical, immunological and histopathological features of MS [75]. This model resembles the pathogenesis of MS, since it is characterized by the induction of a myelin-specific immune response trough subcutaneous injections, for example, of *myelin oligodendrocyte glycoprotein 35–55* (MOG$_{35-55}$) or a syngeneic spinal cord homogenate [76, 77]. The characterization of this model led to important discoveries about the pathogenesis of inflammatory demyelination. The study of hippocampal synaptic plasticity dysfunction occurring during EAE has been conducted by few laboratories, but it represents an important acquisition to understand the course of the disease [13]. Kim Do and colleagues studied the alteration of hippocampal synaptic plasticity during EAE induced in C57/Bl6 mice through immunization against MOG$_{35-55}$ [78]. They showed a synaptic dysfunction in the hippocampal CA1 area, with a selective impairment in the ability to express LTP at two different time points post-immunization (13–16 days and 25–35 days), corresponding approximately to two disability stages (peak and milder). Interestingly, even before motor deficits became evident, mice manifested deficits in spatial learning [78], an evidence also confirmed by other groups [79] consistent with the hypothesis of a latent hippocampal dysfunction during the earlier phases of the disease, just after the beginning of the inflammatory process induced by the administration of the myelin-specific immunological trigger. As an attempt to reverse the observed synaptic deficit, authors fed EAE mice with a ketogenic diet [78]. Interestingly, the ketogenic diet was able to ameliorate the LTP impairment during EAE, in addition to the reduction of CD4$^+$ cells and microglia/macrophages concentration in the CNS during active neuroinflammation, with subsequent reduced production of several pro-inflammatory cytokines (IL-1β, interleukin-6, TNF-α, interleukin-12, interleukin-17) and ROS [78]. These results support the hypothesis that some of the soluble products of inflammation are responsible for the observed hippocampal synaptic plasticity deficit during the earlier phases of the disease. More recently, another research group demonstrated a hippocampal LTP impairment in rats affected by EAE, with *in vivo* electrophysiological recordings [80]. In particular, during the acute phase of EAE (28 hours after mice obtained a disability score of at least 3) the authors described a suppressed LTP induction, probably related to an increased inhibitory GABA-mediated effect [80].

In our laboratory, we found an impaired LTP induction in the hippocampal CA1 area both during the acute inflammatory peak phase of EAE [68] and the later remission phase [58]. As experimental model for MS, we induced EAE in Biozzi ABH mice, which are particularly prone to develop autoimmune responses, by the injection of syngeneic spinal cord homogenate [68]. This model follows a clinical course, reminiscent of relapsing-remitting MS, with acute phases characterized by detectable neurological signs followed by remissions with partial or complete recovery, with a later progressive phase [76]. During the first acute relapse of EAE, the LTP impairment was found to be associated with an intense activation of hippocampal microglia and an increased hippocampal concentration of IL-1β [68]. Such hippocampal synaptic plasticity disruption was associated with changes in the subunit composition of NMDA glutamate receptor in the hippocampus, with a reduced expression of GluN2B-subunit [68]. Several evidences suggested that GluN2B-subunit containing receptors are more prone to favor the induction of LTP in comparison to GluN2A containing ones [81, 82]. These molecular changes could be related to the known effects of IL-1β on gene expression, glutamate signaling and synaptic function [1], ultimately leading to a disruption of hippocampal LTP. Interestingly, synaptic impairment in the CA1 area of the hippocampus was detectable not only during acute EAE phase, but even in the remission phase of the experimental disease. We found that after the resolution of motor deficits, it was still possible to detect a significant impairment of hippocampal LTP and behavioural abnormalities, suggesting a deficit in spatial memory during the open field hole-board test [58]. These abnormalities in remitting EAE mice were associated with a persistent activation of hippocampal CA1 microglia, an increase in hippocampal IL-1β levels and the over expression by microglial cells of a ROS producing enzyme, *nicotinamide adenine dinucleotide phosphate* (NADPH) *oxidase*, as assessed by hippocampal immunohistochemistry and Western blot analyses [58]. The treatment with minocycline, an antibiotic with profound anti-inflammatory properties, was able to significantly reduce hippocampal microglia activation, NADPH oxidase expression and IL-1β levels, and to reverse the previously observed hippocampal LTP impairment and cognitive deficits in remitting EAE mice [58]. As a further support to the role of activated microglia and ROS producing enzymes, we showed that the application of *apocynin*, an inhibitor of NADPH oxidase, was able to rescue hippocampal LTP deficit during the EAE remission phase [58]. Moreover, *apocynin* was also able to block the detrimental effect of IL-1β on synaptic plasticity in control conditions, suggesting an involvement of NADPH oxidase expression in this process [58]. Thus, even after the resolution of motor symptoms in remitting EAE mice, persistent hippocampal microglia activation is associated with the release of inflammatory mediators, such as IL-1β, and the production of ROS through NADPH oxidase, and could be responsible of hippocampal CA1 LTP impairment and related cognitive deficits in spatial learning during MS [58].

Recently, Novkovic and colleagues showed that in the early mild phase of MOG$_{35-55}$ induced EAE (between days 14 and 19 post immunization), there was no impairment of hippocampal synaptic plasticity, while in later phases (between days 40 and 45 post-immunization) hippocampal LTP and LTP-related memory, such as spatial memory, were affected [83]. In their experimental setting they used as control group mice treated with complete Freund's adjuvant (CFA) alone, without MOG$_{35-55}$ [83].

In contrast with the results described above, Nisticò and colleagues found an enhanced hippocampal LTP amplitude in slices obtained by EAE mice, with respect to CFA-treated mice, leading to the hypothesis that the neuro-inflammatory process associated with EAE could also potentiate neuroplastic abilities of the CNS [84] in the utilized experimental setting. This research group utilized MOG$_{35-55}$ induced EAE, and they considered as control group mice treated with an emulsion of CFA. With this experimental protocol, they also showed that the ability of EAE in favouring LTP induction was mimicked by the exposure of control CFA slices to IL-1β [84]. Interestingly, during EAE they found a reduced efficacy of inhibitory GABAergic transmission, coupled with a reduction of hippocampal GABAergic neurons [84]. This effect was mimicked in CFA treated mice slices by the exposure to IL-1β or IL-1β-activated microglial cells [84]. Considering this evidence, the authors suggested that the pathogenic mechanism underlying the enhanced synaptic plasticity during acute phase of EAE was represented by a decreased hippocampal inhibitory neurotransmission [84]. Finally, another research group described a normal hippocampal LTP during the course of EAE. Indeed, Prochnow and colleagues demonstrated that an LTD impairment could be detected in several brain regions during the acute phase of MOG$_{35-55}$ induced EAE, such as the cerebellum and the superior culliculus [85]. Conversely, they did not find abnormalities of synaptic plasticity in the CA1 area of the hippocampus, with a normal expression of LTP and LTD [85].

In conclusion, hippocampal long-term synaptic plasticity during experimental MS has been studied by several research groups with partially contrasting results [13]. The majority of the studies found a reduction of the synapse's ability to express LTP, but reports also describe a normal and even an enhanced LTP during the course of EAE. Unfortunately, the existing differences in experimental models (animal used, modality of EAE induction, CFA treated or untreated mice as control group) and electrophysiological protocols (time points after EAE induction, specific electrophysiological technique, stimulation protocols, clinical severity of EAE symptoms) interfere with the interpretation and comparison of the studies [13]. However, it appears clear that during CNS inflammation there is significant alteration of the neuronal ability to express the main forms of synaptic plasticity, probably due to the effect of activated microglia and soluble products of inflammation (Fig. 3). These abnormalities in synaptic plasticity could be a dynamic process, influenced by the severity of inflammation and the stage of the disease, underlying a progressive functional failure of the brain plastic reserve, possibly contributing to disability progression during human disease. In line with this hypothesis, the ability to express synaptic plasticity has been proposed as a critical factor counteracting disability progression in MS [86]. Mori and colleagues showed that an altered brain ability to express LTP is associated with incomplete symptom recovery after an acute relapse and accumulation of disability [87]. Interestingly, the same group also demonstrated that the ability to express LTP, explored by transcranial magnetic stimulation (TMS) over the primary motor cortex, was still possible in stable relapsing-remitting MS patients, while it was absent in primary progressive MS suggesting that the brain plastic reserve might be crucial to contrast clinical deterioration in MS [88].

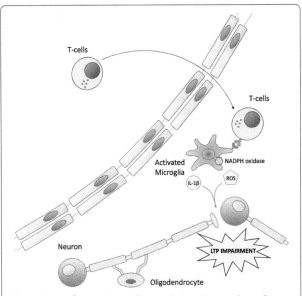

Fig. 3 Neuroinflammation and synaptic impairment. According to a widely accepted pathogenic model for MS and experimental autoimmune encephalomyelitis (EAE), autoreactive B and T cells migrate in the CNS through the blood–brain barrier. At this site, microglial cells participate in the process of T cells reactivation presenting CNS antigens in association with MHC class II molecules. Immune cells trigger the neuroinflammatory process associated with MS and EAE, with the production of cytokines (such as IL-1β and TNF-α) and other soluble products of inflammation (such as ROS) capable to deeply influence neuronal transmission, potentially leading to the disruption of the main form of synaptic plasticity (LTP). In this process, microglial activation is associated with an over-expression of NADPH-oxidase, a ROS producing enzyme, which has been demonstrated to be relevant for synaptic plasticity impairment during neuro-inflammatory processes [58]

Hippocampal involvement during MS

Different histological studies demonstrated that hippocampus is extensively involved during MS, since hippocampal demyelination has been detected in 53% to 79% of post-mortem MS brains [15]. Interestingly, Dutta and colleagues showed that hippocampal demyelination is associated with a pronounced decrease in synaptic density, with minimal neuronal loss, and an altered neuronal expression of genes involved in synaptic plasticity, axonal transport and memory/learning, such as glutamate receptors [16]. This synaptic pauperization could contribute to cognitive dysfunction [16]. During last years, neuroimaging studies showed that hippocampal atrophy is associated with memory dysfunction and depression [18, 29, 89]. In particular, a recent multicentre study used several structural MRI modalities to assess how the involvement of different brain regions links to the specific cognitive deficit suffered by the patient [89]. The authors found that atrophy of left postcentral gyrus and right hippocampus represents one of the best MRI findings useful to discriminate between patients with cognitive deficits and patients cognitively preserved [89].

Together with structural studies, functional MRI highlighted the key role played by the hippocampus in cognitively impaired patients. Hulst and colleagues investigated functional hippocampal activation and its connectivity during specific memory tasks in cognitively preserved and cognitively impaired MS patients [90]. They found that, in addition to a decreased hippocampal volume, patients with memory impairment show a decreased activation of the right hippocampus and an increased functional connectivity of the left hippocampus, mostly in connection with right posterior cingulate region, during cognitive performance [90]. Hippocampus and posterior cingulate region are both included in brain default mode network (DMN), a medial cortical network which has been demonstrated to be impaired during Alzheimer's disease [91, 92]. Interestingly, an increased connectivity between the hippocampus and other brain structures involved in the DMN was linked to cognitive impairment during MS [93]. Hulst and colleagues hypothesized that the increased functional connectivity could represent a maladaptive response of the memory functional pathway to the accumulating damage occurring during MS, possibly related to the disinhibition of the entire DMN [90]. In fact, white matter lesions disseminated throughout the brain could impair functional connectivity between the hippocampus and other brain regions located in the frontal, temporal, parietal lobe and cingulate cortex, ultimately leading to a disconnection syndrome when the compensatory hippocampal circuitries fail. This was the hypothesis raised by Rocca and colleagues, who showed a strong correlation between a high brain T2 lesion volume, reduced

hippocampal resting-state functional connectivity, depressive symptoms and clinical disability in MS patients [17]. A recent study characterized the relationship existing among neuro-inflammation, hippocampal functional connectivity and depressive symptoms during MS, by using positron emission tomography (PET) and functional MRI [94]. The authors measured hippocampal microglia activation in patients with MS using the 18-kDa translocator protein (TSPO) radio ligand [18 F] PBR111, the Beck Depression Inventory (BDI) to assess depressive symptoms, and resting-state functional MRI to study hippocampal functional connectivity [94]. As results, the authors found that intense microglial activation within the hippocampus was correlated with a reduced hippocampal connectivity and severe depression [94]. Moreover, another research group recently quantified the presence of activated macrophages/microglia with simultaneous MR-PET imaging, using the TSPO radio ligand ^{11}C-PBR28, in patients with both relapsing-remitting and secondary progressive MS [95]. Relative to controls, MS subjects exhibited abnormally high brain ^{11}C-PBR28 binding, the greatest increases being in cortex and cortical lesions, thalamus, hippocampus, and normally appearing white matter (NAWM) [95]. Interestingly, the authors found that microglia/macrophages activation correlated with reduced cognitive performances in the investigated cohort. Specifically, increased TSPO levels in the hippocampus, as well as in the thalamus and NAWM were associated with impaired Symbol Digit Modalities Test (SDMT) performances, a measure of information-processing speed [95].

In conclusion, all these studies showed that the hippocampus could be directly and indirectly affected by inflammation/demyelination with a subsequent alteration of synaptic density and neuronal transmission. Moreover, also demyelinating lesions spreading throughout the brain could indirectly determine a disconnection syndrome, affecting normal hippocampal functional connectivity, both during resting condition and memory tasks. Neuro-inflammation, and in particular microglial activation, could contribute to alter normal hippocampal connectivity with other key brain regions involved in the maintenance of a normal affective state and cognition [94, 95].

Conclusions

During the last decades, many studies explored the presence of structural and functional hippocampal changes and their characteristics during neuro-inflammatory processes. A reduction of hippocampal volume was found to be associated to cognitive deficits involving information processing speed and visuo-spatial, verbal and episodic memory during MS [96]. It has been suggested that hippocampal impairment could take place early during the course of MS, not directly relating to the demyelinating lesions [31]. Indeed, a selective bilateral hippocampal CA1 atrophy, exceeding global brain volume loss, was found in patients with relapsing-remitting MS independently from T2-lesion volumes, in association with deficits in memory encoding, but not in the speed of information processing, as assessed with word-list learning test and paced auditory serial addition task (PASAT) [31]. In this scenario, functional hippocampal synaptic plasticity impairment could play a fundamental role in cognitive deficits and symptoms progression during MS. Electrophysiological analysis of synaptic transmission in experimental models of MS showed that hippocampal synaptic plasticity is altered during CNS inflammation, probably due to the activation of microglia and the release of soluble inflammatory products, worsening the performances in hippocampal-related behavioral tests [13]. Accordingly, the presence of active inflammation, represented by isolated gadolinium enhancing lesions at brain MRI, was demonstrated to be associated with poorer cognitive performances in MS patients [97]. An altered synaptic plasticity could affect hippocampal functional connectivity, worsening the disconnection syndrome associated with demyelination and synaptic loss within the hippocampus. In conclusion, the hippocampus emerges as a structure particularly vulnerable to injury during neuro-inflammatory processes. It is affected early during the course of the disease, as assessed by several studies on both experimental animal models of MS and patients suffering with MS. A better understanding of the pathogenic process leading to this selective structural and functional hippocampal impairment appears fundamental to imagine new therapeutic approaches, targeted to preserve cognitive functions and quality of life in people with MS.

Abbreviations

AMPA: α-amino-3-hydroxy-5-methyl-4-isoxazolepropionic acid; AP5: Amino-phosphonovaleric acid; AQP4: Aquaporin-4; BDI: Beck depression inventory; BDNF: Brain derived neurotrophic factor; CA: Cornus ammonis; CaMKII: Calcium/calmodulin-dependent protein kinase II; CFA: Complete freund's adjuvant; CNS: Central nervous system; CNTF: Ciliary neurotrophic factor; CSF: Cerebro-spinal fluid; CX3CR1: Fractalkine; DG: Dentate gyrus; DMN: Default mode network; EAE: Experimental autoimmune encephalomyelitis; EC: Entorhinal cortex; EPSP: Excitatory post-synaptic potential; FGF-2: Fibroblast growth factor 2; GDNF: Glial cell-line derived neurotrophic factor; Glu: Glutamate; GSH: Glutathione; HFS: High frequency stimulation; IAT: Inhibitory avoidance test; IL-1β: Interleukin-1β; LTD: Long-term depression; LTP: Long-term potentiation; MAPK: Mitogen-activated-activated protein kinase; MF: Mossy fibers; MOG_{35-55}: Myelin oligodendrocyte glycoprotein 35–55; MRI: Magnetic resonance imaging; MS: Multiple sclerosis; NADPH: Nicotinamide adenine dinucleotide phosphate; NAWM: Normally appearing white matter; NF-κβ: Nuclear factor-kappa β; NGF: Nerve growth factor; NMDA: N-methyl-D-aspartate; NO: Nitric oxide; PASAT: Paced auditory serial addition task; PET: Positron emission tomography; PKA: Protein kinase A; PP: Performant path; ROS: Reactive oxygen species; SC: Schaffer collaterals; SDMT: Symbol digit modalities test; SUB: Subiculum; TMS: Transcranial magnetic stimulation; TNF-α: Tumor necrosis factor α; TSPO: 18-kDa translocator protein

Acknowledgements

This study was supported by Fondazione Italiana Sclerosi Multipla (FISM) (to P.C., project codes 2010/R/10 and 2011/R/10) and by Ministero della Salute – Ricerca Finalizzata - Bando Giovani Ricercatori (to M.D.F., project code GR-2010–2312924).

Authors' contributions

AM and MDF conceived the review. AM, MDF and AT performed literature review on hippocampal synaptic plasticity in EAE. AM, MDG and LG performed literature review on hippocampal involvement in MS. AM wrote the initial draft of the manuscript. AM and VG prepared the figures. MDF and PC reviewed the manuscript draft. All authors read and approved the final manuscript.

Competing interests

AM received travel grants from Teva and Sanofi Genzyme to attend national conferences. LG received travel grants from Biogen-Idec, Biogen, Novartis, Teva, Genzyme and Almirall to attend national and international conferences. MDF participated to advisory boards of Biogen Idec, Teva, Bayer, and Novartis; received travel grants from Bayer Schering, Biogen Dompé, Biogen Idec, Merck Serono, Novartis and Sanofi Genzyme to attend national and international conferences and speaker and writing honoraria from Biogen Idec, Novartis and Sanofi-Genzyme. MDF received research support from Associazione Italiana Sclerosi Multipla (AISM) and the Italian Minister of Health. MDG received travel grants from Biogen, Novartis, Teva and Merk-Serono to attend national and international conferences. PC received/receives research support from Bayer Schering, Biogen:Dompé, Boehringer Ingelheim, Eisai, Lundbeck, Merck:Serono, Novartis, Sanofi:Aventis, Sigma:Tau and UCB Pharma. PC also receives/received support from Ricerca Corrente IRCCS, Ricerca Finalizzata IRCCS, European Community Grant REPLACES (restorative plasticity at corticostriatal excitatory synapses), the Italian Minister of Health, and AIFA (Agenzia Italiana del Farmaco). AT and VG report no competing interests.

Author details

[1]Clinica Neurologica, Dipartimento di Medicina, Università degli Studi di Perugia, Ospedale Santa Maria della Misericordia, S. Andrea delle Fratte, Perugia 06132, Italy. [2]IRCCS, Fondazione Santa Lucia, via del Fosso di Fiorano 64, Rome 00143, Italy. [3]Sezione di Fisiologia e Biochimica, Dipartimento di Medicina Sperimentale, Università degli Studi di Perugia, S. Andrea delle Fratte, Perugia 06132, Italy. [4]Dipartimento di Filosofia, Scienze Sociali, Umane, e della Formazione, Università degli Studi di Perugia, Perugia, Italy.

References

1. Di Filippo M, Sarchielli P, Picconi B, Calabresi P. Neuroinflammation and synaptic plasticity: theoretical basis for a novel, immune-centred, therapeutic approach to neurological disorders. Trends Pharmacol Sci. 2008;29:402–12.
2. Salter MW, Beggs S. Sublime microglia: expanding roles for the guardians of the CNS. Cell. 2014;158(1):15–24.
3. Morris GP, Clark IA, Zinn R, Vissel B. Microglia: a new frontier for synaptic plasticity, learning and memory, and neurodegenerative disease research. Neurobiol Learn Mem. 2013;105:40–53.
4. Wake H, Moorhouse AJ, Miyamoto A, Nabekura J. Microglia: actively surveying and shaping neuronal circuit structure and function. Trends Neurosci. 2013;36(4):209–17.
5. Bains JS, Oliet SH. Glia: they make your memories stick! Trends Neurosci. 2007;30(8):417–24.

6. Cibelli M, Fidalo AR, Terrando N, Ma D, Monaco C, Feldmann M, Tarata M, Lever IJ, Nanchahal J, Fanselow MS, Maze M. Role of interleukin-1beta in postoperative cognitive dysfunction. Ann Neurol. 2010;68:360–8.

7. Dantzer R, O'Connor JC, Freund GG, Johnson RW, Kelley KW. From inflammation to sickness and depression: when the immune system subjugates the brain. Nat Rev Neurosci. 2008;9:46–56.

8. Konsman JP, Parnet P, Dantzer R. Cytokine-induced sickness behaviour: mechanisms and implications. Trends Neurosci. 2002;25:154–9.

9. Chiaravalloti ND, DeLuca J. Cognitive impairment in multiple sclerosis. Lancet Neurol. 2008;7:1139–51.

10. Rocca MA, Amato MP, De Stefano N, Enzinger C, Geurts JJ, Penner IK, Rovira A, Sumowski JF, Valsasina P, Filippi M. MAGNIMS Study Group. Clinical and imaging assessment of cognitive dysfunction in multiple sclerosis. Lancet Neurol. 2015;14(3):302–17. 2015 Feb 4.

11. Centonze D, Muzio L, Rossi S, Cavasinni F, De Chiara V, Bergami A, Musella A, D'Amelio M, Cavallucci V, Martorana A, Bergamaschi A, Cencioni MT, Diamantini A, Butti E, Comi G, Bernardi G, Cecconi F, Battistini L, Furlan R, Martino G. Inflammation triggers synaptic alteration and degeneration in experimental autoimmune encephalomyelitis. J Neurosci. 2009;29(11):3442–52.

12. Mandolesi G, Gentile A, Musella A, Fresegna D, De Vito F, Bullitta S, Sepman H, Marfia GA, Centonze D. Synaptopathy connects inflammation and neurodegeneration in multiple sclerosis. Nat Rev Neurol. 2015;11(12):711–24.

13. Di Filippo M, de Iure A, Durante V, Gaetani L, Mancini A, Sarchielli P, Calabresi P. Synaptic plasticity and experimental autoimmune encephalomyelitis: implications for multiple sclerosis. Brain Res. 2015;1621:205–13.

14. Pelletier J, Audoin B, Reuter F, Ranjeva J. Plasticity in MS: from functional imaging to rehabilitation. Int MS J. 2009;16(1):26–31.

15. Geurts JJ, Bö L, Roosendaal SD, Hazes T, Daniëls R, Barkhof F, Witter MP, Huitinga I, van der Valk P. Extensive hippocampal demyelination in multiple sclerosis. J Neuropathol Exp Neurol. 2007;66(9):819–27.

16. Dutta R, Chang A, Doud MK, Kidd GJ, Ribaudo MV, Young EA, Fox RJ, Staugaitis SM, Trapp BD. Demyelination causes synaptic alterations in hippocampi from multiple sclerosis patients. Ann Neurol. 2011;69(3):445–54.

17. Rocca MA, Pravatà E, Valsasina P, Radaelli M, Colombo B, Vacchi L, Gobbi C, Comi G, Falini A, Filippi M. Hippocampal-DMN disconnectivity in MS is related to WM lesions and depression. Hum Brain Mapp. 2015; 36(12):5051–63.

18. Gold SM, O'Connor MF, Gill R, Kern KC, Shi Y, Henry RG, Pelletier D, Mohr DC, Sicotte NL. Detection of altered hippocampal morphology in multiple sclerosis-associated depression using automated surface mesh modeling. Hum Brain Mapp. 2014;35(1):30–7.

19. Roosendaal SD, Moraal B, Vrenken H, Castelijns JA, Pouwels PJ, Barkhof F, Geurts JJ. In vivo MR imaging of hippocampal lesions in multiple sclerosis. J Magn Reson Imaging. 2008;27(4):726–31.

20. Longoni G, Rocca MA, Pagani E, Riccitelli GC, Colombo B, Rodegher M, Falini A, Comi G, Filippi M. Deficits in memory and visuospatial learning correlate with regional hippocampal atrophy in MS. Brain Struct Funct. 2015;220(1): 435–44.

21. Scoville WB, Milner B. Loss of recent memory after bilateral hippocampal lesions. J Neurol Neurosurg Psychiatry. 1957;20(1):11–21.

22. Burgess N, Maguire EA, O'Keefe J. The human hippocampus and spatial and episodic memory. Neuron. 2002;35(4):625–41.

23. Eichenbaum H. Hippocampus: cognitive processes and neural representations that underlie declarative memory. Neuron. 2004;44(1):109–20.

24. Di Filippo M, Calabresi P. Ischemic bilateral hippocampal dysfunction during transient global amnesia. Neurology. 2007;69(5):493.

25. O'Keefe J, Nadel L. The hippocampus as a cognitive map. Oxford: Oxford University Press; 1978.

26. Zucker HR, Ranganath C. Navigating the human hippocampus without a GPS. Hippocampus. 2015;25(6):697–703.

27. Bannerman DM, Sprengel R, Sanderson DJ, McHugh SB, Rawlins JN, Monyer H, Seeburg PH. Hippocampal synaptic plasticity, spatial memory and anxiety. Nat Rev Neurosci. 2014;15(3):181–92.

28. Lee DW, Miyasato LE, Clayton NS. Neurobiological bases of spatial learning in the natural environment: neurogenesis and growth in the avian and mammalian hippocampus. Neuroreport. 1998;9(7):R15–27.

29. Sherry DF, Jacobs LF, Gaulin SJ. Spatial memory and adaptive specialization of the hippocampus. Trends Neurosci. 1992;15(8):298–303.

30. Maguire EA, Gadian DG, Johnsrude IS, Good CD, Ashburner J, Frackowiak RS, Frith CD. Navigation-related structural change in the hippocampi of taxi drivers. Proc Natl Acad Sci U S A. 2000;97(8):4398–403.

31. Sicotte NL, Kern KC, Giesser BS, Arshanapalli A, Schultz A, Montag M, Wang H, Bookheimer SY. Regional hippocampal atrophy in multiple sclerosis. Brain. 2008;131(Pt 4):1134–41.

32. Pastalkova E, Serrano P, Pinkhasova D, Wallace E, Fenton AA, Sacktor TC. Storage of spatial information by the maintenance mechanism of LTP. Science. 2006;313(5790):1141–4.

33. Tsien JZ, Huerta PT, Tonegawa S. The essential role of hippocampal CA1 NMDA receptor-dependent synaptic plasticity in spatial memory. Cell. 1996;87(7):1327–38.

34. Neves G, Cooke SF, Bliss TV. Synaptic plasticity, memory and the hippocampus: a neural network approach to causality. Nat Rev Neurosci. 2008;9(1):65–75.

35. Bliss TV, Lomo T. Long-lasting potentiation of synaptic transmission in the dentate area of the anaesthetized rabbit following stimulation of the perforant path. J Physiol. 1973;232(2):331–56.

36. Malenka RC, Nicoll RA. Long-term potentiation, a decade of progress? Science. 1999;285(5435):1870–4.

37. Hebb DO. The organization of behavior. New York: Wiley; 1949.

38. Morris RG. D.O. Hebb: The Organization of Behavior, Wiley: New York; 1949. Brain Res Bull. 1999 Nov-Dec;50(5–6):437.

39. Bliss TV, Collingridge GL. A synaptic model of memory: long-term potentiation in the hippocampus. Nature. 1993;361:31–9.

40. Malenka RC, Bear MF. LTP and LTD: an embarrassment of riches. Neuron. 2004;44(1):5–21.

41. Dudek SM, Bear MF. Homosynaptic long-term depression in area CA1 of hippocampus and effects of N-methyl-D-aspartate receptor blockade. Proc Natl Acad Sci U S A. 1992;89(10):4363–7.

42. Whitlock JR, Heynen AJ, Shuler MG, Bear MF. Learning induces long-term potentiation in the hippocampus. Science. 2006;313(5790):1093–7.

43. Collingridge GL, Kehl SJ, McLennan H. The antagonism of amino acid-induced excitations of rat hippocampal CA1 neurones in vitro. J Physiol. 1983;334:19–31.

44. Morris RG, Anderson E, Lynch GS, Baudry M. Selective impairment of learning and blockade of long-term potentiation by an N-methyl-D-aspartate receptor antagonist, AP5. Nature. 1986;319(6056):774–6.

45. Panatier A, Robitaille R. Astrocytic mGluR5 and the tripartite synapse. Neuroscience. 2016;323:29–34.

46. Clark AK, Gruber-Schoffnegger D, Drdla-Schutting R, Gerhold KJ, Malcangio M, Sandkühler J. Selective activation of microglia facilitates synaptic strength. J Neurosci. 2015;35(11):4552–70.

47. Schafer DP, Lehrman EK, Stevens B. The "quad-partite" synapse: microglia-synapse interactions in the developing and mature CNS. Glia. 2013;61(1):24–36.

48. Miyamoto A, Wake H, Moorhouse AJ, Nabekura J. Microglia and synapse interactions: fine tuning neural circuits and candidate molecules. Front Cell Neurosci. 2013;7:70.

49. Scharfman HE, Binder DK. Aquaporin-4 water channels and synaptic plasticity in the hippocampus. Neurochem Int. 2013;63(7):702–11.

50. Szu JI, Binder DK. The role of astrocytic aquaporin-4 in synaptic plasticity and learning and memory. Front Integr Neurosci. 2016;10:8.

51. Hamilton NB, Attwell D. Do astrocytes really exocytose neurotransmitters? Nat Rev Neurosci. 2010;11(4):227–38.

52. Volterra A, Meldolesi J. Astrocytes, from brain glue to communication elements: the revolution continues. Nat Rev Neurosci. 2005;6(8):626–40.

53. Ota Y, Zanetti AT, Hallock RM. The role of astrocytes in the regulation of synaptic plasticity and memory formation. Neural Plast. 2013;2013:185463.

54. Bélanger M, Magistretti PJ. The role of astroglia in neuroprotection. Dialogues Clin Neurosci. 2009;11(3):281–95.

55. Mayo L, Trauger SA, Blain M, Nadeau M, Patel B, Alvarez JI, Mascanfroni ID, Yeste A, Kivisa P, Kallas K, Ellezam B, Bakshi R, Prat A, Antel JP, Weiner HL, Quintana FJ. Regulation of astrocyte activation by glycolipids drives chronic CNS inflammation. Nat Med. 2014;20(10):1147–56.

56. Rostami A, Ciric B. Astrocyte-derived lactosylceramide implicated in multiple sclerosis. Nat Med. 2014;20(10):1092–3.

57. Laurier-Laurin ME, De Montigny A, Attiori Essis S, Cyr M, Massicotte G. Blockade of lysosomal acid ceramidase induces GluN2B-dependent Tau phosphorylation in rat hippocampal slices. Neural Plast. 2014;2014:196812.

58. Di Filippo M, de Iure A, Giampà C, Chiasserini D, Tozzi A, Orvietani PL, Ghiglieri V, Tantucci M, Durante V, Quiroga-Varela A, Mancini A, Costa C, Sarchielli P, Fusco FR, Calabresi P. Persistent activation of microglia and NADPH oxidase drive hippocampal dysfunction in experimental multiple sclerosis. Sci Rep. 2016;6:20926.

59. Aguzzi A, Barres BA, Bennett ML. Microglia: scapegoat, saboteur, or something else? Science. 2013;339(6116):156–61.

60. Davalos D, Grutzendler J, Yang G, Kim JV, Zuo Y, Jung S, Littman DR, Dustin ML, Gan WB. ATP mediates rapid microglial response to local brain injury in vivo. Nat Neurosci. 2005;8(6):752–8.

61. Nimmerjahn A, Kirchhoff F, Helmchen F. Resting microglial cells are highly dynamic surveillants of brain parenchyma in vivo. Science. 2005;308(5726): 1314–8.

62. Kaindl AM, Koppelstaetter A, Nebrich G, Stuwe J, Sifringer M, Zabel C, Klose J, Ikonomidou C. Brief alteration of NMDA or GABAA receptor-mediated neurotransmission has long term effects on the developing cerebral cortex. Mol Cell Proteomics. 2008;7(12):2293–310.

63. Paolicelli RC, Bolasco G, Pagani F, Maggi L, Scianni M, Panzanelli P, Giustetto M, Ferreira TA, Guiducci E, Dumas L, Ragozzino D, Gross CT. Synaptic pruning by microglia is necessary for normal brain development. Science. 2011; 333(6048):1456–8.

64. Parkhurst CN, Yang G, Ninan I, Savas JN, Yates 3rd JR, Lafaille JJ, Hempstead BL, Littman DR, Gan WB. Microglia promote learning-dependent synapse formation through brain-derived neurotrophic factor. Cell. 2013;155(7):1596–609.

65. Goshen I, Kreisel T, Ounallah-Saad H, Renbaum P, Zalzstein Y, Ben-Hur T, Levy-Lahad E, Yirmiya R. A dual role for interleukin-1 in hippocampal-dependent memory processes. Psychoneuroendocrinology. 2007;32(8–10): 1106–15.

66. Vereker E, O'Donnell E, Lynch MA. The inhibitory effect of interleukin-1beta on long-term potentiation is coupled with increased activity of stress-activated protein kinases. J Neurosci. 2000;20(18):6811–9.

67. Katsuki H, Nakai S, Hirai Y, Akaji K, Kiso Y, Satoh M. Interleukin-1 beta inhibits long-term potentiation in the CA3 region of mouse hippocampal slices. Eur J Pharmacol. 1990;181:323–6.

68. Di Filippo M, Chiasserini D, Gardoni F, Viviani B, Tozzi A, Giampà C, Costa C, Tantucci M, Zianni E, Boraso M, Siliquini S, de Iure A, Ghiglieri V, Colcelli E, Baker D, Sarchielli P, Fusco FR, Di Luca M, Calabresi P. Effects of central and peripheral inflammation on hippocampal synaptic plasticity. Neurobiol Dis. 2013;52:229–36.

69. Bellinger FP, Madamba S, Siggins GR. Interleukin 1 beta inhibits synaptic strength and long-term potentiation in the rat CA1 hippocampus. Brain Res. 1993;628:227–34.

70. Murray CA, Lynch MA. Evidence that increased hippocampal expression of the cytokine interleukin-1 beta is a common trigger for age- and stress-induced impairments in longterm potentiation. J Neurosci. 1998;18:2974–81.

71. Schneider H, Pitossi F, Balschun D, Wagner A, del Rey A, Besedovsky HO. A neuromodulatory role of interleukin-1beta in the hippocampus. Proc Natl Acad Sci U S A. 1998;95:7778–83.

72. Avital A, Goshen I, Kamsler A, Segal M, Iverfeldt K, Richter-Levin G, Yirmiya R. Impaired interleukin-1 signaling is associated with deficits in hippocampal memory processes and neural plasticity. Hippocampus. 2003;13:826–34.

73. Rossi S, Studer V, Motta C, Germani G, Macchiarulo G, Buttari F, Mancino R, Castelli M, De Chiara V, Weiss S, Martino G, Furlan R, Centonze D. Cerebrospinal fluid detection of interleukin-1β in phase of remission predicts disease progression in multiple sclerosis. J Neuroinflammation. 2014;11:32.

74. Jones RS, Lynch MA. How dependent is synaptic plasticity on microglial phenotype? Neuropharmacology. 2015;96(Pt A):3–10.

75. Fletcher JM, Lalor SJ, Sweeney CM, Tubridy N, Mills KH. T cells in multiple sclerosis and experimental autoimmune encephalomyelitis. Clin Exp Immunol. 2010;162:1–11.

76. Amor S, Smith PA, Hart B, Baker D. Biozzi mice: of mice and human neurological diseases. J Neuroimmunol. 2005;165:1–10.

77. Baker D, Jackson SJ. Models of multiple sclerosis. ACNR. 2007;6:10–2.

78. Kim do Y, Hao J, Liu R, Turner G, Shi FD, Rho JM. Inflammation-mediated memory dysfunction and effects of a ketogenic diet in a murine model of multiple sclerosis. PLoS One. 2012;7(5):e35476.

79. Dutra RC, Moreira EL, Alberti TB, Marcon R, Prediger RD, Calixto JB. Spatial reference memory deficits precede motor dysfunction in an experimental autoimmune encephalomyelitis model: the role of kallikrein-kinin system. Brain Behav Immun. 2013;33:90–101.

80. Mosayebi G, Soleyman MR, Khalili M, Mosleh M, Palizvan MR. Changes in synaptic transmission and long-term potentiation induction as a possible mechanism for learning disability in an animal model of multiple sclerosis. Int Neurourol J. 2016;20(1):26–32.

81. Gardoni F, Mauceri D, Malinverno M, Polli F, Costa C, Tozzi A, Siliquini S, Picconi B, Cattabeni F, Calabresi P, Di Luca M. Decreased NR2B subunit synaptic levels cause impaired long-term potentiation but not long-term depression. J Neurosci. 2009;29:669–77.

82. Foster KA, McLaughlin N, Edbauer D, Phillips M, Bolton A, Constantine-Paton M, Sheng M. Distinct roles of NR2A and NR2B cytoplasmic tails in long-term potentiation. J Neurosci. 2010;30:2676–85.

83. Novkovic T, Shchyglo O, Gold R, Manahan-Vaughan D. Hippocampal function is compromised in an animal model of multiple sclerosis. Neuroscience. 2015;309:100–12.

84. Nisticò R, Mango D, Mandolesi G, Piccinin S, Berretta N, Pignatelli M, Feligioni M, Musella A, Gentile A, Mori F, Bernardi G, Nicoletti F, Mercuri NB, Centonze D. Inflammation subverts hippocampal synaptic plasticity in experimental multiple sclerosis. PLoS One. 2013;8(1):e54666.

85. Prochnow N, Gold R, Haghikia A. An electrophysiologic approach to quantify impaired synaptic transmission and plasticity in experimental autoimmune encephalomyelitis. J Neuroimmunol. 2013;264(1–2):48–53.

86. Weiss S, Mori F, Rossi S, Centonze D. Disability in multiple sclerosis: when synaptic long-term potentiation fails. Neurosci Biobehav Rev. 2014;43:88–99.

87. Mori F, Kusayanagi H, Nicoletti CG, Weiss S, Marciani MG, Centonze D. Cortical plasticity predicts recovery from relapse in multiple sclerosis. Mult Scler. 2014;20(4):451–7.

88. Mori F, Rossi S, Piccinin S, Motta C, Mango D, Kusayanagi H, Bergami A, Studer V, Nicoletti CG, Buttari F, Barbieri F, Mercuri NB, Martino G, Furlan R, Nisticò R, Centonze D. Synaptic plasticity and PDGF signaling defects underlie clinical progression in multiple sclerosis. J Neurosci. 2013;33(49): 19112–9.

89. Preziosa P, Rocca MA, Pagani E, Stromillo ML, Enzinger C, Gallo A, Hulst HE, Atzori M, Pareto D, Riccitelli GC, Copetti M, De Stefano N, Fazekas F, Bisecco A, Barkhof F, Yousry TA, Arévalo MJ, Filippi M. MAGNIMS study group. Structural MRI correlates of cognitive impairment in patients with multiple sclerosis: a multicenter study. Hum Brain Mapp. 2016;37(4):1627–44.

90. Hulst HE, Schoonheim MM, Van Geest Q, Uitdehaag BM, Barkhof F, Geurts JJ. Memory impairment in multiple sclerosis: relevance of hippocampal activation and hippocampal connectivity. Mult Scler. 2015;21(13):1705–12.

91. Greicius MD, Srivastava G, Reiss AL, Menon V. Default mode network activity distinguishes Alzheimer's disease from healthy aging: Evidence from functional MRI. Proc Natl Acad Sci U S A. 2004;101:4637–42.

92. Kenny ER, Blamire AM, Firbank MJ, O'Brien JT. Functional connectivity in cortical regions in dementia with Lewy bodies and Alzheimer's disease. Brain. 2012;135:569–81.

93. Hawellek DJ, Hipp JF, Lewis CM, Corbetta M, Engel AK. Increased functional connectivity indicates the severity of cognitive impairment in multiple sclerosis. Proc Natl Acad Sci U S A. 2011;108:19066–71.

94. Colasanti A, Guo Q, Giannetti P, Wall MB, Newbould RD, Bishop C, Onega M, Nicholas R, Ciccarelli O, Muraro PA, Malik O, Owen DR, Young AH, Gunn RN, Piccini P, Matthews PM, Rabiner EA. Hippocampal neuroinflammation, functional connectivity, and depressive symptoms in multiple sclerosis. Biol Psychiatry. 2015. S0006-3223(15)01025-2.

95. Herranz E, Giannì C, Louapre C, Treaba CA, Govindarajan ST, Ouellette R, Loggia ML, Sloane JA, Madigan N, Izquierdo-Garcia D, Ward N, Mangeat G, Granberg T, Klawiter EC, Catana C, Hooker JM, Taylor N, Ionete C, Kinkel RP, Mainero C. Neuroinflammatory component of gray matter pathology in multiple sclerosis. Ann Neurol. 2016;80(5):776–90.

96. Koenig KA, Sakaie KE, Lowe MJ, Lin J, Stone L, Bermel RA, Beall EB, Rao SM, Trapp BD, Phillips MD. Hippocampal volume is related to cognitive decline and fornicial diffusion measures in multiple sclerosis. Magn Reson Imaging. 2014;32(4):354–8.

97. Bellmann-Strobl J, Wuerfel J, Aktas O, Dörr J, Wernecke KD, Zipp F, Paul F. Poor PASAT performance correlates with MRI contrast enhancement in multiple sclerosis. Neurology. 2009;73(20):1624–7.

16

The heritage of glatiramer acetate and its use in multiple sclerosis

Giancarlo Comi[1*], Maria Pia Amato[2], Antonio Bertolotto[3], Diego Centonze[4,5], Nicola De Stefano[6], Cinthia Farina[7], Paolo Gallo[8], Angelo Ghezzi[9], Luigi Maria Grimaldi[10], Gianluigi Mancardi[11], Maria Giovanna Marrosu[12], Enrico Montanari[13], Francesco Patti[14], Carlo Pozzilli[15], Leandro Provinciali[16], Marco Salvetti[17], Gioacchino Tedeschi[18] and Maria Trojano[19]

Abstract

Multiple sclerosis (MS) is a chronic and progressively debilitating disease of the central nervous system. Treatment of MS involves disease-modifying therapies (DMTs) to reduce the incidence of relapses and prevent disease progression. Glatiramer acetate (Copaxone®) was the first of the currently approved DMTs to be tested in human subjects, and it is still considered a standard choice for first-line treatment. The mechanism of action of glatiramer acetate appears to be relatively complex and has not been completely elucidated, but it is likely that it involves both immunomodulating and neuroprotective properties. The efficacy of glatiramer acetate 20 mg/mL once daily as first-line treatment in relapsing-remitting MS is well established, with ample evidence of efficacy from both placebo-controlled and active-comparator controlled clinical trials as well as real-world studies. There is also a considerable body of evidence indicating that the efficacy of glatiramer acetate is maintained in the long term. Clinical trial and real-world data have also consistently shown glatiramer acetate to be safe and well tolerated. Notably, glatiramer acetate has a good safety profile in women planning a pregnancy, and is not associated with foetal toxicity. Until recently, glatiramer acetate was only approved as 20 mg/mL once daily, but a new formulation with less frequent administration, 40 mg/mL three times weekly, has been developed and is now approved in many countries, including Italy. This review examines the mechanism of action, clinical efficacy, safety and tolerability of glatiramer acetate to provide suggestions for optimizing the use of this drug in the current MS therapeutic scenario.

Keywords: Multiple sclerosis, Glatiramer acetate, Disease-modifying therapy, Pregnancy, Clinically isolated syndrome

Background

Multiple sclerosis (MS) is a chronic, progressively debilitating disease affecting the central nervous system (CNS). It is characterised by multifocal inflammation leading to demyelination, axonal damage and impaired nerve conduction; MS is usually thought to be an inflammatory, immune-mediated condition in the relapsing phase, but in the chronic progressive phase a neurodegenerative component is predominant [1]. The definition of clinically isolated syndrome (CIS) [2] is used to recognize the first clinical presentation of a disease that could be MS, but has yet to fulfil criteria of dissemination in time.

Several disease-modifying therapies (DMTs) are currently available to effectively treat MS, with the aim of abolishing/reducing the number of relapses and preventing disease progression [3]. Due to the chronic nature of the disease, when assessing/exploring the profile of a putative treatment both efficacy and safety have to be examined in the long term [4].

Glatiramer acetate (GA, Copaxone®) was the first of the currently approved drugs to be tested in human subjects with MS [5, 6]. However, the approval of GA by the European Medicines Agency (EMA), at the dose of 20 mg/mL once daily, subcutaneously administered, dates to 2001, when it joined interferon-beta (IFN-β) in the therapeutic armamentarium. The therapeutic indications are the following: first-line treatment of ambulatory patients with RRMS according to McDonald criteria and treatment of patients who have experienced a CIS and are considered

* Correspondence: comi.giancarlo@hsr.it
[1]Department of Neurology, INSPE, San Raffaele Scientific Institute, Via Olgettina 48, 20132 Milan, Italy
Full list of author information is available at the end of the article

at high risk of developing clinically definite multiple sclerosis (CDMS) [7].

Very recently, with the availability of a new GA formulation (40 mg/mL, injected three times weekly), that was demonstrated to be equally effective as the 20 mg/mL once daily dose in patients with RRMS [8] and was approved both by the EMA and the Food and Drug Administration (FDA), a substantial gain in patients' quality of life has been achieved. The aim of this review is examining the mechanism of action, clinical efficacy, safety and tolerability profiles of GA to provide suggestions for optimizing the use of this drug in the current MS therapeutic scenario.

Mechanism of action

The mechanism of action of GA in MS is complex, likely involving an interplay of immunomodulating and neuroprotective properties, with details still to be fully elucidated [9–13] (Fig. 1).

GA was originally designed by researchers at the Weizmann Institute in Israel as a synthetic analogue of myelin basic protein (MBP, an autoantigen implicated in the pathogenesis of MS), with the aim of using it as a molecular mimic of MBP to study the biology of experimental autoimmune encephalomyelitis (EAE), an animal model of MS [14]. GA is a standardised mixture of polypeptides randomly polymerized from four L-amino acids,

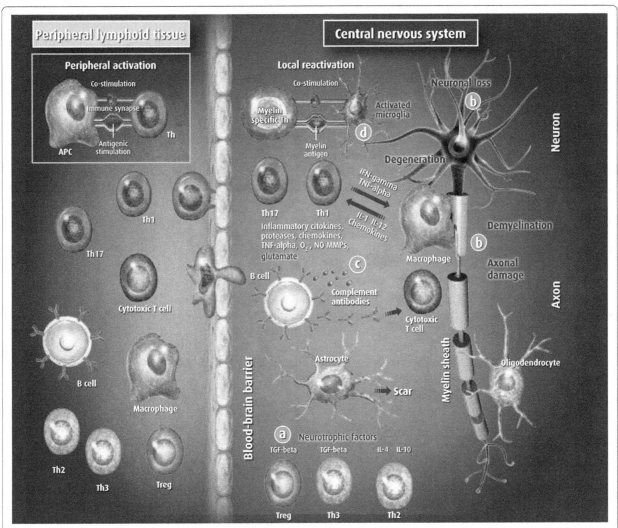

Fig. 1 Immune-mediated pathological and modulatory pathways in multiple sclerosis (MS) and possible neuroprotective actions of glatiramer acetate (GA). GA has been shown to increase levels of neurotrophic factors (**a**), which are reduced in the serum and the cerebrospinal fluid of MS patients and whose actions include protection of neurons against pathological insults. By inducing specific populations of Th2 cells in the periphery, GA may promote neural growth and inhibit inflammatory demyelination resulting in loss of axons, neurons and oligodendrocytes (**b**). GA has also been shown to oppose glutamate excitotoxicity by restoring normal kinetic properties of glutamate-mediated synaptic transmission in the striatum (**c**). GA may produce this effect by blocking synaptic alterations due to TNF-alpha released by activated microglia (**d**). APC, antigen presenting cell; IFN, interferon; IL, interleukin; MMP, matrix metalloproteinase; TGF, transforming growth factor; Th, T helper; TNF, tumor necrosis factor; Treg, regulatory T cell (Modified with permission from [11])

L-glutamic acid, L-lysine, L-alanine and L-tyrosine, in a defined molar residue ratio of 0.14:0.34:0.43:0.09. The same ratio is found in the amino acid sequence of MBP. The molecular mass of the constituent polypeptides of GA ranges from 4.7 to 11 KDa.

The researchers found that, surprisingly, the synthesised analogue did not induce EAE, but instead suppressed its development after exposure to crude myelin preparations [15]. This finding encouraged studies focussing on potential competition between GA and MBP in various immune cell-related events, especially in binding to major histocompatibility complex (MHC) molecules and T-cell antigen receptors [16, 17]. However, it should be noted that these results were mostly obtained using in vitro test systems, and their relevance to the mechanism of action of GA in vivo is uncertain. Aharoni and colleagues also reported that GA can block the proliferation of MBP-reactive T lymphocytes [18], but this finding was not reliably reproduced in subsequent studies. In fact, more recently, it has been shown that GA does not alter the proliferation of MBP-reactive T cells, but some GA-reactive T cells (specifically the Th2 cells) can respond to MBP by secreting protective cytokines [19]. GA-specific T cells, being able to cross the blood-brain barrier (while the drug itself is not) mediate the activity of GA in the central nervous system (CNS). Moreover GA-activated T cells are able to suppress EAE induced not only by MBP, but also by other encephalitogens, such as proteolipid protein (PLP) and myelin oligodendrocyte glycoprotein (MOG): this so-called "bystander suppression mechanism" is considered an essential component of the mechanism of action of GA [20].

An important immunomodulatory effect of GA – and possibly the primary mechanism behind its activity – is the induction of a shift in the phenotype of reactive T cells from a mostly pro-inflammatory Th1 pattern of cytokine secretion to a mostly anti-inflammatory Th2 pattern involving the production of IL-4, IL-5, IL-13, IL-10 and TGF-β [19, 21–27]. However, even if this is probably the most important mechanism of action of GA, other biological effects have been reported.

The role of Th17 cells (a subset of T cells that produce a distinct profile of proinflammatory cytokines, including interleukin [IL]-17, IL-6, IL-9, IL-21, IL-22, IL-23, IL-26 and tumour necrosis factor-α [TNF-α]) in the immunopathogenesis of MS and EAE has recently been elucidated [28–30]. GA was found to reduce Th-17-related neuroinflammation and levels of IL-17 and IL-6 in EAE mice [31, 32].

Studies have shown that, in addition to Th17 cells, GA acts on regulatory T (Treg) cells, whose role in suppressing autoimmunity is well recognized [33]. Patients with RRMS have an impaired CD4+ CD25+ Treg cells-related suppressive capacity [34], and functional alterations of Treg cells in RRMS may be associated with decreased expression of scurfin, a product of the transcription factor forkhead box P3 (Foxp3) [35]. GA can increase Foxp3 expression, and in vitro studies have shown that exposure of peripheral CD4+ T cells from healthy humans or GA-immunized mice to GA results in an increase in regulatory T cells, via activation of Foxp3 [36]. A similar finding was reported in a small study in RRMS patients, in which treatment with GA for up to 6 months increased total Treg numbers and reversed the Treg defect [37].

Additionally, it has been demonstrated that GA may act to cause a switch in the B cell phenotype of patients with MS, leading to the development of low but significant titres of GA-reactive IgG4 antibodies [38]. Because the isotype switch to IgG4 in B cells requires IL-4, an important anti-inflammatory cytokine, this finding further supports the anti-inflammatory action of GA in treated patients.

There is also evidence to suggest that GA, in addition to its action on the adaptive immune system, acts on the innate immune system by directly modulating the activity of myeloid cells, in particular monocytes and dendritic cells [39–42]. The properties of monocytes of RRMS patients undergoing treatment with GA have been compared with those of untreated patients and of healthy controls, showing that monocyte reactivity was inhibited in the treated patients. This study is important since it was the first to demonstrate this effect in human subjects treated with GA [43].

A number of studies have also addressed the question of the possible neuroprotective effects of GA. The results of in vitro and animal model studies have shed some light on the possible mechanisms of these effects. In addition to inducing an anti-inflammatory milieu in the CNS through the action of reactive T cells, GA has been shown to increase levels of neurotrophic factors such as brain-derived neurotrophic factor (BDNF), the actions of which include protection of neurons against pathological insults [11, 44]. Another possible neuroprotective action of GA, against glutamate excitotoxicity, was recently reported in a mouse model of MS [45]: GA was found to restore normal kinetic properties of glutamate-mediated synaptic transmission in the striatum of treated animals, contrasting the excessive glutamate action on postsynaptic receptors. GA produces this effect (independently of its immunomodulatory action) possibly by blocking synaptic alterations induced by activated microglia-released TNF-α.

The induction of specific populations of Th2 cells in the periphery by GA may lead to an environment favouring axonal protection, neural growth and remyelination, as reported in an in vitro and in vivo study by Skihar and colleagues [46]. Exposure of mouse embryonic forebrain cells in culture to GA-reactive T cells resulted in increased levels of insulin-like growth factor-1 (IGF-1) and promoted the formation of oligodendrocyte precursor cells (OPC). Subsequently, mice subjected to induced demyelination of the spinal cord were treated with GA; after 7 days, increased OPC generation and remyelination were observed, associated with higher levels of IGF-1 and BDNF in the spinal cord.

Some observations from clinical trials seem to support such effects. In a substudy of the PreCISe trial, patients treated with GA had increased brain concentrations of the neuronal integrity marker N-acetylaspartate, and an improvement in brain neuronaxonal integrity, whereas patients receiving placebo did not [47]. Also, magnetic resonance imaging (MRI) studies have demonstrated the ability of GA to reduce the proportion of new T1 hypointense lesions evolving into permanent black holes (markers of irreversible axonal loss), therefore supporting the neuroprotective scenario [48, 49].

Clinical efficacy

Subcutaneous GA has a long history of use for the treatment of RRMS. The initially approved dose, on the basis of animal studies, is 20 mg/mL once daily; still widely considered as standard, it was a keystone for all later drug development. Attempts to explore higher weekly doses (40 mg/mL once daily) showed no additive benefit [50, 51]. Recent results of the GALA study [8] indicate that maintaining a similar weekly dose, but with a different dosing regimen (40 mg/mL three times a week), provides advantages in clinical use without impacting on efficacy.

The feasibility of oral administration of GA was tested in the placebo-controlled CORAL trial [52]. Patients with RRMS received 50 mg or 5 mg of GA or placebo daily for 14 months. Neither dose of GA affected the primary endpoint (relapse rate) or any other clinical and MRI endpoint. Thus, further development of oral administration was discontinued. GA has been tested in progressive MS with negative results.

Once-daily formulation
In relapsing-remitting multiple sclerosis
The efficacy of GA 20 mg/mL once daily as first-line treatment in RRMS is well established in many phase II, III and IV studies.

Placebo-controlled trials The efficacy of GA on clinical and MRI-assessed outcomes has been demonstrated in two major pivotal placebo-controlled trials – the US Glatiramer Acetate trial [53] and the European/Canadian MRI study [54], and supported by an initial small study in 50 patients [55] (Table 1). This latter study provided the first clinical evidence supporting GA in RRMS, with 2 years of treatment with GA 20 mg/mL daily resulting in a significant difference in the proportion of patients experiencing no relapses versus placebo

(56 % vs. 26 %; $p = 0.045$) [55]. The first pivotal trial, the US Glatiramer Acetate phase III study, provided clear evidence for the efficacy of GA, demonstrating a significant 29 % reduction favouring GA in annualised relapse rate (ARR) (0.59 vs. 0.84 for placebo; $p = 0.007$), supported by trends in the proportion of relapse-free patients (33.6 % vs. 27.0 %, respectively), and the median time to first relapse (287 vs. 198 days, respectively), after 2 years of treatment [53] (Table 1). In this study MRI measures were not used. A second study, the European/Canadian MRI trial, was planned in order to better define the profile of efficacy and safety of GA. It provided for the first time MRI evidence of the beneficial effect of GA; 9 months of therapy resulted in significant differences favouring GA versus placebo for most endpoints: mean total number of enhancing lesions on T1-weighted images (primary endpoint; 25.96 vs. 36.80; $p = 0.003$), number of new enhancing lesions (17.4 vs. 26.0; $p < 0.003$) and their change of volume ($p < 0.01$), number of new lesions detected on T2-weighted images (9.4 vs. 13.5, respectively; $p < 0.003$) and their change of volume ($p = 0.001$). Moreover, a significant reduction of the relapse rate was reported in the GA group versus placebo (33 %; $p = 0.012$) (Table 1). A later study that analysed MRI data from the European-Canadian trial using a fully automated, normalized method also showed a significant ($p = 0.037$ at 18 months) reduction in the development of brain atrophy in the GA group versus placebo [56]. A noteworthy finding of the European/Canadian MRI study was a reduction in severity of tissue disruption in newly-formed lesions with GA [48]: the percentage of new lesions evolving into permanent black holes was significantly lower in patients treated with GA than in those receiving placebo at 7 months (18.9 % vs. 26.3 %, respectively; $p = 0.04$) and at 8 months (15.6 % vs. 31.4 %, respectively; $p = 0.002$) after lesion appearance.

Active comparator-controlled trials GA has been compared head-to-head with high-dose subcutaneous IFN-β1a or -1b in two double blind trials in patients with RRMS: REGARD [57] and BECOME [58] (Table 1). Both showed comparable efficacy between GA and IFN-β1a or -1b. Moreover in the REGARD trial, GA was found to better protect against brain-volume loss (−1.07 % vs. −1.24 %; $p = 0.018$). These data were confirmed by two trials in which GA was used as reference comparator. In the BEYOND trial [59], two arms receiving IFN-β1b (250 μg and 500 μg) were included, along with a third arm receiving GA: no significant differences were found between groups either in the primary endpoint (ARR: 0.33 for IFN-β1b 500 μg, 0.36 for IFN-β1b 250 μg and 0.34 for GA; p = ns for all comparisons) and in all other clinical outcomes (Table 1). The CONFIRM trial [60] compared two doses of dimethyl fumarate versus placebo, again with a third

Table 1 Clinical trials

Study	Number of patients	Trial length	Key outcomes
Placebo-controlled trials			
Johnson et al. 1995 [53]	251 randomised 1:1 GA:PBO	2 years	Mean relapse rate: GA 1.19 versus PBO 1.68; $p = 0.007$ (29 % reduction) (ARR: GA 0.59 versus PBO 0.84)
Comi et al. 2001 [54]	239 randomised 1:1 GA:PBO	9 months	Mean reduction in total enhancing lesions GA vs PBO -10.8 (95 % CI -18.0 to -3.7; $p = 0.003$; 29 % reduction.
Bornstein et al. 1987 [55]	50 randomised 1:1 GA:PBO	2 years	Proportion of relapse-free patients GA 56 % vs 26 % PBO; $p = 0.045$
Active comparator-controlled trials			
Mikol et al. 2008 [57] (REGARD)	764 randomised 1:1 GA:IFNβ-1a	96 weeks	No between-group difference in time to first relapse (HR 0.94; 95 % CI 0.74–1.21; $p = 0.64$)
Cadavid et al. 2009 [58] (BECOME)	75 randomised 1:1 GA: INF-β1b	2 years	Similar median (75th percentile) CAL count per scan in months 1–12, of 0.58 (2.45) vs 0.63 (2.76)
O'Connor et al. 2009 [59] (BEYOND)	2447 randomised 2:2:1 250 μg IFNβ-1b:500 μg IFNβ-1b:GA	3.5 years	No between-group differences in relapse risk or EDSS progression
Fox et al. 2012 [60] (CONFIRM)	Randomised 1:1:1:1 PBO: BG-12 twice daily:BG-12 three times daily:GA	96 weeks	ARR significantly lower with twice-daily BG-12 (0.22), three times-daily BG-12 (0.20), and GA (0.29) than PBO (0.40) (RR GA 29 %, $P = 0.01$).
Combination trials			
Goodman et al. 2009 [85] (GLANCE)	110 randomised 1:1 GA + NTZ versus GA alone	6 months	Mean rate of development of new active lesions over the 24-week study lower with combination therapy (0.03) vs GA alone (0.11; $p = 0.031$)
Lindsey et al. 2012 [116] (CombiRx)	1008 randomised 2:1:1 IFN + GA: IFN: GA	3 years	No difference in ARR between combination group and GA group (0.12 vs. 0.11). Both combination and GA alone superior to IFN group (0.16; $p = 0.022$ for combination group and $p = 0.027$ for GA group)
Clinically isolated syndrome			
Comi et al. 2009 [86] (PreCISe)	481 randomised 1:1 GA:PBO	36 months	GA reduced risk of CDMS by 45 % versus PBO (HR 0.55, 95 % CI 0.40–0.77; $p = 0.0005$)

95 % CI 95 % confidence interval, *ARR* Annualised relapse rate, *CAL* Combined active lesions, *CDMS* Clinically definite multiple sclerosis, *EDSS* Expanded disability status scale, *GA* Glatiramer acetate, *HR* Hazard ratio, *IFN* Interferon, *NTZ* natalizumab, *PBO* Placebo, *RR* Relative risk

arm with GA as a reference comparator. Even if the design of the trial did not allow a comparison between the two active treatments, both drugs proved to be significantly superior to placebo in all clinical and MRI outcomes (Table 1). In particular, GA significantly reduced the ARR versus placebo by 29 % ($p = 0.01$), thus confirming the results of the pivotal trials in a very large population sample (over 1400 patients). A post hoc subgroup analysis reported numerically similar relapse-related outcomes between the two dimethyl fumarate arms and the GA arm in most patient subgroups [61].

A systematic review summarising data from five randomised studies comparing IFN-β with GA in patients with RRMS confirmed a similar efficacy after 2 years of treatment [62].

Long-term and real-word data Even with all the limitations of long-term extension studies, due to potential selection bias, available data suggest that the efficacy of GA is maintained over time [63–71]. Moreover, there have been no reports of rebound effect or delayed disease reactivation after treatment

discontinuation in extensions of clinical trials or post-marketing studies [63, 70, 72, 73].

The first follow-up of the US Glatiramer Acetate trial presented 15-year data [63]. Patients continuing in the study (100 of the initial 232) showed a reduced ARR (0.25 ± 0.34 per year vs. 1.12 ± 0.82 at baseline); 57 % had stable or improved Expanded Disability Status Scale (EDSS) scores (change ≤0.5 points) and 67 % showed stable disease, without transitioning to secondary progressive MS. The most frequently reported reasons for treatment discontinuation were patient perception of disease worsening ($n = 29$), a desire to switch or combine therapies ($n = 26$) and difficulty, inability, or unwillingness to adhere to the study protocol ($n = 32$). Twenty-year results are now available for the long-term extension of this study [64]. Of the initial 232 patients, 74 remain in the trial and have been continuously treated for a mean of 19.3 years. Very long-term use of GA appears to be associated with stable disease activity (cumulative ARR = 0.2; 24.3 % of patients remained free of relapse for the entire period) and low levels of accumulated disability (mean EDSS score 3.1 vs. 2.4 at baseline).

The extension of the European/Canadian MRI study offers serial long-term MRI data for a large cohort of patients treated with GA [70]. After the 9-month double-blind, placebo-controlled phase, all patients entered an open-label, active treatment phase in which they received GA 20 mg/mL once daily for a further 9 months, with a long-term follow-up visit (LTFU) scheduled at least five years after study entry. Overall, MRI results show that the effects of GA on MS activity are sustained (number of active lesions 0.9 at LTFU vs. 3.4 at baseline; percentage brain volume change −5.02 vs. baseline). Moreover, MRI results in the patients that were shifted from placebo to GA showed a significant reduction of MRI measures of disease activity, paralleling what was observed in the patients that received GA from the start. A notable finding is that the proportion of patients requiring walking aids at the LTFU was significantly lower ($p = 0.034$) in the group that received GA from the start of the study compared with delayed treatment, suggesting that early treatment may have a positive impact on long-term disease outcomes.

A 5-year brain MRI retrospective open study provides some evidence of the efficacy of GA in reducing brain volume loss [74]: smaller reductions in brain volume were observed in patients with RRMS treated with subcutaneous GA than with high-dose IFN-β regimens (percentage change in brain volume −2.27 % vs. −3.21 %; $p < 0.0001$).

Various studies report real-world data for GA treatment in RRMS [72, 73, 75, 76], confirming the efficacy profile of GA observed in the clinical studies. A significant impact of the treatment with GA on health-related quality of life has also been reported [77, 78], with beneficial effects including significant reductions in fatigue and in days of absence from work.

Controlled studies of MS treatments in children and adolescents are still lacking, but some published evidence, albeit retrospective, points to the efficacy of GA in this population. In an Italian cohort, 14 patients with a mean age of 13.1 years were treated for a mean of 5 years or more; these patients had a reduction in relapse rate, from about 3 per year before treatment initiation to 0.2–0.4 per year during the treatment period [79]. A small study of seven patients with RRMS who had disease onset at 9–16 years of age and began GA before 18 years of age showed that 24 months of treatment resulted in two of seven patients remaining relapse free over the study period, and three of seven patients having stable disability scores as measured by the EDSS [80].

Switching to glatiramer acetate Several trials have evaluated switching to GA from other MS therapies for safety and efficacy reasons [81–83]. For patients not responding to first line therapies GA can be offered as an alternative to so-called second line medications if there are concerns of tolerability/adverse events with the latter therapies. Most studies describe switches from IFNβ-1a or -1b to GA, reporting reductions in mean ARR after switching [81–83]. However, in those situations when the shift is due to failure of the previous treatment, results should be interpreted with caution because the regression to the mean phenomenon is a major concern. Therefore, randomised, controlled trials are needed to confirm these results.

Combination treatment trials Two important combination therapy trials are the CombiRx trial [84] and the GLANCE trial [85] (Table 1). In CombiRx, patients were randomised to GA 20 mg/mL once daily plus IFN-β1a 30 µg once weekly or to monotherapy with one of these medications plus placebo for 3 years. For the primary outcome of ARR, the combination therapy was significantly superior to IFN-β, reducing the relapse rate by 25 % ($p = 0.022$), while there was no significant difference between the combination therapy and GA. It should be noted that the study design allowed for the first time a comparison between intramuscular IFN-β and GA, with GA resulting superior (relapse rate reduction by 31 % compared with IFN-β; $p = 0.027$). The GLANCE study compared combination therapy with GA 20 mg/mL once daily plus intravenous natalizumab 300 mg every 4 weeks versus monotherapy with GA 20 mg/mL once daily plus placebo every 4 weeks. At 24 weeks, the combination therapy was superior on major MRI disease activity measures.

In clinically isolated syndrome
Early treatment with GA in patients with CIS has been shown to delay onset of CDMS in the placebo-controlled study PreCISe [86] (Table 1) and during its subsequent open-label extension period [87]. The study enrolled 481 patients with one unifocal neurological event and a positive MRI scan (defined as the presence of at least two cerebral lesions ≥6 mm in diameter on T2-weighted images). Patients were randomised to GA 20 mg/mL once daily or placebo for up to 36 months or until conversion to MS. GA was associated with a 45 % reduction in risk of conversion to MS (primary endpoint; $p = 0.0005$) and a delay in the time to conversion compared with placebo (336 days vs. 722 days, respectively). GA was associated with a 58 % reduction in number of new T2 lesions and a smaller volume of T2 lesions. During the extension phase (total 5 years' duration) the efficacy of GA was sustained, with a 41 % reduction in risk of conversion to MS in those treated with GA from the start compared with delayed treatment; in the GA group, there was a delay of 972 days before conversion to MS, a 42 % reduction in new T2 lesions per year ($p < 0.0001$) and a 22 % reduction in T2-

lesion volume (p = 0.0005). In the extension phase patients treated with GA from study entry showed a significant 28 % reduction (p = 0.0209) in brain volume loss compared with patients initially randomised to placebo, confirming the neuroprotective effects of GA. This is the first trial to demonstrate that early treatment with GA reduces brain atrophy versus delayed treatment in this setting.

In progressive forms of multiple sclerosis

GA was assessed in primary progressive forms of MS, with negative results. The PROMiSe study [88] was a randomised, double-blind, placebo-controlled, multicentre, international study that investigated the effect of GA on disability progression in 943 patients with progressive MS. After 3 years of treatment, the time to sustained accumulated disability was similar between GA- and placebo-treated patients (hazard ratio [HR] 0.87; 95 % CI 0.71 to 1.07; p = 0.1753). A post hoc analysis showed a possible effect in slowing clinical progression in male patients (HR 0.71; 95 % CI 0.53 to 0.95; p = 0.0193) [88], but a subsequent analysis of these results did not demonstrate an impact of gender on the efficacy of GA [89]. An additional study investigating metabolite ratios as determined by MRI in a subset of 58 patients from the PROMISe study showed no difference between the GA and placebo groups [90]. However, it should be noted that the PROMISe study was terminated early due to lack of effect, and that the low rate of disability progression and the high rate of premature discontinuations led to a decrease in power of the study, hampering the determination of a treatment effect [88].

Three times weekly formulation

The first trial to evaluate a high-dose regimen of GA was the phase III FORTE study [51] that compared the 40 mg/mL once daily dose with the standard 20 mg/mL once daily dose in patients with RRMS. Both doses showed similar effects on efficacy measures and no difference in the safety profile. Post-hoc analyses revealed potential benefits of the 40 mg/mL dose in some subgroups (for example, in the "frequent MRI cohort" patients treated with 40 mg/mL showed a slight numerical advantage in the reduction of the mean number of gadolinium-enhancing lesions at various timepoints vs. baseline). After this study the development of the high-dose once daily regimen was discontinued, but it provided a starting point for subsequent research on the high-dose, lower-frequency regimen (40 mg/mL three times weekly).

The efficacy of subcutaneous GA 40 mg/mL three times weekly in patients with RRMS was shown in the 1-year, double blind, placebo-controlled GALA study, involving about 1400 patients [8]. Significant reductions compared with placebo in relapse rate (34.0 %; p < 0.0001),

cumulative number of gadolinium-enhancing T1 lesions (44.8 %; p < 0.0001) and new or enlarged T2 lesions (34.7 %; p < 0.0001) were reported; the numerical values of these parameters were very similar to those observed in the pivotal studies with the 20 mg/mL once daily dose. Three-year results of the open-label extension of the GALA study demonstrated sustained efficacy on ARR and MRI parameters of disease activity [91]. Patients switched from placebo to GA after the double blind phase reported significant gains in efficacy, but those treated with GA from study entry showed a significantly lower relapse rate (ARR 0.23 vs 0.30, respectively, p = 0.0052) and significantly fewer enhancing T1 lesions and new or enlarged T2 lesions (RR = 0.660, p = 0.0005 for T1; RR = 0.680, p < 0.0001 for T2) compared with patients with delayed treatment.

An important finding from a recent post hoc MRI analysis of data from the GALA study is that GA 40 mg/mL three times weekly (cumulative weekly dose of 120 mg) shares the ability of the standard formulation (cumulative weekly dose of 140 mg) to reduce conversion of new active lesions into black holes, markers of permanent damage and disability progression, with a significant 24 % reduction compared with placebo (p = 0.006) in the odds of conversion from new lesions at month 6 to black holes at month 12 [49].

In the absence of head-to-head studies comparing GA 20 mg/mL once daily and 40 mg/mL three times weekly, indirect comparisons have also shown very similar efficacy of the two doses [92, 93].

On the same lines, the GLACIER study, in which patients were asked to report the personal experience of shifting from the 20 mg/mL once daily dose to the 40 mg/mL three times weekly dose, demonstrated a favourable convenience profile and patient satisfaction when converting from the once-daily formulation [94].

Safety

After 20 years' continuous clinical use and more than 2 million patient-years' exposure, the safety profile of GA is well established. No evidence of any association of GA with immunosuppression or with malignant and autoimmune disease has been reported after 10 and 15 years follow-up [63, 65]. GA was not associated with psychiatric or mood disorders and in some studies a significant improvement in fatigue was observed, even in patients switching from other DMTs [78]. In a study of patients with RRMS and spasticity, switching from IFN-β to GA improved spasm frequency, muscle tone and pain after 3 months of treatment; these improvements were maintained over 6 months of treatment with GA [95]. A few cases of hepatotoxicity during treatment with GA have recently been reported [96–98], with no such cases reported in clinical trials, hence it is unclear at present if liver function monitoring is warranted. It should be noted, though, that because some of the patients reporting this AE had concurrent autoimmune conditions, it is impossible to disentangle the potential contribution of GA treatment and the underlying condition to hepatotoxicity. IgE-mediated allergic reactions have also been described [99, 100].

Both formulations of GA appear equivalent from the safety standpoint [64, 91, 94]. In the GALA study AEs associated with administration of GA 40 mg/mL three times a week were found to be consistent with the known safety profile of GA 20 mg/mL once daily. Moreover, no new AEs emerged during treatment with high-dose GA [8, 91].

At present there are no controlled studies of DMTs in children and adolescents with MS, but published evidence, mostly retrospective studies, support a similar safety profile of GA in this population [79, 80]. GA, along with IFN-β, has been recommended as the standard treatment for paediatric RRMS in two position papers, one produced by European experts [101] and the other one by the International paediatric MS Study [102]. Since paediatric onset MS is characterized by high disease burden, early treatment, although off-label, should be promptly started after confirmation of the diagnosis. The favourable tolerability profile of GA should be considered when making a therapeutic choice [101, 102].

No limitations to concomitant administration of GA and other drugs have been identified; the medication is not linked to blood test abnormalities that require monitoring.

Pregnancy

Animal reproduction studies have failed to demonstrate a risk of GA treatment to the foetus, and post-marketing studies support the absence of foetal toxicity [103–108]. For these reasons GA has been classified as FDA Class B during pregnancy [109]. Most of the other drugs approved for the treatment of MS are categorized by the FDA as Class C, with the exception of mitoxantrone, classified as Class D (positive evidence of human foetal risk), and teriflunomide, classified as Class X (foetal toxicity) [104, 109]. GA can be continued right up until conception, unlike other DMTs for which a washout period is recommended prior to trying to conceive [104]. GA may also be used as bridging therapy in women planning a pregnancy who are receiving treatments requiring a washout period, if it exposes women to the risk of MS reactivation, and offers some advantages in women risking unplanned pregnancies.

While it is currently recommended that, as for any other DMT, GA should be discontinued after confirmed evidence of pregnancy and until childbirth, available evidence suggests GA could be continued at least throughout the first trimester, while further continuation of GA

treatment may be assessed on a case-by-case basis [104]. An Italian retrospective study showed that the mother's exposure to GA when the drug was suspended within 4 weeks from conception was not associated with an increased frequency of spontaneous abortion nor with other negative pregnancy and foetal outcomes compared with women in whom the medication was suspended 4 weeks or more from conception, or who were untreated [107]. These findings confirm those of a previous observational study [106] suggesting that GA and the IFNs do not represent a significant risk for prenatal developmental toxicity. Relapse rate decreases during pregnancy, with a well-known increase in the first three months after childbirth [110] that sometimes requires second-line therapy to be controlled [103–105].

Tolerability

The tolerability of GA 20 mg/mL once daily has consistently been reported as good versus both placebo and active treatment in the previously mentioned clinical trials [54, 57, 59, 86], and the nature and frequency of treatment-related AEs were similar between short- and long-term treatment periods [63–65, 67]. The most common (>1/10) treatment-related AEs are transient injection-site reactions, occurring occasionally in about two thirds of patients [7]. These include injection site bruising, erythema, pain, pruritus and induration. Rarer cases of localized lipoatrophy and skin necrosis at injection sites have been reported during post-marketing [111, 112]. One peculiar injection-related tolerability issue with GA is the occurrence of immediate post-injection reactions (IPIR) that present immediately or a few minutes after the injection, consisting in flushing, chest tightness, palpitation, dyspnoea and intense anxiety. The crisis resolves spontaneously in a few minutes [53]. These reactions are unpredictable, affecting about 15 % of patients and seldom recurring more than once. The intensity of the reaction is not connected to any real risk to patients.

The tolerability of GA 40 mg/mL three times weekly has been shown to be similar to that of the 20 mg/mL once-daily formulation [8, 91]. Importantly, in the GLACIER study [94], three times weekly GA was found to be better tolerated than the once-daily formulation in terms of injection-related adverse events (IRAEs): the adjusted mean annualized rate of IRAEs was reduced by 50 % in patients receiving the new formulation (35.3 events per year vs. 70.4 events per year, respectively; $p = 0.0006$), while the rate of moderate/severe events was reduced by 60 % (0.9 events per year vs. 2.2 events per year, respectively; $p = 0.0021$). Furthermore, treatment convenience, as measured by the Treatment Satisfaction Questionnaire for Medication-9 (TSQM-9) convenience subscale, was improved for patients switching from GA 20 mg/mL once daily to the three times weekly formulation

[94]. Recently, results from the extension phase of the GLACIER study confirm the safety profile of the 40 mg/mL three times weekly formulation, in terms of both IRAEs and convenience [113].

Conclusions

The availability of multiple drugs has totally changed the scenario of MS treatment. Treatment choices became much more complicated and decisions should be based on the combination of the efficacy and safety profiles. From this point of view GA associates a favourable efficacy profile, confirmed by more than 20 years of clinical use, with an excellent safety and tolerability profile. The burden of daily injections has been recently reduced by the availability of the new 40 mg/mL three times a week formulation, which has been shown to share the same efficacy of the 20 mg/mL once daily formulation, but with obvious advantages in terms of patient convenience.

GA has been classified as a first-line drug for the treatment of RRMS in Europe, with a clear indication both in naïve patients and in patients who discontinue other therapies for safety or tolerability issues. The recent evidence of the importance of personalized treatment implies that the assessment of the individual prognostic profile should drive treatment decisions, at the same time considering also patients' preference and convenience. Patients with a good prognostic profile as indicated by low disease activity – revealed by low brain lesion burden and few or absent active lesions at the time of treatment onset – may have a high probability of responding to first-line therapies, including GA. On the contrary, patients with very active disease in the early phases tend to require an induction approach to obtain a positive response to treatment.

Considering the choice among first-line therapies, GA offers an obvious advantage in young, potentially fertile women for the favourable safety profile in this population, as discussed above [107]. Patients with CIS are also expected to benefit from GA, given the evidence of efficacy in such patients, supported by extension studies showing clear protection from brain atrophy [86, 87]. Another possible use of GA is as maintenance treatment in patients who start with an induction approach because of a negative prognostic profile. Induction therapy has often the advantage of "reshaping" the immune system, which can then be maintained by GA [114, 115].

The classification of MS clinical courses [2] defines the importance of disease activity not only in RRMS, but also in patients with a progressive disease course. The presence of disease activity represents a clear target for DMTs. Among them, the use of GA should be considered because of the long-term safety and absence of negative impact on spasticity, a frequent AE of IFN-β treatment in this population. It should be noted, however, that conclusive data from

clinical trials demonstrating the efficacy of GA in these patients are currently lacking.

We anticipate that the new 40 mg/mL three times weekly regimen might increase compliance and adherence. Therefore it is recommended that, in all consenting patients currently treated with the once daily formulation, the switch to the new formulation should be considered. An early start of GA treatment should be considered in the light of data on brain atrophy from the PreCISe study [87]: there was a significant (-28%; $p = 0.0209$) difference when comparing early GA treatment versus delayed GA treatment.

In conclusion, clinical trials and real-life studies have consistently shown the efficacy and safety of both formulations of GA in the first-line treatment of patients with RRMS and for delaying the onset of clinically definite MS in patients with CIS. Overall, data suggest that while many types of patients can be expected to benefit from GA, the "ideal" subject would be one with RR disease or newly-diagnosed, young and active, wanting to lead a normal life. The use of GA for more than two decades shows a reassuring safety profile and optimal tolerability. The major concern may be the frequency of administration, an issue that the new formulation can be expected to minimize, contributing to the use of this drug. Besides patient convenience, the fact that no complex clinical monitoring is required during treatment clearly represents another strong point of the clinical use of GA.

Abbreviations

ARR: Annualized relapse rate; BDNF: Brain derived neurotrophic factor; CDMS: Clinically definite multiple sclerosis; CIS: Clinically isolated syndrome; CNS: Central nervous system; DMTs: Disease-modifying therapies; EDSS: Expanded disability status scale; GA: Glatiramer acetate; IFN: Interferon; IRAEs: Injection-related adverse events; LTFU: Long-term follow up; MBP: Myelin basic protein; MHC: Major histocompatibility complex; MRI: Magnetic resonance imaging; MS: Multiple sclerosis; RRMS: Relapsing-remitting multiple sclerosis; TNF: Tumour necrosis factor; TSQM-9: Treatment satisfaction questionnaire for medication-9.

Competing interests

GC has received honoraria as a consultant and for lecturing at scientific meetings from Novartis, Teva, Sanofi-Aventis, Genzyme, Merck Serono, Biogen, Bayer, Serono Symposia International Foundation, Excemed, Roche, Almirall, Chugai, Receptos and Forward Pharma.
AB has received honoraria for serving in the scientific advisory boards of Almirall, Bayer, Biogen, Genzyme, with approval by the Director of AOU San Luigi University Hospital, and has received speaker honoraria from Biogen, Genzyme, Novartis, Teva; his institution has received grant support from Bayer, Biogen, Merck, Novartis, Teva, from the Italian Multiple Sclerosis Society, Fondazione Ricerca Biomedica ONLUS and San Luigi ONLUS.
DC is an Advisory Board member of Almirall, Bayer Schering, Biogen, Genzyme, GW Pharmaceuticals, Merck Serono, Novartis, Teva and received honoraria for speaking or consultation fees from Almirall, Bayer Schering, Biogen Idec, Genzyme, GW Pharmaceuticals, Merck Serono, Novartis, Sanofi-Aventis, Teva. He is also an external expert consultant of the European Medicine Agency (EMA), and the principal investigator in clinical trials for Bayer Schering, Biogen Idec, Merck Serono, Mitsubishi, Novartis, Roche, Sanofi-Aventis, Teva. His preclinical and clinical research was supported by grants from Bayer, Biogen, Merck Serono, Novartis and Teva.

NDS has received honoraria or consultation fees from Novartis, Merck Serono, Biogen Idec, La Roche; has been member of Advisory Boards for Novartis, Merck Serono, Biogen Idec; has participated in company-sponsored speaker's bureau for Novartis, Merck Serono, Biogen Idec; has received travel reimbursements from Novartis, Merck Serono and Biogen Idec.
CF has received grants and personal fees from Teva, and grants from Merck Serono, Novartis and Fondazione Italiana Sclerosi Multipla.
AG serves on scientific advisory boards or as consultant for Merck Serono, Teva, Novartis, Biogen Idec; he has received honoraria for lecturing from Merck Serono, Biogen Idec, Novartis, Teva, Genzyme, Almirall.
PG is an Advisory Board member of Almirall, Biogen Italy, Sanofi-Genzyme, GW Pharmaceuticals, Merck Serono, Novartis, Teva and received honoraria for speaking or consultation fees from Almirall, Biogen Idec, Genzyme, GW Pharmaceuticals, Merck Serono, Novartis, Sanofi-Aventis, Teva. He is also an external expert consultant of the European Medicine Agency (EMA), and has been the principal investigator in clinical trials for Biogen Idec, Merck Serono, Novartis, Roche, Sanofi-Aventis, Teva, Almirall. His preclinical and clinical research was supported by grants from Bayer-Shering, Biogen-Idec, Merck-Serono, Novartis and Teva.
GLM has received honoraria for lecturing, travel expenses reimbursements for attending meetings, and financial support for research from Bayer Schering, Biogen Idec, Genzyme, Merck Serono, Novartis, Sanofi-Aventis and Teva.
EM has received grants from Teva and Novartis and speaker honoraria from Biogen.
FP has received fees for speaking and advisory board activities by Almirall, Bayer, Biogen, Merck, Novartis, Sanofi-Genzyme and Teva.
CP has served on scientific advisory boards for Novartis, Merck Serono, Biogen Idec, Sanofi-Aventis, Genzyme, Almirall and Bayer, has received funding for travel and speaker honoraria from Sanofi-Aventis, Biogen Idec, Bayer, Teva, Merck Serono, Almirall, Genzyme, Actelion and Novartis, and receives research support from Novartis, Merck Serono, Biogen Idec, Bayer and Sanofi-Aventis.
MS receives research support and has received fees as speaker from Sanofi-Aventis, Biogen, Bayer Schering and Merck Serono.
GT has received grants and personal fees from Teva, Novartis, Merck Serono, Abbvie and Abbott.
MT has served on scientific Advisory Boards for Biogen Idec, Novartis, Almirall, Roche and Genzyme; has received speaker honoraria from Biogen Idec, Bayer-Schering, Sanofi Aventis, Merck Serono, Teva, Genzyme, Almirall and Novartis; has received research grants for her Institution from Biogen Idec, Merck Serono and Novartis.
The other Authors declare no conflicts of interest.

Authors' contributions
All the authors critically contributed to the draft and subsequent reviews of the manuscript and approved the final version before submission.

Acknowledgments
We wish to thank Marie Cheeseman who provided medical writing assistance on behalf of Springer Healthcare Communications. This assistance was funded by Teva.

Author details
[1]Department of Neurology, INSPE, San Raffaele Scientific Institute, Via Olgettina 48, 20132 Milan, Italy. [2]Department NEUROFARBA, Section Neurosciences, University of Florence, Florence, Italy. [3]Neurology 2-CRESM (Multiple Sclerosis Regional Reference Center), AOU San Luigi Gonzaga, Orbassano, TO, Italy. [4]Clinica Neurologica, Dipartimento di Medicina dei Sistemi, Università Tor Vergata, Rome, Italy. [5]IRCCS Istituto Neurologico Mediterraneo (INM) Neuromed Pozzilli, Pozzilli, IS, Italy. [6]Department of Neurological and Behavioural Sciences, University of Siena, Siena, Italy. [7]Department of Neuroscience, INSPE, San Raffaele Scientific Institute, Milan, Italy. [8]Department of Neurosciences DNS, The Multiple Sclerosis Centre - Veneto Region (CeSMuV), University Hospital of Padova, Padova, Italy. [9]Multiple Sclerosis Study Center, Hospital of Gallarate, Gallarate, VA, Italy. [10]Neurology Unit, Fondazione Istituto San Raffaele "G. Giglio" di Cefalù, Cefalù, PA, Italy. [11]Department of Neuroscience, Rehabilitation, Ophthalmology, Genetics, Maternal and Child Health, University of Genoa, Genoa, Italy. [12]Department of Medical Sciences, Multiple Sclerosis Center, University of Cagliari, Cagliari, Italy. [13]Neurology Unit, AUSL Parma – Fidenza Hospital, Fidenza, PR, Italy. [14]Department of Medical and Surgical Sciences and Advanced Technologies, G.F. Ingrassia, Multiple Sclerosis Center, University of Catania, Catania, Italy. [15]Department of Neurology and Psychiatry, Sapienza University of Rome, Rome, Italy. [16]Department of Experimental and Clinical Medicine, 1 Neurological Clinic, Marche Polytechnic University, Ancona, Italy. [17]Centre for Experimental Neurological Therapies (CENTERS), S. Andrea Hospital Site, Sapienza University of Rome, Rome, Italy. [18]Department of Medical, Surgical, Neurological, Metabolic and Aging Sciences, Second University of Naples, Naples, Italy. [19]Department of Basic Medical Sciences, Neuroscience and Sense Organs, University of Bari, Bari, Italy.

References

1. Nylander A, Hafler DA. Multiple sclerosis. J Clin Invest. 2012;122(4):1180–8. doi:10.1172/JCI58649.
2. Lublin FD. New multiple sclerosis phenotypic classification. Eur Neurol. 2014; 72 Suppl 1:1–5. doi:10.1159/000367614.
3. Cohen JA, Rae-Grant A. Handbook of Multiple Sclerosis. 2nd ed. London: Springer Healthcare; 2012.
4. Richards RG, Sampson FC, Beard SM, Tappenden P. A review of the natural history and epidemiology of multiple sclerosis: implications for resource allocation and health economic models. Health Technol Assess. 2002;6(10):1–73.
5. Abramsky O, Teitelbaum D, Arnon R. Effect of a synthetic polypeptide (COP 1) on patients with multiple sclerosis and with acute disseminated encephalomeylitis. Preliminary report. J Neurol Sci. 1977;31(3):433–8.
6. Bornstein MB, Miller AI, Teitelbaum D, Arnon R, Sela M. Multiple sclerosis: trial of a synthetic polypeptide. Ann Neurol. 1982;11(3):317–9. doi:10.1002/ana.410110314.
7. Teva Pharmaceuticals Ltd. Copaxone ® 20 mg/ml Solution for Injection, Pre-filled Syringe 2003. http://www.mhra.gov.uk/home/groups/par/documents/websiteresources/con025676.pdf. Accessed 14 Apr 2016.
8. Khan O, Rieckmann P, Boyko A, Selmaj K, Zivadinov R. Three times weekly glatiramer acetate in relapsing-remitting multiple sclerosis. Ann Neurol. 2013;73(6):705–13. doi:10.1002/ana.23938.
9. Aharoni R. The mechanism of action of glatiramer acetate in multiple sclerosis and beyond. Autoimmun Rev. 2013;12(5):543–53. doi:10.1016/j.autrev.2012.09.005.
10. Arnon R, Aharoni R. Mechanism of action of glatiramer acetate in multiple sclerosis and its potential for the development of new applications. Proc Natl Acad Sci U S A. 2004;101 Suppl 2:14593–8. doi:10.1073/pnas.0404887101.
11. Arnon R, Aharoni R. Neurogenesis and neuroprotection in the CNS–fundamental elements in the effect of Glatiramer acetate on treatment of autoimmune neurological disorders. Mol Neurobiol. 2007;36(3):245–53. doi:10.1007/s12035-007-8002-z.
12. Farina C, Weber MS, Meinl E, Wekerle H, Hohlfeld R. Glatiramer acetate in multiple sclerosis: update on potential mechanisms of action. Lancet Neurol. 2005;4(9):567–75. doi:10.1016/S1474-4422(05)70167-8.
13. Messina S, Patti F. The pharmacokinetics of glatiramer acetate for multiple sclerosis treatment. Expert Opin Drug Metab Toxicol. 2013;9(10):1349–59. doi:10.1517/17425255.2013.811489.
14. Arnon R. The development of Cop 1 (Copaxone), an innovative drug for the treatment of multiple sclerosis: personal reflections. Immunol Lett. 1996; 50(1-2):1–15.
15. Teitelbaum D, Meshorer A, Hirshfeld T, Arnon R, Sela M. Suppression of experimental allergic encephalomyelitis by a synthetic polypeptide. Eur J Immunol. 1971;1(4):242–8. doi:10.1002/eji.1830010406.
16. Teitelbaum D, Aharoni R, Arnon R, Sela M. Specific inhibition of the T-cell response to myelin basic protein by the synthetic copolymer Cop 1. Proc Natl Acad Sci U S A. 1988;85(24):9724–8.
17. Teitelbaum D, Milo R, Arnon R, Sela M. Synthetic copolymer 1 inhibits human T-cell lines specific for myelin basic protein. Proc Natl Acad Sci U S A. 1992;89(1):137–41.
18. Aharoni R, Teitelbaum D, Arnon R, Sela M. Copolymer 1 acts against the immunodominant epitope 82-100 of myelin basic protein by T cell receptor antagonism in addition to major histocompatibility complex blocking. Proc Natl Acad Sci U S A. 1999;96(2):634–9.
19. Neuhaus O, Farina C, Yassouridis A, Wiendl H, Then Bergh F, Dose T, et al. Multiple sclerosis: comparison of copolymer-1- reactive T cell lines from

treated and untreated subjects reveals cytokine shift from T helper 1 to T helper 2 cells. Proc Natl Acad Sci U S A. 2000;97(13):7452–7.

20. Aharoni R, Teitelbaum D, Sela M, Arnon R. Bystander suppression of experimental autoimmune encephalomyelitis by T cell lines and clones of the Th2 type induced by copolymer 1. J Neuroimmunol. 1998;91(1-2):135–46.

21. Duda PW, Schmied MC, Cook SL, Krieger JI, Hafler DA. Glatiramer acetate (Copaxone) induces degenerate, Th2-polarized immune responses in patients with multiple sclerosis. J Clin Invest. 2000;105(7):967–76. doi:10.1172/JCI8970.

22. Farina C, Then Bergh F, Albrecht H, Meinl E, Yassouridis A, Neuhaus O, et al. Treatment of multiple sclerosis with Copaxone (COP): Elispot assay detects COP-induced interleukin-4 and interferon-gamma response in blood cells. Brain. 2001;124(Pt 4):705–19.

23. Farina C, Wagenpfeil S, Hohlfeld R. Immunological assay for assessing the efficacy of glatiramer acetate (Copaxone) in multiple sclerosis. A pilot study. J Neurol. 2002;249(11):1587–92. doi:10.1007/s00415-002-0904-0.

24. Miller A, Shapiro S, Gershtein R, Kinarty A, Rawashdeh H, Honigman S, et al. Treatment of multiple sclerosis with copolymer-1 (Copaxone): implicating mechanisms of Th1 to Th2/Th3 immune-deviation. J Neuroimmunol. 1998; 92(1-2):113–21.

25. Chen M, Gran B, Costello K, Johnson K, Martin R, Dhib-Jalbut S. Glatiramer acetate induces a Th2-biased response and crossreactivity with myelin basic protein in patients with MS. Mult Scler. 2001;7(4):209–19.

26. Chen M, Conway K, Johnson KP, Martin R, Dhib-Jalbut S. Sustained immunological effects of Glatiramer acetate in patients with multiple sclerosis treated for over 6 years. J Neurol Sci. 2002;201(1-2):71–7.

27. Oreja-Guevara C, Ramos-Cejudo J, Aroeira LS, Chamorro B, Diez-Tejedor E. TH1/TH2 Cytokine profile in relapsing-remitting multiple sclerosis patients treated with Glatiramer acetate or Natalizumab. BMC Neurol. 2012;12:95. doi: 10.1186/1471-2377-12-95.

28. Becher B, Segal BM. T(H)17 cytokines in autoimmune neuro-inflammation. Curr Opin Immunol. 2011;23(6):707–12. doi:10.1016/j.coi.2011.08.005.

29. Jadidi-Niaragh F, Mirshafiey A. Th17 cell, the new player of neuroinflammatory process in multiple sclerosis. Scand J Immunol. 2011; 74(1):1–13. doi:10.1111/j.1365-3083.2011.02536.x.

30. Tzartos JS, Friese MA, Craner MJ, Palace J, Newcombe J, Esiri MM, et al. Interleukin-17 production in central nervous system-infiltrating T cells and glial cells is associated with active disease in multiple sclerosis. Am J Pathol. 2008;172(1):146–55. doi:10.2353/ajpath.2008.070690.

31. Aharoni R, Eilam R, Stock A, Vainshtein A, Shezen E, Gal H, et al. Glatiramer acetate reduces Th-17 inflammation and induces regulatory T-cells in the CNS of mice with relapsing-remitting or chronic EAE. J Neuroimmunol. 2010;225(1-2):100–11. doi:10.1016/j.jneuroim.2010.04.022.

32. Begum-Haque S, Sharma A, Kasper IR, Foureau DM, Mielcarz DW, Haque A, et al. Downregulation of IL-17 and IL-6 in the central nervous system by glatiramer acetate in experimental autoimmune encephalomyelitis. J Neuroimmunol. 2008;204(1-2):58–65. doi:10.1016/j.jneuroim.2008.07.018.

33. Miyara M, Gorochov G, Ehrenstein M, Musset L, Sakaguchi S, Amoura Z. Human FoxP3+ regulatory T cells in systemic autoimmune diseases. Autoimmun Rev. 2011;10(12):744–55. doi:10.1016/j.autrev.2011.05.004.

34. Viglietta V, Baecher-Allan C, Weiner HL, Hafler DA. Loss of functional suppression by CD4 + CD25+ regulatory T cells in patients with multiple sclerosis. J Exp Med. 2004;199(7):971–9. doi:10.1084/jem.20031579.

35. Huan J, Culbertson N, Spencer L, Bartholomew R, Burrows GG, Chou YK, et al. Decreased FOXP3 levels in multiple sclerosis patients. J Neurosci Res. 2005;81(1):45–52. doi:10.1002/jnr.20522.

36. Hong J, Li N, Zhang X, Zheng B, Zhang JZ. Induction of CD4 + CD25+ regulatory T cells by copolymer-I through activation of transcription factor Foxp3. Proc Natl Acad Sci U S A. 2005;102(18):6449–54. doi:10.1073/pnas. 0502187102.

37. Haas J, Korporal M, Balint B, Fritzsching B, Schwarz A, Wildemann B. Glatiramer acetate improves regulatory T-cell function by expansion of naive CD4(+)CD25(+)FOXP3(+)CD31(+) T-cells in patients with multiple sclerosis. J Neuroimmunol. 2009;216(1-2):113–7. doi:10.1016/j.jneuroim.2009.06.011.

38. Farina C, Vargas V, Heydari N, Kumpfel T, Meinl E, Hohlfeld R. Treatment with glatiramer acetate induces specific IgG4 antibodies in multiple sclerosis patients. J Neuroimmunol. 2002;123(1-2):188–92.

39. Vieira PL, Heystek HC, Wormmeester J, Wierenga EA, Kapsenberg ML. Glatiramer acetate (copolymer-1, copaxone) promotes Th2 cell development and increased IL-10 production through modulation of dendritic cells. J Immunol. 2003;170(9):4483–8.

40. Kim HJ, Ifergan I, Antel JP, Seguin R, Duddy M, Lapierre Y, et al. Type 2 monocyte and microglia differentiation mediated by glatiramer acetate therapy in patients with multiple sclerosis. J Immunol. 2004;172(11):7144–53.

41. Carpintero R, Brandt KJ, Gruaz L, Molnarfi N, Lalive PH, Burger D. Glatiramer acetate triggers PI3Kdelta/Akt and MEK/ERK pathways to induce IL-1 receptor antagonist in human monocytes. Proc Natl Acad Sci U S A. 2010; 107(41):17692–7. doi:10.1073/pnas.1009443107.

42. Weber MS, Prod'homme T, Youssef S, Dunn SE, Rundle CD, Lee L, et al. Type II monocytes modulate T cell-mediated central nervous system autoimmune disease. Nat Med. 2007;13(8):935–43. doi:10.1038/nm1620.

43. Weber MS, Starck M, Wagenpfeil S, Meinl E, Hohlfeld R, Farina C. Multiple sclerosis: glatiramer acetate inhibits monocyte reactivity in vitro and in vivo. Brain. 2004;127(Pt 6):1370–8. doi:10.1093/brain/awh163.

44. Aharoni R, Kayhan B, Eilam R, Sela M, Arnon R. Glatiramer acetate-specific T cells in the brain express T helper 2/3 cytokines and brain-derived neurotrophic factor in situ. Proc Natl Acad Sci U S A. 2003;100(24):14157–62. doi:10.1073/pnas.2336171100.

45. Gentile A, Rossi S, Studer V, Motta C, De Chiara V, Musella A, et al. Glatiramer acetate protects against inflammatory synaptopathy in experimental autoimmune encephalomyelitis. J Neuroimmune Pharmacol. 2013;8(3):651–63. doi:10.1007/s11481-013-9436-x.

46. Skihar V, Silva C, Chojnacki A, Doring A, Stallcup WB, Weiss S, et al. Promoting oligodendrogenesis and myelin repair using the multiple sclerosis medication glatiramer acetate. Proc Natl Acad Sci U S A. 2009; 106(42):17992–7. doi:10.1073/pnas.0909607106.

47. Arnold DL, Narayanan S, Antel S. Neuroprotection with glatiramer acetate: evidence from the PreCISe trial. J Neurol. 2013;260(7):1901–6. doi:10.1007/s00415-013-6903-5.

48. Filippi M, Rovaris M, Rocca MA, Sormani MP, Wolinsky JS, Comi G. Glatiramer acetate reduces the proportion of new MS lesions evolving into "black holes". Neurology. 2001;57(4):731–3.

49. Zivadinov R, Dwyer M, Barkay H, Steinerman JR, Knappertz V, Khan O. Effect of glatiramer acetate three-times weekly on the evolution of new, active multiple sclerosis lesions into T1-hypointense "black holes": a post hoc magnetic resonance imaging analysis. J Neurol. 2015;262(3):648–53. doi:10.1007/s00415-014-7616-0.

50. Cohen JA, Rovaris M, Goodman AD, Ladkani D, Wynn D, Filippi M. Randomized, double-blind, dose-comparison study of glatiramer acetate in relapsing-remitting MS. Neurology. 2007;68(12):939–44. doi:10.1212/01.wnl. 0000257109.61671.06.

51. Comi G, Cohen JA, Arnold DL, Wynn D, Filippi M. Phase III dose-comparison study of glatiramer acetate for multiple sclerosis. Ann Neurol. 2011;69(1):75–82. doi:10.1002/ana.22316.

52. Filippi M, Wolinsky JS, Comi G. Effects of oral glatiramer acetate on clinical and MRI-monitored disease activity in patients with relapsing multiple sclerosis: a multicentre, double-blind, randomised, placebo-controlled study. Lancet Neurol. 2006;5(3):213–20. doi:10.1016/S1474-4422(06)70327-1.

53. Johnson KP, Brooks BR, Cohen JA, Ford CC, Goldstein J, Lisak RP, et al. Copolymer 1 reduces relapse rate and improves disability in relapsing-remitting multiple sclerosis: results of a phase III multicenter, double-blind placebo-controlled trial. Neurology. 1995;45(7):1268–76.

54. Comi G, Filippi M, Wolinsky JS. European/Canadian multicenter, double-blind, randomized, placebo-controlled study of the effects of glatiramer acetate on magnetic resonance imaging–measured disease activity and burden in patients with relapsing multiple sclerosis. European/Canadian Glatiramer Acetate Study Group. Ann Neurol. 2001;49(3):290–7.

55. Bornstein MB, Miller A, Slagle S, Weitzman M, Crystal H, Drexler E, et al. A pilot trial of Cop 1 in exacerbating-remitting multiple sclerosis. N Engl J Med. 1987;317(7):408–14. doi:10.1056/NEJM198708133170703.

56. Sormani MP, Rovaris M, Valsasina P, Wolinsky JS, Comi G, Filippi M. Measurement error of two different techniques for brain atrophy assessment in multiple sclerosis. Neurology. 2004;62(8):1432–4.

57. Mikol DD, Barkhof F, Chang P, Coyle PK, Jeffery DR, Schwid SR, et al. Comparison of subcutaneous interferon beta-1a with glatiramer acetate in patients with relapsing multiple sclerosis (the REbif vs Glatiramer Acetate in Relapsing MS Disease [REGARD] study): a multicentre, randomised, parallel, open-label trial. Lancet Neurol. 2008;7(10):903–14. doi:10.1016/S1474-4422(08)70200-X.

58. Cadavid D, Wolansky LJ, Skurnick J, Lincoln J, Cheriyan J, Szczepanowski K, et al. Efficacy of treatment of MS with IFNbeta-1b or glatiramer acetate by monthly

brain MRI in the BECOME study. Neurology. 2009;72(23):1976–83. doi:10.1212/01. wnl.0000345970.73354.17.

59. O'Connor P, Filippi M, Arnason B, Comi G, Cook S, Goodin D, et al. 250 microg or 500 microg interferon beta-1b versus 20 mg glatiramer acetate in relapsing-remitting multiple sclerosis: a prospective, randomised, multicentre study. Lancet Neurol. 2009;8(10):889–97. doi:10.1016/S1474-4422(09)70226-1.

60. Fox RJ, Miller DH, Phillips JT, Hutchinson M, Havrdova E, Kita M, et al. Placebo-controlled phase 3 study of oral BG-12 or glatiramer in multiple sclerosis. N Engl J Med. 2012;367(12):1087–97. doi:10.1056/NEJMoa1206328.

61. Hutchinson M, Fox RJ, Miller DH, Phillips JT, Kita M, Havrdova E, et al. Clinical efficacy of BG-12 (dimethyl fumarate) in patients with relapsing-remitting multiple sclerosis: subgroup analyses of the CONFIRM study. J Neurol. 2013; 260(9):2286–96. doi:10.1007/s00415-013-6968-1.

62. La Mantia L, Di Pietrantonj C, Rovaris M, Rigon G, Frau S, Berardo F, et al. Comparative efficacy of interferon beta versus glatiramer acetate for relapsing-remitting multiple sclerosis. J Neurol Neurosurg Psychiatry. 2015; 86(9):1016–20. doi:10.1136/jnnp-2014-309243.

63. Ford C, Goodman AD, Johnson K, Kachuck N, Lindsey JW, Lisak R, et al. Continuous long-term immunomodulatory therapy in relapsing multiple sclerosis: results from the 15-year analysis of the US prospective open-label study of glatiramer acetate. Mult Scler. 2010;16(3):342–50. doi:10.1177/1352458509358088.

64. Ford C, Ladkani D, editors. Twenty years of continuous treatment of multiple sclerosis with glatiramer acetate 20 mg daily: long-term clinical results of the US open-label extension study. 29th Congress of the European Committee for Treatment and Research in Multiple Sclerosis and 18th Annual Conference of Rehabilitation in Multiple Sclerosis; 2013 October 2-5; Copenhagen, Denmark

65. Ford CC, Johnson KP, Lisak RP, Panitch HS, Shifronis G, Wolinsky JS. A prospective open-label study of glatiramer acetate: over a decade of continuous use in multiple sclerosis patients. Mult Scler. 2006;12(3):309–20.

66. Johnson KP, Brooks BR, Cohen JA, Ford CC, Goldstein J, Lisak RP, et al. Extended use of glatiramer acetate (Copaxone) is well tolerated and maintains its clinical effect on multiple sclerosis relapse rate and degree of disability. Copolymer 1 Multiple Sclerosis Study Group. Neurology. 1998;50(3):701–8.

67. Johnson KP, Brooks BR, Ford CC, Goodman AD, Lisak RP, Myers LW, et al. Glatiramer acetate (Copaxone): comparison of continuous versus delayed therapy in a six-year organized multiple sclerosis trial. Mult Scler. 2003;9(6):585–91.

68. Johnson KP, Ford CC, Lisak RP, Wolinsky JS. Neurologic consequence of delaying glatiramer acetate therapy for multiple sclerosis: 8-year data. Acta Neurol Scand. 2005;111(1):42–7. doi:10.1111/j.1600-0404.2004.00351.x.

69. Wolinsky JS, Narayana PA, Johnson KP. United States open-label glatiramer acetate extension trial for relapsing multiple sclerosis: MRI and clinical correlates. Multiple Sclerosis Study Group and the MRI Analysis Center. Mult Scler. 2001;7(1):33–41.

70. Rovaris M, Comi G, Rocca MA, Valsasina P, Ladkani D, Pieri E, et al. Long-term follow-up of patients treated with glatiramer acetate: a multicentre, multinational extension of the European/Canadian double-blind, placebo-controlled, MRI-monitored trial. Mult Scler. 2007;13(4):502–8. doi:10.1177/1352458506070704.

71. Wolinsky JS, Comi G, Filippi M, Ladkani D, Kadosh S, Shifroni G. Copaxone's effect on MRI-monitored disease in relapsing MS is reproducible and sustained. Neurology. 2002;59(8):1284–6.

72. Arnal-Garcia C, Amigo-Jorrin Mdel C, Lopez-Real AM, Lema-Devesa C, Llopis N, Sanchez-de la Rosa R. Long-term effectiveness of glatiramer acetate in clinical practice conditions. J Clin Neurosci. 2014;21(12):2212–8. doi:10.1016/j.jocn.2014.05.045.

73. Kalincik T, Jokubaitis V, Izquierdo G, Duquette P, Girard M, Grammond P, et al. Comparative effectiveness of glatiramer acetate and interferon beta formulations in relapsing-remitting multiple sclerosis. Mult Scler. 2015;21(9):1159–71. doi:10.1177/1352458514559865.

74. Khan O, Bao F, Shah M, Caon C, Tselis A, Bailey R, et al. Effect of disease-modifying therapies on brain volume in relapsing-remitting multiple sclerosis: results of a five-year brain MRI study. J Neurol Sci. 2012;312(1-2):7–12. doi:10.1016/j.jns.2011.08.034.

75. Bergvall N, Makin C, Lahoz R, Agashivala N, Pradhan A, Capkun G, et al. Comparative effectiveness of fingolimod versus interferons or glatiramer acetate for relapse rates in multiple sclerosis: a retrospective US claims

database analysis. Curr Med Res Opin. 2013;29(12):1647–56. doi:10.1185/03007995.2013.847411.

76. Gobbi C, Zecca C, Linnebank M, Muller S, You X, Meier R, et al. Swiss analysis of multiple sclerosis: a multicenter, non-interventional, retrospective cohort study of disease-modifying therapies. Eur Neurol. 2013;70(1-2):35–41. doi:10.1159/000346761.

77. Jongen PJ, Lehnick D, Sanders E, Seeldrayers P, Fredrikson S, Andersson M, et al. Health-related quality of life in relapsing remitting multiple sclerosis patients during treatment with glatiramer acetate: a prospective, observational, international, multi-centre study. Health Qual Life Outcomes. 2010;8:133. doi:10.1186/1477-7525-8-133.

78. Ziemssen T, Hoffman J, Apfel R, Kern S. Effects of glatiramer acetate on fatigue and days of absence from work in first-time treated relapsing-remitting multiple sclerosis. Health Qual Life Outcomes. 2008;6:67. doi:10.1186/1477-7525-6-67.

79. Ghezzi A, Amato MP, Annovazzi P, Capobianco M, Gallo P, La Mantia L, et al. Long-term results of immunomodulatory treatment in children and adolescents with multiple sclerosis: the Italian experience. Neurol Sci. 2009; 30(3):193–9. doi:10.1007/s10072-009-0083-1.

80. Kornek B, Bernert G, Balassy C, Geldner J, Prayer D, Feucht M. Glatiramer acetate treatment in patients with childhood and juvenile onset multiple sclerosis. Neuropediatrics. 2003;34(3):120–6. doi:10.1055/s-2003-41274.

81. Caon C, Din M, Ching W, Tselis A, Lisak R, Khan O. Clinical course after change of immunomodulating therapy in relapsing-remitting multiple sclerosis. Eur J Neurol. 2006;13(5):471–4. doi:10.1111/j.1468-1331.2006.01273.x.

82. Zwibel HL. Glatiramer acetate in treatment-naive and prior interferon-beta-1b-treated multiple sclerosis patients. Acta Neurol Scand. 2006;113(6):378–86. doi:10.1111/j.1600-0404.2006.00627.x.

83. Ziemssen T, Bajenaru OA, Carra A, de Klippel N, de Sa JC, Edland A, et al. A 2-year observational study of patients with relapsing-remitting multiple sclerosis converting to glatiramer acetate from other disease-modifying therapies: the COPTIMIZE trial. J Neurol. 2014;261(11):2101–11. doi:10.1007/s00415-014-7446-0.

84. Lublin FD, Cofield SS, Cutter GR, Conwit R, Narayana PA, Nelson F, et al. Randomized study combining interferon and glatiramer acetate in multiple sclerosis. Ann Neurol. 2013;73(3):327–40. doi:10.1002/ana.23863.

85. Goodman AD, Rossman H, Bar-Or A, Miller A, Miller DH, Schmierer K, et al. GLANCE: results of a phase 2, randomized, double-blind, placebo-controlled study. Neurology. 2009;72(9):806–12. doi:10.1212/01.wnl.0000343880.13764.69.

86. Comi G, Martinelli V, Rodegher M, Moiola L, Bajenaru O, Carra A, et al. Effect of glatiramer acetate on conversion to clinically definite multiple sclerosis in patients with clinically isolated syndrome (PreCISe study): a randomised, double-blind, placebo-controlled trial. Lancet. 2009;374(9700):1503–11. doi:10.1016/S0140-6736(09)61259-9.

87. Comi G, Martinelli V, Rodegher M, Moiola L, Leocani L, Bajenaru O, et al. Effects of early treatment with glatiramer acetate in patients with clinically isolated syndrome. Mult Scler. 2013;19(8):1074–83. doi:10.1177/1352458512469695.

88. Wolinsky JS, Narayana PA, O'Connor P, Coyle PK, Ford C, Johnson K, et al. Glatiramer acetate in primary progressive multiple sclerosis: results of a multinational, multicenter, double-blind, placebo-controlled trial. Ann Neurol. 2007;61(1):14–24. doi:10.1002/ana.21079.

89. Wolinsky JS, Shochat T, Weiss S, Ladkani D. Glatiramer acetate treatment in PPMS: why males appear to respond favorably. J Neurol Sci. 2009;286(1-2):92–8. doi:10.1016/j.jns.2009.04.019.

90. Sajja BR, Narayana PA, Wolinsky JS, Ahn CW. Longitudinal magnetic resonance spectroscopic imaging of primary progressive multiple sclerosis patients treated with glatiramer acetate: multicenter study. Mult Scler. 2008; 14(1):73–80. doi:10.1177/1352458507079907.

91. Khan O, Rieckmann P, Boyko A, Selmaj K, Ashtamker N, Davis M, et al. Efficacy and safety of a three-times weekly dosing regimen of glatiramer acetate in relapsing–remitting multiple sclerosis patients: 3-year results of the Glatiramer Actetate Low-frequency Administration (GALA) open-label extension study [abstract]. Presented at the 67th American Academy of Neurology Annual Meeting. Washington, DC. April 18-24, 2015. Neurology. 2015;84(14 Suppl):P7.273.

92. Cutter G, Wolinsky JS, Comi G, Ladkani D, Knappertz V, Vainstein A, et al. Comparable clinical and MRI efficacy of glatiramer acetate 40 mg/mL TIW and 20 mg/mL QD: results of a systematic review and meta-analysis [abstract no. P053]. Mult Scler. 2014;20 Suppl 1:90–1.

93. Cutter G, Wolinsky JS, Comi G, Ladkani D, Knappertz V, Vainstein A, et al. Indirect comparison of glatiramer acetate 40 mg/mL TIW and 20 mg/mL QD dosing regimen effects on relapse rate: results of a predictive statistical model [abstract no. P100]. Mult Scler. 2014;20 Suppl 1:112.

94. Wolinsky JS, Borresen TE, Dietrich DW, Wynn D, Sidi Y, Steinerman JR, et al. GLACIER: An open-label, randomized, multicenter study to assess the safety and tolerability of glatiramer acetate 40 mg three-times weekly versus 20 mg daily in patients with relapsing-remitting multiple sclerosis. Mult Scler Relat Disord. 2015;4(4):370–6. doi:10.1016/j.msard.2015.06.005.

95. Meca-Lallana JE, Balseiro JJ, Lacruz F, Guijarro C, Sanchez O, Cano A, et al. Spasticity improvement in patients with relapsing-remitting multiple sclerosis switching from interferon-beta to glatiramer acetate: the ESCALA Study. J Neurol Sci. 2012;315(1-2):123–8. doi:10.1016/j.jns.2011.11.010.

96. Makhani N, Ngan BY, Kamath BM, Yeh EA. Glatiramer acetate-induced acute hepatotoxicity in an adolescent with MS. Neurology. 2013;81(9):850–2. doi: 10.1212/WNL.0b013e3182a2cc4a.

97. Antezana A, Herbert J, Park J, Kister I. Glatiramer acetate-induced acute hepatotoxicity in an adolescent with MS. Neurology. 2014;82(20):1846–7. doi:10.1212/01.wnl.0000450224.37865.80.

98. La Gioia S, Bacis G, Sonzogni A, Frigeni B, Conti MZ, Vedovello M, et al. Glatiramer acetate-induced hepatitis in a young female patient with multiple sclerosis. Mult Scler Relat Disord. 2014;3(6):732–4. doi:10.1016/j.msard.2014.08.001.

99. Rauschka H, Farina C, Sator P, Gudek S, Breier F, Schmidbauer M. Severe anaphylactic reaction to glatiramer acetate with specific IgE. Neurology. 2005;64(8):1481–2. doi:10.1212/01.WNL.0000158675.01711.58.

100. Corominas M, Postigo I, Cardona V, Lleonart R, Romero-Pinel L, Martinez J. IgE-mediated allergic reactions after the first administration of glatiramer acetate in patients with multiple sclerosis. Int Arch Allergy Immunol. 2014; 165(4):244–6. doi:10.1159/000371418.

101. Ghezzi A, Banwell B, Boyko A, Amato MP, Anlar B, Blinkenberg M, et al. The management of multiple sclerosis in children: a European view. Mult Scler. 2010;16(10):1258–67. doi:10.1177/1352458510375568.

102. Chitnis T, Tenembaum S, Banwell B, Krupp L, Pohl D, Rostasy K, et al. Consensus statement: evaluation of new and existing therapeutics for pediatric multiple sclerosis. Mult Scler. 2012;18(1):116–27. doi:10.1177/1352458511430704.

103. Amato MP, Portaccio E. Fertility, pregnancy and childbirth in patients with multiple sclerosis: impact of disease-modifying drugs. CNS Drugs. 2015;29(3): 207–20. doi:10.1007/s40263-015-0238-y.

104. Fragoso YD. Glatiramer acetate to treat multiple sclerosis during pregnancy and lactation: a safety evaluation. Expert Opin Drug Saf. 2014;13(12):1743–8. doi:10.1517/14740338.2014.955849.

105. Ghezzi A, Annovazzi P, Portaccio E, Cesari E, Amato MP. Current recommendations for multiple sclerosis treatment in pregnancy and puerperium. Expert Rev Clin Immunol. 2013;9(7):683–91. doi:10.1586/1744666X.2013.811046. quiz 92.

106. Weber-Schoendorfer C, Schaefer C. Multiple sclerosis, immunomodulators, and pregnancy outcome: a prospective observational study. Mult Scler. 2009;15(9):1037–42. doi:10.1177/1352458509106543.

107. Giannini M, Portaccio E, Ghezzi A, Hakiki B, Pasto L, Razzolini L, et al. Pregnancy and fetal outcomes after glatiramer acetate exposure in patients with multiple sclerosis: a prospective observational multicentric study. BMC Neurol. 2012;12:124. doi:10.1186/1471-2377-12-124.

108. Fragoso YD, Finkelsztejn A, Kaimen-Maciel DR, Grzesiuk AK, Gallina AS, Lopes J, et al. Long-term use of glatiramer acetate by 11 pregnant women with multiple sclerosis: a retrospective, multicentre case series. CNS Drugs. 2010;24(11):969–76. doi:10.2165/11538960-000000000-00000.

109. US Food and Drug Administration. Content and format of labeling for human prescription drug and biological products: requirements for pregnancy and lactation labeling. 2015. http://www.fda.gov/downloads/aboutfda/reportsmanualsforms/reports/economicanalyses/ucm427798.pdf. Accessed 21 Oct 2015.

110. Confavreux C, Hutchinson M, Hours MM, Cortinovis-Tourniaire P, Moreau T. Rate of pregnancy-related relapse in multiple sclerosis. Pregnancy in Multiple Sclerosis Group. N Engl J Med. 1998;339(5):285–91. doi:10.1056/NEJM199807303390501.

111. Balak DM, Hengstman GJ, Cakmak A, Thio HB. Cutaneous adverse events associated with disease-modifying treatment in multiple sclerosis: a systematic review. Mult Scler. 2012;18(12):1705–17. doi:10.1177/1352458512438239.

112. Watkins CE, Litchfield J, Youngberg G, Leicht SS, Krishnaswamy G. Glatiramer acetate-induced lobular panniculitis and skin necrosis. Cutis. 2015;95(3):E26–30.

113. Wynn DS, Kolodny S, Rubinchick S, Steinerman J, Knappertz V, Wolinsky J. Patient experience with glatiramer acetate 40 mg/1 mL three-times weekly treatment for relapsing–remitting multiple sclerosis: results from the GLACIER extension study [abstract]. Presented at the 67th American Academy of Neurology Annual Meeting. Washington, DC. April 18-24, 2015. Neurology. 2015;84(14 Suppl):P7.218.

114. Arnold DL, Campagnolo D, Panitch H, Bar-Or A, Dunn J, Freedman MS, et al. Glatiramer acetate after mitoxantrone induction improves MRI markers of lesion volume and permanent tissue injury in MS. J Neurol. 2008;255(10): 1473–8. doi:10.1007/s00415-008-0911-x.

115. Vollmer T, Panitch H, Bar-Or A, Dunn J, Freedman MS, Gazda SK, et al. Glatiramer acetate after induction therapy with mitoxantrone in relapsing multiple sclerosis. Mult Scler. 2008;14(5):663–70. doi:10.1177/1352458507085759.

116. Lindsey JW, Scott TF, Lynch SG, Cofield SS, Nelson F, Conwit R, et al. The CombiRx trial of combined therapy with interferon and glatiramer acetate in relapsing remitting MS: Design and baseline characteristics. Mult Scler Relat Disord. 2012;1(2):81–6. doi:10.1016/j.msard.2012.01.006.

17

Disease modifying treatments and symptomatic drugs for cognitive impairment in multiple sclerosis: where do we stand?

Claudia Niccolai*⊙, Benedetta Goretti and Maria Pia Amato

Abstract

Cognitive dysfunction is frequent in multiple sclerosis patients and has important and negative consequences for daily activities and quality of life of subjects. Disease modifying treatments for multiple sclerosis reduce the incidence of relapses and may prevent disease progression, but the influence on cognitive impairment is unclear, due to several limitations of the available studies. Moreover, symptomatic drugs for the improvement of already established cognitive deficits have been tested in small pilot studies, providing conflicting or mainly negative results. Currently, specific pharmacological therapies for the management of cognitive deficits in MS have not yet been developed. We will provide an updated overview of available evidence of pharmacological approaches for ameliorating cognitive deficits, based either on disease modifying treatments or symptomatic drugs.

Keywords: Pharmacological treatment, Cognitive impairment, Multiple sclerosis

Background

Cognitive impairment (CI) in multiple sclerosis (MS) affects about 40–70% of patients. It involves all the disease subtypes, sometimes from the early stages of the disease, also independently from physical disability. It has a negative impact on patient daily life, employment and on the capacity to benefit from in-patient rehabilitation [1]. Therefore, to improve patient function and quality of life, interventions to ameliorate or reduce CI are of paramount importance, through pharmacological and/or rehabilitation approaches. We will review available evidence on pharmacological approaches for CI in MS, based either on disease modifying treatments (DMT) or symptomatic drugs.

Disease modifying treatments

Since 1990s, DMTs are usually employed in clinical practice to reduce the incidence of relapses and disability progression in MS. The possible positive effect on cognitive outcomes can be due to the decrease of the ongoing

inflammatory activity, which may contribute to better cognitive performances. DMTs can also positively influence the cognitive performances, by acting on some key pathogenic mechanisms of MS-related cognitive impairment. In particular, all the approved DMTs reduce the accumulation of T2 and T1 lesions in the brain, and some of them also reduce the progression of brain atrophy. Moreover, some of the DMTs may also produce a neuroprotective effect via different mechanisms of action, such as through the delivery of neurotrophic factors or newer mechanism of action for newer drugs [2]. However, the interpretation of available data is complicated, due to methodological problems of study design and execution [1].

The bulk of available evidence for the effects of DMTs on cognitive outcomes in MS has been collected with the interferons (IFNB-1a and IFNB-1b).

Fisher et al. [3] have published an extensive study, exploring the effects of IFN b-1a on cognition, assessed by Multiple Sclerosis Functional Composite (MSFC) administered to 166 relapsing-remitting multiple sclerosis (RRMS) patients, in the context of a multicenter, 2-year, phase III randomized clinical trial. After two years,

* Correspondence: claunicco@libero.it
Department of NEUROFARBA, University of Florence, Viale Pieraccini 6, Florence 50134, Italy

adjusting for baseline performance, IFN b-1a showed a significant beneficial effect on tests of information processing speed, learning and memory, as well as a positive trend on tests of visuospatial abilities and problem solving. Although it is difficult to generalize the trial results to everyday practice, due to the extensive neuropsychological assessment, the trial showed an improvement in cognitive performance in both arms, possibly due to "practice effects", which was however significantly more pronounced in the treatment group. The treatment arm also exhibited a significantly increased time to sustained deterioration in the performance on the Paced Auditory Serial Addition Test (PASAT).

The BENEFIT (Betaferon/Betaseron in Newly Emerging MS for Initial Treatment) trial and its extension at 3 and 5 years [4–6], underline the effect of IFNB-1b on cognition in patients with clinically isolated syndromes (CIS). In these trials, patients were randomized to receive IFNB-1b immediately after the clinical event or at the end of the trial. The results showed an improvement on cognitive performance in the PASAT over the five years, whose scores were in the normal range in the majority of the subjects at baseline. Improvement on the PASAT was significantly more pronounced in the early treatment group compared with the delayed treatment group after five years, suggesting an effect of early treatment in maintaining an intact cognitive functioning [7]. No cognitive data have been published from the IFNB trials in persons with secondary and primary progressive MS [8–12].

Most of the existing post-marketing observational studies involving interferons and cognition in MS, have been non-randomized, so we should interpreted their results with caution. We are reviewing only studies that have included at least 100 patients.

The effects IFN b-1a on cognitive function in early, mildly disabled RRMS patients were addressed in the Italian multicenter, post-marketing COGIMUS (Cognitive Impairment in Multiple Sclerosis) study [13]. This prospective cohort study included 459 early RRMS patients treated with IFN b-1a s.c. 22 or 44 mcg in everyday clinical practice. The patients were assessed through the Brief Repeatable Neuropsychological Battery (BRNB) and the Stroop test at baseline and at 12 monthly intervals for three years for a total of four cognitive assessments. At baseline there were no differences between the two groups in demographic and clinical characteristics and in the proportions of patients impaired on more than three tests. Data on cognitive performance at baseline and 3 years were available for 318 patients of the original cohort (72.1%; 22 mcg, n = 153; 44 mcg, n = 165) and showed a 32% risk reduction of developing impairment in three or more tests for patients on high dose compared with those on the lower dose.

The effect of glatiramer acetate (GA) on cognition was evaluated as part of a phase III trial on RRMS where patients were randomized to receive GA (20 mg subcutaneously every day) or placebo [14]. Two hundred forty-eight patients were assessed by the BRNB at baseline and after 1–2 years using. Both treatment groups showed a significant improvement in cognitive performance because of "practice effects". The absence of an effect of GA on cognitive profile, could be explain by the low level of baseline cognitive abnormalities and the short-term observation period. No cognitive data have been published in primary progressive MS, although the MSFC was included in a phase III trial of GA [15]. The impact of natalizumab on cognitive profile was investigated in a phase III clinical trials of RRMS patients -the AFFIRM (Natalizumab Safety and Efficacy in Relapsing Remitting Multiple Sclerosis) and SENTINEL (Safety and Efficacy of Natalizumab in Combination with Interferon Beta-1a in Patients with Relapsing Remitting Multiple Sclerosis) [16, 17]. Both studies showed a positive effect on cognition in all the subjects treated with natalizumab, although the cognitive outcome was evaluated only by the PASAT.

Iaffaldano et al. [18] have examined the effects of natalizumab on cognitive performance in an uncontrolled observational study, by the BRNB and the Stroop test, calculating a global score, defined Cognitive Impairment Index (CII) every 12 months, that allowing the evaluation of changes in cognitive performances independently by the number of cognitive tests failed, using the mean and SD from the normative sample of Rao's battery and the Stroop Test. One hundred and 53 patients completed 1 and 2 year-natalizumab treatment, respectively, at the standard dose of 300 mg every 4 weeks intravenously. After 1 year of treatment the percentage of cognitively impaired patients decreased from 29% at baseline to 19% and the mean baseline values of the CII and fatigue scores were significantly reduced. These significant effects were confirmed in the subgroup of patients treated up to 2 years.

Stephenson et al. [19] have conducted a prospective, uncontrolled study in 333 patients on the effect of natalizumab in patient-reported outcomes measures. After 12 months of pharmacological treatment, 69% to 88% of patients reported an improvement in quality of life assessed by the SF-12v2 [20], the MSIS-29 [21], the FS [22], the DS scale [23], fatigue assessed by the MFIS [24] and cognition assessed by the MOS-Cog [25]. Reduction of self-reported fatigue assessed by the Fatigue Scale for Motor and Cognitive functions (FSMC) was also reported in the large uncontrolled TYNERGY study [26, 27].

Although the above studies showed positive influence of natalizumab treatment on cognition, there are limits in the validity of results, due to observational, non-randomized studies design and the absence of a control group.

In the FREEDOMS trial, a 24 month, RCT of oral fingolimod compared with placebo in patients with RRMS, a significant effect on the MSFC was observed in both groups compared with the placebo group (Cohen et al., 2010) [28]. Trials on newer oral and biologic DMTs have included the PASAT in the context of the MFSC, although no cognitive results have been published so far.

In conclusion, all these study limitations do not allow to achieve firm conclusions. In fact, the studies with DMTs have shown weak positive effects on cognition and the methodological limitations reduce the strength of the results. The majority of randomized controlled trials on DMT are not appropriate to detect cognitive changes. Cognition is not the primary outcome and often the only explorative measure of cognition is the PASAT, in the context of the MSFC [29]. Observational studies on DMT are non-randomized, have included small sample of patients with different clinical characteristics, used heterogeneous cognitive assessment tools and outcome measures and have not considered the patients' cognitive status at baseline. We can only speculate that early treatment may be the most effective way to preserve intact cognitive functioning and delay the development of cognitive impairment, on the basis of studies focusing on CIS and early RRMS patients. Future trials should assess cognition more systematically, to better understand the potential effect of the new DMT on the patient cognitive performance [1].

Symptomatic drugs

Due to frequent association between fatigue and cognitive impairment in MS patients and the hypothesis of a shared pathophysiologic basis, it has been speculated that drugs used for the symptomatic management of fatigue in MS may be beneficial also for cognitive functioning [30]. Studies on symptomatic drugs in MS have focused on improving performance in specific, impaired cognitive domains, typically involved in the profile of neuropsychological deficits in MS, such as information processing speed and complex attention or episodic memory. Most of these studies show a few methodological limitations, in particular small sample sizes, the study design, not inclusion of impaired cognition and heterogeneity of cognitive outcomes. The main features of these studies are synthesized in Table 1.

Geisler et al. [31] evaluated 45 MS patients treated with amantadine, pemoline, or placebo for 6 week. Fatigue did not significantly correlate with any of the neuropsychological outcome measures at baseline or after treatment and there were no significant differences in cognitive performance between amantadine, pemoline, and placebo patients. The neuropsychological

measures were tests of attention (Digit Span, Trail Making Test, and Symbol Digit Modalities Test), verbal memory (Selective Reminding Test), nonverbal memory (Benton Visual Retention Test), and motor speed (Finger Tapping Test). All groups improved on tests of attention, verbal memory and motor speed, probably due to "practice effects".

Studies with patients treated with modafinil, have done uncertain results. Moller et al. [32] conducted a double-blind, placebo-controlled randomized trial involving 121 patients with MS and fatigue, finding that modafinil had no great effects on fatigue or cognitive dysfunction. Another study with modafinil suggested a positive treatment effect on other neuropsychological tests, but this study was not placebo-controlled [33]. In a double-blind, placebo-controlled study conducted by Bruce et al. [34], 23 patients with MS had significantly improved delayed memory on a list-learning task after they took modafinil, but no improvement on other cognitive domains or self-reported fatigue. Recently, Ford-Johnson et al. [35] showed no effect of modafinil on learning and memory performance. However, participants showed improvement in working memory task administered, the Wechsler Adult Intelligence Scale-III (WAIS-III) Letter-Number Sequencing task, as compared with those on placebo.

Acetylcholinesterase inhibitors (AChEIs) used in Alzheimer's disease have been tested for improving cognition in other neurological disorders. Specifically, in MS, it is hypothesized that disruption of cholinergic pathways and impaired axonal transport of acetylcholine may produce a reduction of cholinergic drive that might underlie at least in part cognitive dysfunction [1]. Parry et al. [36] have suggested that rivastigmine, a central cholinesterase inhibitor, can perform an acute modulation of potentially adaptive functional changes in cognitive functioning. They studied ten patients with MS and 11 healthy controls using a functional MRI (fMRI) during the execution of Stroop task. All the participants took the drug. In five out of ten MS patients there were a relative normalization of the abnormal Stroop-associated pattern of brain activation, although no change in brain activation was found in any of four healthy controls taking the drug. Cader et al. [37] showed the administration of rivastigmine significantly enhanced fMRI activation in the prefrontal regions for the Stroop task, in a group of 15 MS patients. In this small study, there were no significant changes in the neuropsychological task performance, 11 of 15 patients showed improvements, whereas 4 of 15 patients showed decline. Shaygannejad et al. [38] enrolled 60 MS patients with cognitive impairment in a 3-month single-center, double-blind, placebo-controlled clinical trial. Patients were randomly allocated

Table 1 Overview of the main studies on symptomatic treatments for cognitive impairment in multiple sclerosis

Authors, year	Drug	Number treated	Design	Duration	Cognitive results
Geisler et al., 1996 [31]	Amantadine, pemoline	16	DB, PC, RCT	6 weeks	No improv.
Moller et al., 2011 [32]	Modafinil	62	DB, PC, RCT	8 weeks	No improv.
Lange et al., 2009 [52]	Modafinil	8	DB, PC, RCT	8 weeks	Improvement
Stankoff et al., 2005 [53]	Modafinil	59	DB, PC, RCT	5 weeks	No improv.
Wilken et al., 2008 [33]	Modafinil	23	Randomized, evaluator blind	4 months	Improvement
Bruce et al., 2012 [34]	Armodafinil	16	DB, PC, CO	1 week	Improvement
Ford-Johnson et al., 2016 [35]	Modafinil	16	DB, CO	5 weeks	Improvement
Shaygannejad et al. [38]	Rivastigmine	30	DB, PC, RCT	12 weeks	No improvement
Parry et al., 2003 [36]	Rivastigmine	10	OLT	4–6 weeks	Improvement
Cader et al., 2009 [37]	Rivastigmine	15	CO, SB	4–6 weeks	No improv.
Krupp et al., 2004 [39]	Donepezil	35	DB, PC, RCT	24 weeks	Improvement
Krupp et al., 2011 [40]	Donepezil	61	DB, PC, RCT	24 weeks	No Improv.
Lovera et al., 2010 [41]	Memantina	58	DB, PC, RCT	16 weeks	No improv.
Villoslada et al., 2009 [54]	Memantina	19	DB, PC, CO	12 months	No improv.
Peyro Saint Paul et al., 2016 [42]	Memantina	50	DB, PC, PG, RCT	52 weeks	No improv.
Benedict et al., 2008 [43]	l-amphetamine	19	Counterbalanced, within-subject	4x single doses	Improvement
Morrow et al., 2009 [44]	l-amphetamine	108	DB, PC, RCT	4 weeks	No improv.
Sumowki et al., 2011 [45] (re-analysis of 66)	l-amphetamine	108	DB, PC, RCT	4 weeks	Improvement
Harel et al., 2009 [46]	Methylphenidate	14	DB, PC, RCT	Single dose	Improvement
Lovera et al., 2007 [55]	Ginkgo biloba	20	DB, PC, RCT	12 weeks	No improv.
Lovera et al., 2012 [56]	Ginkgo biloba	61	DB, PC, RCT	12 weeks	No improv.
Johnson et al., 2006 [57]	Ginkgo biloba	12	DB, PC, PG	4 weeks	Improvement variable responses
Magnin et al., 2015 [48]	Fampridine	50	OLT	4 weeks	Improvement
Pavsic et al., 2015 [49]	Fampridine	30	OLT	4 weeks	No improv.
Jensen et al., 2014 [50]	Fampridine	108	OLT	26–28 days	Improvement
Romero et al., 2015 [47]	Cannabis	20	PG	Single dose	No improv.

DB double blind, *PC* placebo controlled, *RCT* randomized controlled trial, *CO* crossover, *SB* single blind, *OLT* open label trial, *PG* parallel group

to receive a 12-week treatment course of either rivastigmine (1.5 mg once a day increment over 4 weeks to 3 mg twice daily) or placebo. Response to treatment was assessed by the Wechsler Memory Scale (WMS) at baseline and 12 weeks after the start of therapy. They observed a significant memory improvement occurred in both groups, possibly due to "practice effects" and the average WMS general memory score at the end of trial did not change between rivastigmine and placebo group.

The effects of Donepezil on cognitive function in MS have also investigated. Krupp et al. [39] conducted a randomized, double-blind, placebo-controlled, single-center clinical trial of 69 patients with MS who were selected for initial memory difficulties and randomly assigned to receive a 24-week treatment course of either donepezil (10 mg daily) or placebo. Donepezil improved memory performance on the Selective Reminding Test (SRT)

when compared with placebo and this benefit remained significant after controlling for several demographic and clinical covariates. Patients in the donepezil group were significantly more likely to self-report memory improvement than those receiving placebo. More recently, Krupp et al. [40], investigated the effects of 10 mg daily of donepezil ($n = 61$) versus 10 mg of placebo ($n = 59$) in 120 cognitively impaired MS patients. After 24 weeks, there were no improvements in memory performance on SRT in the donepezil group, although the subgroup of patients exhibiting more severe degrees of cognitive dysfunction.

Lovera et al. [41] conducted a multicenter double-blind placebo-controlled clinical trial in MS patients with cognitive impairment. Fifty-eight patients were treated with memantine at 20 mg daily and 68 controls were tested. The results showed that patients treated had no improvements in cognitive performance assessed by PASAT and California Verbal Learning Test-II (CVLT-II) Long Delay Free Recall (LDFR). Recently, Peyro Saint Paul et al. [42] conducted a study for examining the efficacy and safety of a long-term administration of memantine as a symptomatic treatment for cognitive disorders in 50 patients. In this double-blind, placebo-controlled, parallel group, randomized trial, the participants were assigned to receive memantine (20 mg/day) or a placebo for 52 weeks. No differences between the placebo and memantine groups were observed in the PASAT score, used as primary neuropsychological outcome.

It is reasonable to consider in this overview also CNS stimulants for MS patients and their influence on cognitive profile. In a pilot double-blind, placebo-controlled study involving 19 MS patients [43], single 45 mg doses of L-amphetamine sulfate in MS were associated with improved performance on information processing speed. Morrow et al. [44] tested 151 clinically definite MS patients randomized to L-amphetamine or to placebo in a 6-week. The trial results did not confirm any significant improvement on Symbol Digit Modalities Test (SDMT) or on the subjective ratings of cognition. In a re-analysis of the study conducted by Sumowski et al. [45], the Authors suggested the drug may act by improving hippocampal function. In fact, there was a significant effect of L-amphetamine sulfate on auditory/verbal and visual/spatial memory in the cognitively impaired MS patients. Harel et al. studied the effect of methylphenidate on 26 MS patients with impaired attention in a double-blind placebo-controlled trial [46]. The patients were randomized to receive a single dose of 10 mg methylphenidate or placebo. Attention was assessed using PASAT-3" and PASAT-2" at baseline and one hour after drug/placebo administration. Methylphenidate significantly improved performance of both PASAT-3" and PASAT-2" tests by 22.8 and 25.6% respectively, while no significant changes were observed in placebo treated patients.

Recently the use of the cannabis has been approved for the symptomatic treatment of spasticity. Romero et al. [47] conducted a study on the effect of cannabis on cognition. They examined 20 MS patients who smoke cannabis for symptom relief, and 19 matched non-cannabis-smoking MS patients. Patients were evaluated by the BRNB and structural MRI scans. Results showed that decreased regional brain volume was associated with poorer performance on all neuropsychological tests in MS patients who smoked cannabis. Specially cannabis-smoking MS patients showed significantly lower performance on the 10/36 spatial recall test and the PASAT.

Few studies have preliminarily explored the impact of fampridine (4-aminopyridine) on motor and cognitive parameters. Results from a trial conducted by Magnin et al. [48] with 50 MS patients, showed that verbal fluencies were significantly improved after fampridine treatment. Pavsic et al. [49] conducted a non-randomized study including 30 patients with different types of MS, treated with 10 mg of fampridine twice daily. They obtained a gait performance of 56.7% and after 28 days of treatment, significant improvement among responders occurred in total MSFC score. However, there was no statistically significant improvement of PASAT.

Jensen et al. performed another open-label study of 108 MS patients treated with fampridine 10 mg BID. After 26–28 days of treatment, results showed significant improvements on quantitative tests of upper and lower limb functions as well as the SDMT [50].

We can summarize that, taking together, all these weak results do not support the use of any of the above symptomatic drugs for improving MS-related cognitive impairments.

Conclusions

Over the past two decades MS-related cognitive dysfunction has received growing attention. Validated brief and extensive batteries for the neuropsychological assessment of MS patients are now available [1]. The approach to cognitive assessment should be extensive, taking into account possible confounding factors. Among these, fatigue, depression, comorbidities and also the possible harmful effect of symptomatic medications on cognition, such as benzodiazepines, antiepileptic drugs, anticholinergic drugs used for bladder dysfunction [1].

Despite the great availability of pharmacological drugs for reducing disease activity in MS, no effective symptomatic treatment has been established for cognitive impairment. The results of studies are inconsistent or negative and the few positive findings have not been confirmed in successive trials. Pharmacological therapies of comorbidities that can contribute to poor cognitive performance, such as depression or fatigue, may also provide cognitive benefits, but currently there are not consistent evidences in this area. The use of cognitive enhancer agents could have a positive effect in contrasting the side effects of other drugs (such as benzodiazepines, baclofen, alpha lytic, etc.) which are currently used to treat other participating symptoms. The research in this field must be considered preliminary. The findings that we already have are controversial and not sufficiently strong to currently recommend the clinical use of these classes of medications for treating CI. Further studies in this field could combine older and newer pharmacological strategies with cognitive rehabilitation and, possibly, physical exercise [51].

Abbreviations

AchEIS: Acetylcholinesterase inhibitors; AFFIRM: Natalizumab safety and efficacy in relapsing remitting multiple sclerosis; BRNB: Brief repeatable neuropsychological battery; CI: Cognitive impairment; CII: Cognitive impairment index; CIS: Clinically isolated syndrome; COGIMUS: Cognitive impairment in multiple sclerosis; CVLT-II: California Verbal Learning Test-II; DMT: Disease modifying treatment; DS: Disease step; fMRI: Functional magnetic resonance imaging; FS: Functional status; FSMC: Fatigue scale for motor and cognitive functions; GA: Glatiramer acetato; LDFR: Long delay free recall; MFIS: Modified fatigue impact scale; MOS-Cog: Medical outcome scale cognitive functioning; MS: Multiple sclerosis; MSFC: Multiple sclerosis functional composite; MSIS-29: Multiple sclerosis impact scale; PASAT: Paced auditory serial addition test; RRMS: Relapsing remitting multiple sclerosis; SDMT: Symbol digit modalities test; SENTINEL: Safety and Efficacy of Natalizumab in Combination with Interferon Beta-1a in Patients with Relapsing Remitting Multiple Sclerosis; SF-12v2: Short form 12 version 2; SRT: Selective reminding test; WAIS-III: Wechsler Adult Intelligence Scale-III; WMS: Wechsler memory scale; BENEFIT: (Betaferon/Betaseron in Newly Emerging MS for Initial Treatment)

Acknowledgements

Not applicable.

Funding

Not applicable.

Authors' contributions

All authors wrote the manuscript. MPA drafted/revised the manuscript. All authors read and approved the final manuscript.

Competing interests

CN and BG have no competing interests. MPA received grants/research supports from Biogen, Teva, Merck Serono, Novartis; received honoraria from Merck Serono, Biogen, Teva, Novartis, Almirall.

References

1. Amato MP, Langdon D, Montalban X, Benedict RH, DeLuca J, Krupp LB, et al. Treatment of cognitive impairment in multiple sclerosis: position Paper. J Neurol. 2013;260(6):1452–68.
2. Gold R, Wolinsky JS, Amato MP, Comi G. Evolving expectations around early management of multiple sclerosis. Ther Adv Neurol Disord. 2010;3(6):351–67.
3. Fischer JS, Priore RL, Jacobs LD, Cookfair DL, Rudick RA, Herndon RM, et al. Neuropsychological effects of interferon beta-1a in relapsing multiple sclerosis. Multiple Sclerosis Collaborative Research Group. Ann Neurol. 2000; 48:885–92.
4. Kappos L, Polman CH, Freedman MS, Edan G, Hartung HP, Miller DH, et al. Treatment with interferon beta-1b delays conversion to clinically definite and McDonald MS in patients with clinically isolated syndromes. Neurology. 2006;67(7):1242–9.
5. Kappos L, Freedman MS, Polman CH, Montalbán X, Hartung HP, Hemmer B, et al. Effect of early versus delayed interferon beta-1b treatment on disability after a first clinical event suggestive of multiple sclerosis: a 3-year follow-up analysis of the BENEFIT study. Lancet. 2007;370(9585):389–97.
6. Kappos L, Freedman MS, Polman CH, Kappos L, Freedman MS, Polman CH, et al. Long-term effect of early treatment with interferon beta-1b after a first clinical event suggestive of multiple sclerosis: 5-year active treatment extension of the phase 3 BENEFIT trial. Lancet Neurol. 2009; 8(11):987–97.
7. Penner IK, Stemper B, Calabrese P, Freedman MS, Polman CH, Edan G, et al. Effects of interferon beta-1b on cognitive performance in patients with a first event suggestive of multiple sclerosis. Mult Scler. 2012;18(10):1466–71.
8. Kappos L, Polman C, Pozzilli C, Thompson A, Beckmann K, Dahlke F. European Study Group in Final analysis of the European multicenter trial on IFNbeta-1b in secondary-progressive MS Interferon beta-1b in Secondary-Progressive MS. Neurology. 2001;57(11):1969 75.
9. Panitch H, Miller A, Paty D, Weinshenker B. North American Study Group on Interferon beta-1b in Secondary Progressive MS Interferon beta-1b in secondary progressive MS: results from a 3-year controlled study. Neurology. 2004;63(10):1788–95.
10. Cohen JA, Cutter GR, Fischer JS, Goodman AD, Heidenreich FR, Kooijmans MF, et al. Benefit of interferon beta-1a on MSFC progression in secondary progressive MS. Neurology. 2002;59:679–87.
11. Leary SM, Miller DH, Stevenson VL, Brex PA, Chard DT, Thompson AJ. Interferon beta-1a in primary progressive MS: an exploratory, randomize Cohen, J.d, controlled trial. Neurology. 2003;60(1):44–51.
12. Montalban X, Sastre-Garriga J, Filippi M, Khaleeli Z, Téllez N, Vellinga MM. Primary progressive multiple sclerosis diagnostic criteria: a reappraisal. Mult Scler. 2009;15(12):1459–65.
13. Patti F, Amato MP, Bastianello S, Caniatti L, Di Monte E, Ferrazza P, et al. Effects of immunomodulatory treatment with subcutaneous interferon beta-1a on cognitive decline in mildly disabled patients with relapsing-remitting multiple sclerosis. Mult Scler. 2010;16:68–77.
14. Weinstein A, Scwid SI, Schiffer RB, McDermott MP, Giang DW, Goodman AD. Neuropsychologic status in multiple sclerosis after treatment with glatiramer. Arch Neurol. 1999;56:319–24.
15. Wolinsky JS, Narayana PA, O'Connor P, Coyle PK, Ford C, Johnson K, et al. Glatiramer acetate in primary progressive multiple sclerosis: results of a multinational, multicenter, double-blind, placebo-controlled trial. Ann Neurol. 2007;61(1):14–24.
16. Polman CH, O'Connor PW, Havrdova E, Hutchinson M, Kappos L, Miller DH, et al. A randomized, placebo-controlled trial of natalizumab for relapsing multiple sclerosis. N Engl J Med. 2006;354(9):899–910.
17. Rudick RA, Stuart WH, Calabresi PA, Confavreux C, Galetta SL, Radue EW, et al. Natalizumab plus interferon beta-1a for relapsing multiple sclerosis. N Engl J Med. 2006;354(9):911–23.
18. Iaffaldano P, Viterbo RG, Paolicelli D, Lucchese G, Portaccio E, Goretti B, et al. Impact of natalizumab on cognitive performances and fatigue in relapsing multiple sclerosis: a prospective, open-label, two years observational study. PLoS One. 2012;7(4):e35843.
19. Stephenson JJ, Kern DM, Agarwal SS, Zeidman R, Rajagopalan K, Kamat SA, et al. Impact of natalizumab on patient-reported outcomes in multiple sclerosis: a longitudinal study. Health Qual Life Outcomes. 2012;27:155.
20. Ware Jr J, Kosinski M, Keller SD. A 12-Item Short-Form Health Survey: construction of scales and preliminary tests of reliability and validity. Med Care. 1996;34(3):220–33.
21. Hobart J, Lamping D, Fitzpatrick R, Riazi A, Thompson A. The Multiple Sclerosis Impact Scale (MSIS-29): a new patient-based outcome measure. Brain. 2001;124(Pt 5):962–73.
22. Goodin DS. A questionnaire to assess neurological impairment in multiple sclerosis. Mult Scler. 1998;4(5):444–51.
23. Hohol MJ, Orav EJ, Weiner HL. Disease steps in multiple sclerosis: a simple approach to evaluate disease progression. Neurology. 1995;45(2):251–5.
24. Stewart AL, Ware JE. Measuring functioning and well-being: the medical outcomes study approach. Durham: Duke University Press; 1992.
25. Ritvo PG. The Consortium of Multiple Sclerosis Centers Health Services Research Subcommittee. MSQLI Multiple Sclerosis Quality of Life Inventory: a user's manual. New York: National Multiple Sclerosis Society; 1997.
26. Penner IK, Sivertsdotter EC, Celius EG, Fuchs S, Schreiber K, Berkö S. et al., TYNERGY trial investigators.Improvement in Fatigue during Natalizumab Treatment is Linked to Improvement in Depression and Day-Time Sleepiness. Front Neurol. 2015;23(6):18.
27. Svenningsson A, Falk E, Celius EG, Fuchs S, Schreiber K, Berkö S, et al. Natalizumab treatment reduces fatigue in multiple sclerosis. Results from the TYNERGY trial; a study in the real life setting. PLoS One. 2013;8(3):e58643.
28. Cohen JA, Barkhof F, Comi G, Hartung HP, Khatri BO, Montalban X, et al. Oral fingolimod or intramuscular interferon for relapsing multiple sclerosis. N Engl J Med. 2010;362(5):402–15.
29. Rudick R, Antel J, Confavreux C, Cutter G, Ellison G, Fischer J, et al. Recommendations from the national multiple sclerosis society clinical outcomes assessment task force. Ann Neurol. 1997;42:379–82.
30. Tur C. Fatigue management in multiple sclerosis. Curr Treat Options Neurol. 2016;18(6):26.
31. Geisler MW, Sliwinski M, Coyle PK, Masur DM, Doscher C, Krupp LB. The effects of amantadine and pemoline on cognitive functioning in multiple sclerosis. Arch Neurol. 1996;53(2):185–8.

32. Moller F, Poettgen J, Broemel F, Neuhaus A, Daumer M, Heesen C. HAGIL (Hamburg Vigil Study): a randomized placebo-controlled double-blind study with modafinil for treatment of fatigue in patients with multiple sclerosis. Mult Scler. 2011;17(8):1002–9.

33. Wilken JA, Sullivan C, Wallin M, Rogers C, Kane RL, Rossman H, et al. Treatment of multiple sclerosis-related cognitive problems with adjunctive modafinil: rationale and preliminary supportive data. Int J MS Care. 2008;10:1–10.

34. Bruce J, Hancock L, Roberg B, Brown A, Henkelman E, Lynch S. Impact of armodafinil on cognition in multiple sclerosis: a randomized, double-blind crossover pilot study. Cogn Behav Neurol. 2012;25(3):107–14.

35. Ford-Johnson L, DeLuca J, Zhang J, Elovic E, Lengenfelder J, Chiaravalloti ND. Cognitive effects of modafinil in patients with multiple sclerosis: A clinical trial. Rehabil Psychol. 2016;61(1):82–91.

36. Parry AM, Scott RB, Palace J, Smith S, Matthews PM. Potentially adaptive functional changes in cognitive processing for patients with multiple sclerosis and their acute modulation by rivastigmine. Brain. 2003;126(Pt 12):2750–60.

37. Cader S, Palace J, Matthews PM. Cholinergic agonism alters cognitive processing and enhances brain functional connectivity in patients with multiple sclerosis. J Psychopharmaco. 2009;23(6):686–96.

38. Shaygannejad V, Janghorbani M, Ashtari F, Zanjani HA, Zakizade N. Effects of rivastigmine on memory and cognition in multiple sclerosis. Can J Neurol Sci. 2008;35(4):476–81.

39. Krupp LB, Christodoulou C, Melville P, Scherl WF, MacAllister WS, Elkins LE. Donepezil improved memory in multiple sclerosis in a randomized clinical trial. Neurology. 2004;63:1579–85.

40. Krupp LB, Christodoulou C, Melville P, Scherl WF, Pai L-Y, Muenz LR, et al. Multicenter randomized clinical trial of donepezil for memory impairment in multiple sclerosis. Neurology. 2011;76:1500–7.

41. Lovera JF, Frohman E, Brown TR, Bandari D, Nguyen L, Yadav V, et al. Memantine for cognitive impairment in multiple sclerosis: a randomized placebo-controlled trial. Mult Scler. 2010;16(6):715–23.

42. Peyro Saint Paul L, Creveuil C, Heinzlef O, De Seze J, Vermersch P, Castelnovo G, et al. Efficacy and safety profile of memantine in patients with cognitive impairment in multiple sclerosis: A randomized, placebo-controlled study. J Neurol Sci. 2016;363:69–76.

43. Benedict RH, Munschauer F, Zarevics P, Erlanger D, Rowe V, Feaster T, et al. Effects of L-amphetamine sulfate on cognitive function in multiple sclerosis patients. J Neurol. 2008;255:848–52.

44. Morrow SA, Kaushik T, Zarevics P, Erlanger D, Mark F, Munschauer BE, et al. The effects of L-amphetamine sulfate on cognition in MS patients: results of a randomized controlled trial. J Neurol. 2009;256:1095–102.

45. Sumowski JF, Chiaravalloti N, Erlanger D, Kaushik T, Benedict RH, Deluca J. L-amphetamine improves memory in MS patients with objective memory impairment. Mult Scler. 2011;17(9):988. 1141–45.

46. Harel Y, Appleboim N, Lavie M, Achiron A. Single dose of methylphenidate improves cognitive performance in multiple sclerosis patients with impaired attention process. J Neurol Sci. 2009;15:38–40.

47. Romero K, Pavisian B, Staines WR, Feinstein A. Multiple sclerosis, cannabis and cognition: A structural MRI study. Neuroimage Clin. 2015;9(8):140–7.

48. Magnin E, Sagawa Jr Y, Chamard L, Berger E, Moulin T, Decavel P. Verbal fluencies and fampridine treatment in multiple sclerosis. Eur Neurol. 2015; 74:243–50.

49. Pavsic K, Pelicon K, Ledinek AH, Sega S. Short-term impact of fampridine on motor and cognitive functions, mood and quality of life among multiple sclerosis patients. Clin Neurol Neurosurg. 2015;139:35–40.

50. Jensen H, Ravnborg M, Mamoei S, Dalgas U, Stenager E. Changes in cognition, arm function and lower body function after slow-release Fampridine treatment. Mult Scler. 2014;20(14):1872–80.

51. Feinstein A, Dalgas U. The benefits of exercise in progressive MS: some cautious optimism. Mult Scler. 2014;20(3):269–70.

52. Lange R, Volkmer M, Heesen C, Liepert J. Modafinil effects in multiple sclerosis patients with fatigue. J Neurol, 2009;256:645–50.

53. Stankoff B, Waubant E, Confavreux C, Edan G, Debouverie M, Rumbach L, et al. Modafinil for fatigue in MS: a randomized placebo-controlled double-blind study. Neurology. 2005;64:1139–43.

54. Villoslada P, Arrondo G, Sepulcre J, Alegre M, Artieda J. Memantine induces reversible neurologic impairment in patients with MS. Neurology. 2009; 72(19):1630–3.

55. Lovera J, Bagert B, Smoot K, Morris CD, Frank R, Bogardus K, et al. Ginkgo biloba for the improvement of cognitive performance in multiplesclerosis: a randomized, placebo-controlled trial. Mult Scler. 2007;13:376–85.

56. Lovera JF, Kim E, Heriza E, Fitzpatrick M, Hunziker J, Turner AP, Adams J, et al. Ginkgo biloba does not improve cognitive function in MS: a randomized placebo-controlled trial. Neurology. 2012;79(12):1278–84.

57. Johnson SK, Diamond BJ, Rausch S, Kaufman M, Shiflett SC, Graves L. The effect of Ginkgo biloba on functional measures in multiple sclerosis: a pilot randomized controlled trial. Explore (NY). 2006;2:19.

18

Use of rituximab and risk of re-hospitalization for children with neuromyelitis optica spectrum disorder

Sabrina Gmuca[1][*] ⓘ, Rui Xiao[2], Pamela F. Weiss[1], Amy T. Waldman[3] and Jeffrey S. Gerber[2,4]

Abstract

Background: Treatment algorithms for neuromyelitis optica spectrum disorder (NMOSD) vary, and sparse data exist regarding the impact of initial treatments on disease course. We aimed to determine whether administration of rituximab during first hospitalization reduces 1-year readmission rates.

Methods: We conducted a retrospective cohort study of subjects with NMOSD using the Pediatric Health Information System database from 2005 to 2015. Subjects were ages 1 to 21 years who received glucocorticoids and an ICD-9-CM code indicating neuromyelitis optica (NMO) during first hospitalization. All subjects had at least 12 months of continuous enrollment. The primary exposure was ≥1 rituximab dose during first hospitalization. We tested for the association of rituximab use with all-cause re-hospitalization, the primary outcome, using survival analysis. Re-hospitalization was considered if a hospital admission occurred > 30 days after initial discharge with exclusion of admissions with re-dosing of rituximab and data were censored at 12 months. Secondary outcomes included time to and median duration of re-hospitalization using 25th percentiles of survival time and the Wilcoxon-rank sum test, respectively.

Results: Of 180 subjects who met inclusion criteria, 71.7% were female and the median age was 13 years (IQR: 10, 15). Fifty-two subjects (28.9%) received rituximab during first hospitalization, and there was an increasing trend in rituximab use over time ($p < 0.01$). Overall, 36.7% of children were readmitted and time to readmission was a median of 365 days (IQR: 138, 365). Rituximab exposure was not associated with re-hospitalization (adjusted HR: 0.71: 95% CI: 0.38, 1.34) nor a reduced time to re-hospitalization. Median duration of re-hospitalization was 2 days shorter in the rituximab exposed group ($p = 0.02$). Receipt of physical therapy, a surrogate marker for neurologic impairment, during first hospitalization was associated with re-admission within 12 months (adjusted HR: 4.81; 95% CI: 1.14, 20.29).

Conclusions: Among children with NMOSD, first-line administration of rituximab was not associated with risk of or time to re-hospitalization. Rituximab use was found to be associated with a shorter duration of re-hospitalization. Need for physical therapy during first hospitalization was independently associated with an increased risk of re-admission.

Keywords: Autoimmune, Demyelinating, Neuromyelitis optica, Rituximab

* Correspondence: gmucas@email.chop.edu
[1]Division of Rheumatology, Center for Pediatric Clinical Effectiveness,
Children's Hospital of Philadelphia, Philadelphia, PA, USA
Full list of author information is available at the end of the article

Background

Neuromyelitis optica spectrum disorder (NMOSD) is a rare, immune-mediated inflammatory disorder of the central nervous system. This chronic astrocytopathy preferentially targets the optic nerves and spinal cord, resulting in severe and potentially devastating sequelae such as paralysis and blindness. Despite the life-threatening consequences of uncontrolled disease activity, there are no validated treatment strategies for NMOSD [1–3].

NMOSD is rare among children and adolescents, with pediatric onset NMOSD accounting for approximately 3–5% of all cases [4]. However, early recognition and initiation of treatment is critical for preventing disease relapses in children with NMOSD. Therapeutic management of pediatric NMOSD is largely based on Class IV evidence, extrapolated from studies of adults [5–10]. Immunotherapeutic agents targeting T and B cell functions and reducing pro-inflammatory molecules from the peripheral blood circulation have been shown to attenuate disease progression in NMOSD [11]. Rituximab is a chimeric, murine/human monoclonal antibody directed against the CD20 antigen that results in depletion of B cells. Although small, open label [12] and retrospective studies [5] have reported benefits of rituximab in NMOSD, the effectiveness and safety of rituximab for NMOSD remains unclear [3, 13]. We sought to determine the impact of rituximab on all-cause re-hospitalization for children and young adults with NMOSD. We hypothesized that subjects who received rituximab during their first hospitalization were less likely to be re-admitted within 12 months.

Methods

We conducted a retrospective cohort study of subjects with NMOSD in the Pediatric Health Information System (PHIS) from January 2005 until December 2015. PHIS is an administrative database of 46 children's hospitals across the United States and represents 85% of all pediatric hospitalizations at freestanding tertiary care pediatric facilities. All subjects with at least 12 months of continuous enrollment and ≤ 21 years of age [14] at the time of initial documentation of an ICD-9-CM code for NMO (341.0) were included. The index date was the date of the first admission with an ICD-9-CM code for NMO. We excluded patients less than 1 year of age at the time of diagnosis (because NMOSD is unlikely to present within the first year of life) [15]; or who had an ICD-9-CM code for multiple sclerosis (MS), as this is a distinct disease from NMOSD. We also excluded subjects who did not receive glucocorticoids, which are frequently administered intravenously for optic neuritis or spinal cord deficits in NMOSD. Subjects with an ICD-9-CM code for NMOSD but without glucocorticoid exposure likely did not have active neurologic disease and

were less likely to be incident cases. The primary exposure was defined as billing for ≥1 dose of rituximab during the initial hospitalization. The primary outcome was all-cause re-hospitalization (binary), a surrogate marker for disease and treatment related morbidity. Re-hospitalization was considered if a hospital admission occurred > 30 days after initial discharge with exclusion of re-hospitalizations with re-dosing of rituximab and data were censored at 12 months. Secondary outcomes included time to first re-hospitalization and duration of re-hospitalization.

Demographics were summarized by standard descriptive statistics including frequencies and percentages for categorical variables (e.g. sex, race) and by range, median, and interquartile range (IQR) for continuous or count variables. Characteristics between the rituximab exposed and unexposed groups were compared by Wilcoxon rank sum test for medians, and chi-squared test or Fisher's exact test for proportions as appropriate. Time to hospitalization was calculated in days from the initial hospitalization until the first readmission and survival analysis was used to calculate 25th percentiles of time to re-hospitalization based on rituximab exposure. Kaplan-Meier survival curves of re-hospitalization were generated for the rituximab exposed and unexposed groups and compared using the log-rank test. The proportional hazards assumption for the primary exposure was met (Shoenfeld residuals $p = 0.58$). The univariate Cox proportional hazard regression model was used to evaluate the marginal effect of each covariate on the outcome, including demographics, glucocorticoid type, level of care, physical therapy, plasma exchange (PLEX) and duration of initial hospital stay. Covariates with a p-value less than 0.2 were considered in forward selection using the likelihood ratio test to build a multivariable cox regression model with certain variables of interest forced into the model. The proportional hazards assumption was met using Schoenfeld residuals with global test $p = 0.31$. According to Cox-Snell residuals, the final model fit the data well. We did not assess competing risks because the data source did not include mortality data. The trend in the proportion of children with NMOSD who received first-line rituximab therapy per calendar year was tested by 'nptrend' command implemented in Stata. All tests considered were two-sided and a significance level of 0.05 was applied. Data analyses were performed using STATA 14 (STATA Corp, College Station TX).

Results

Of the 351 eligible subjects with at least one code for NMO, 180 subjects met study inclusion and exclusion criteria (Fig. 1). Table 1 shows patient characteristics. The majority of subjects were female (71.7%) and a little

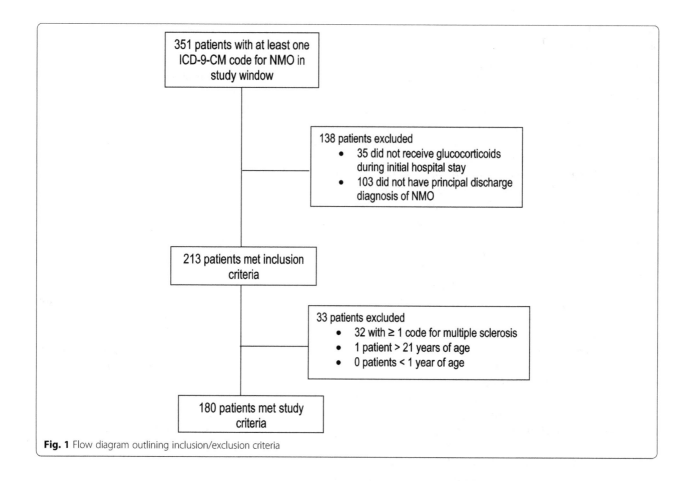

Fig. 1 Flow diagram outlining inclusion/exclusion criteria

less than half were Caucasian (40.0%). Median age at time of first hospitalization was 13 years (IQR: 10.0, 15.0) and median duration of initial hospitalization was 6 days (IQR: 3.0, 12.0). Only 3 subjects had a concomitant systemic rheumatologic condition. A total of 16 subjects (8.9%) received oral glucocorticoids only; 76 (42.2%) received methylprednisolone only; and 88 (48.9%) received a combination of oral and intravenous glucocorticoids. Table 2 lists the proportion of subjects who received each of the glucocorticoid sparing therapies administered during initial hospitalization. The most common were plasma exchange (PLEX) (31.1%), rituximab (28.9%), and intravenous immunoglobulin (IVIg) (18.3%); 61 subjects (33.9%) did not receive any glucocorticoid sparing therapies. Of those subjects who received rituximab ($n = 52$), 20 subjects (38.5%) also received plasma exchange and 23 subjects (44.2%) received rituximab without any other non-glucocorticoid immunosuppressive therapy.

Fifty-two subjects (28.9%) received rituximab during their first hospitalization with an increasing trend over time ($p < 0.01$) (Fig. 2). Comparing subjects in the rituximab exposed to unexposed, the proportion of non-Caucasian subjects in the rituximab group was

greater than in the unexposed group (70.2% vs. 42.0%). Overall, 36.7% of subjects were re-hospitalized at least once within the first year after diagnosis (Table 1). Kaplan-Meier estimates comparing the probability of re-hospitalization for children with NMOSD treated with rituximab versus those treated with alternative therapies showed no statistically significant difference between groups (log-rank test $p = 0.76$) (Fig. 3). Median duration of re-hospitalization was 2 days (IQR: 1.0, 4.0) in subjects administered first-line rituximab compared to 4 days (IQR: 2.0, 6.0) in those subjects who did not receive rituximab ($p = 0.02$). 25% of rituximab exposed subjects were re-hospitalized within 137 days (95% CI: 65, 295) and 25% of rituximab unexposed were re-hospitalized within 134 days (95% CI: 92, 192), indicating a similar time to re-hospitalization irrespective of rituximab exposure.

In univariate Cox regression modeling, the relative hazard of all-cause re-hospitalization in the first 12 months was 1.08 (95% CI: 0.64, 1.83) for those treated with rituximab compared to those not treated with rituximab ($p = 0.77$). In the final multivariate model (Table 3), the hazard ratio (HR) of re-hospitalization within 12 months was 0.71 (95% CI: 0.38, 1.34) for those children who received rituximab compared to those

Table 1 Patient characteristics

	Total (n = 180)	Rituximab exposed (n = 52)	Rituximab unexposed (n = 128)
Demographics			
Female, n (%)	129 (71.7)	43 (82.7)	86 (67.2)
Age, median (IQR)	13.0 (10.0, 15.0)	13.0 (10.0, 16.0)	12.5 (9.0, 15.0)
Caucasian[a], n (%)	72 (48.9)	14 (29.8)	58 (58.0)
Region, n (%)			
Northeast	29 (16.1)	9 (17.3)	20 (15.6)
Midwest	29 (16.1)	8 (15.4)	21 (16.4)
South	98 (54.4)	30 (57.7)	68 (53.1)
West	24 (13.3)	5 (9.6)	19 (14.8)
Systemic lupus erythematosus, n (%)	2 (1.1)	2 (3.9)	0 (0.0)
Sjögren syndrome, n (%)	1 (0.6)	1 (1.9)	0 (0.0)
ICU status, n (%)	31 (17.2)	11 (21.2)	20 (15.6)
Length of stay (days), median (IQR)	6 (3.0, 12.0)	7.0 (3.0, 17.0)	6.0 (3.0, 11.0)
Primary outcome			
Re-hospitalization in 12 months, n (%)	66 (36.7)	20 (38.5)	46 (35.9)
Secondary outcomes			
Length of re-hospitalization (days), median (IQR)	3.0 (1.0, 5.0)	2.0 (1.0, 4.0)	4.0 (2.0, 6.0)
Time to re-hospitalization (days), median (IQR)	365 (138, 365)	365 (138, 365)	365 (137, 365)

ICU intensive care unit, IQR interquartile range

[a]Race was missing for 33 subjects. Rituximab exposure was defined as having received at least one dose of rituximab during initial hospitalization with a documented ICD-9-CM code for neuromyelitis optica (341.0)

who did not ($p = 0.29$). Receipt of physical therapy was independently associated with an increased risk of re-hospitalization within the first 12 months (HR: 4.82; 95% CI: 1.14, 20.29).

Discussion

Using a database of 46 freestanding children's hospitals, we assessed the impact of first-line rituximab use on children and adolescents with NMOSD. We did not observe an association between rituximab use and risk of

Table 2 Proportion of subjects administered non-glucocorticoid treatment regimens during first hospitalization (n = 180)

Treatment	n, (%)
Plasma exchange (PLEX)[a]	56 (31.1)
Rituximab[b]	52 (28.9)
Intravenous immunoglobulin (IVIg)[c]	33 (18.3)
Mycophenolate mofetil	23 (12.8)
Azathioprine	15 (8.3)
Cyclophosphamide	10 (5.6
Methotrexate	1 (0.6)

Legend. Subjects were able to contribute to more than one treatment regimen therefore total does not equal 100%

[a]PLEX + rituximab (n = 20)

[b]Rituximab only, without any of the above listed non-glucocorticoid agent (n = 23)

[c]IVIg + rituximab (n = 8)

all-cause re-hospitalization or time to all-cause re-hospitalization. Although first-line rituximab use was associated with a shorter duration of re-hospitalization, the clinical significance of this is unclear. Receipt of physical therapy was independently associated with an increased risk of re-hospitalization.

This study, to our knowledge, comprises the largest cohort of pediatric subjects with NMOSD administered rituximab first-line. Previous work has largely focused on the use of rituximab as maintenance therapy in the treatment of NMOSD, with a limited number of studies examining the efficacy of first-line rituximab use [1, 5, 16]. Zephir et al. reported a retrospective analysis of 32 adults with NMOSD who received first-line rituximab and found that at the end of the follow-up period (mean 28.7 months), 84.3% were relapse free [1]. Olivieri et al. described the case of a 9-year-old girl who received rituximab along with administration of methylprednisolone and plasma exchange and had a slow but full neurologic recovery [16]. Longoni et al. performed a retrospective cohort study of 5 pediatric subjects (all aquaporin-4 antibody positive) with NMOSD treated with first-line rituximab; 60% (3/5) had a relapse of their disease within 12 months of initial rituximab therapy but relapses were reportedly less severe than prior to treatment and all patients demonstrated neurologic improvements by the end of the follow-up period [5].

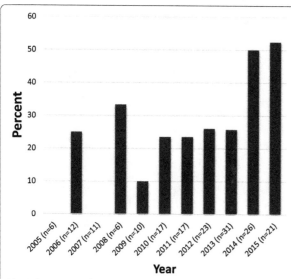

Fig. 2 Proportion of subjects with NMOSD administered first-line rituximab per year (*n* = 180)

Our findings did not show a statistically significant reduction in risk of all-cause re-hospitalization with first-line rituximab use. However, it is possible that our study was underpowered or did not fully account for residual confounding by indication, resulting in negative findings. We did find that the duration of re-hospitalization, however, was statistically significantly shorter among those subjects who received rituximab therapy upfront. This suggests, similar to the findings of Longoni et al., that even for rituximab exposed children who experienced disease flares within 12 months, the severity of their flares was less. Therefore, in light of the potential for significant morbidity and mortality in children with newly diagnosed NMOSD, first-line rituximab should be carefully considered.

Receipt of physical therapy during initial hospitalization was found to be an independent predictor of re-hospitalization within 12 months. Likely, those children necessitating physical therapy during their initial hospital encounter, had a more severe presentation of their NMOSD. Children with physical therapy services likely incurred significant morbidity such as paralysis and for this reason alone would be more likely to have subsequent complications leading to re-admissions. Unfortunately, such insults cannot be reversed even with first-line rituximab use.

With respect to demographics, we found that non-Caucasian subjects were more likely to receive rituximab during their first hospitalization. Previous research has shown that certain races, specifically Afro-Caribbeans, have greater relapse rates [17]. This may drive providers to treat non-Caucasian patients more aggressively and favor first-line rituximab in this patient population.

This study has limitations. First, there is a possibility of misclassification bias because the NMO ICD-9-CM code has not been validated. However, given the specificity of language for this code and the rarity of this disease, we believe it would be unlikely for practitioners to incorrectly assign patients an ICD-9-CM code for NMO. We also attempted to increase the specificity of the code by requiring receipt of glucocorticoids and excluding subjects with codes for MS. We may, however, have failed to capture all patients with NMOSD.

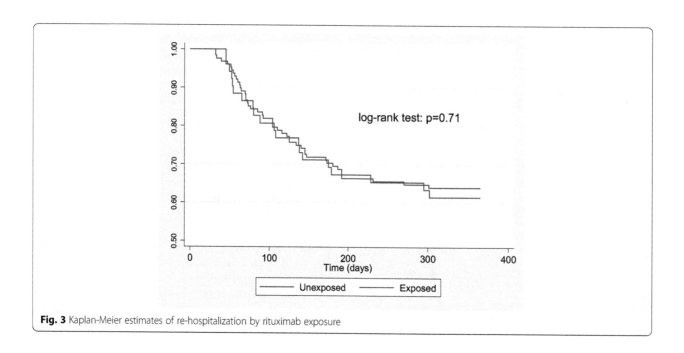

Fig. 3 Kaplan-Meier estimates of re-hospitalization by rituximab exposure

Table 3 Multivariate Cox proportional hazards for re-hospitalization within 12 months

Covariate	Adjusted HR	95% CI	P-value
Rituximab exposure	0.71	0.38, 1.34	0.29
Male gender	0.68	0.35, 1.32	1.32
Caucasian	0.90	0.50, 1.61	0.72
Region (reference: Midwest)			
Northeast	0.74	0.28, 1.91	0.53
South	0.70	0.33, 1.47	0.35
West	1.09	0.40, 2.95	0.87
Length of Initial Stay (days)	0.98	0.94, 1.03	0.41
ICU status	1.41	0.61, 3.25	0.43
Receipt of PT	4.81	1.14, 20.29	0.03
Receipt of PLEX	1.01	0.49, 2.08	0.98
Glucocorticoid (reference: oral only)			
Intravenous only	0.88	0.28, 2.72	0.82
Oral + intravenous	1.72	0.57, 5.18	0.33

Physical therapy (PT) exposure defined as at least one procedure code for PT during initial hospitalization. Oral glucocorticoids defined as at least one billing code for dexamethasone, hydrocortisone, prednisone or prednisolone
CI confidence interval, *ICU* intensive care unit, *PLEX* plasma exchange

Additionally, the relatively recent discovery of the anti-myelin oligodendrocyte glycoprotein (MOG) antibodies [18–20] could lead to misclassification bias in our study. During the study interval, testing for MOG would not have been available to providers and would not affect treatment decision making; however, subjects with NMOSD who are seropositive for anti-MOG, have more favorable outcomes and tend to be glucocorticoid responsive [19]. Therefore, dependent on the number of subjects with anti-MOG positivity in this study, this could bias our primary outcome towards the null and, in part, explain our study's negative findings. Second, we likely did not identify all outcomes of interest by using retrospective data; however, by only including patients with 12 months of available follow-up time in the database we aimed to minimize any outcome bias. Third, by using claims data we were limited in our ability to assess clinical severity or aquaporin-4 antibody status in this cohort of patients with NMOSD. Of note, laboratory detection of aquaporin-4 antibodies is a send-out test for most institutions with a turn-around-time of 5–8 days; thus most providers make treatment decisions for a patient's initial attack prior to receiving the test results. Fourth, there may have been residual confounding by indication. However, we attempted to address confounding by indication by adjusting for receipt of PLEX, receipt of PT, duration of initial hospitalization, and ICU status in our final multivariate logistic regression model. We did not find that these indicators of disease severity were independently associated with re-hospitalization.

Conclusions

Among children with NMOSD, first-line rituximab therapy was not associated with a decreased risk of or time to all-cause re-hospitalization within 12 months. However, first-line rituximab use was associated with a decreased duration of re-hospitalization, suggesting its possible role in mitigating the severity of subsequent disease relapses. Further research is warranted to determine the long-term effects of first-line rituximab on morbidity and mortality, which will help guide the optimal treatment regimen for NMOSD taking into consideration disease progression, adverse events, and re-admissions.

Abbreviations
HR: Hazard ratio; ICU: Intensive care unit; IVIg: Intravenous immunoglobulin; MS: Multiple sclerosis; NMO: Neuromyelitis optica; NMOSD: Neuromyelitis optica spectrum disorder; PHIS: Pediatric health information system; PLEX: Plasma exchange; SLE: Systemic lupus erythematosus

Acknowledgements
The authors thank Emily R. Schriver for her assistance with data management.

Funding
Dr. Gmuca is supported by the National Institute of Health Rheumatology Research Training Grant T32-AR007442-29. Dr. Waldman has received funding from the National Institute of Neurologic Disorders and Stroke Grant K23-NS069806. This study was funded by the Children's Hospital of Philadelphia Center for Pediatric Clinical Effectiveness (CPCE) Pilot Grant Program.

Authors' contributions
SG, PW, AW, JG are responsible for the conception and design of the work. SG is responsible for data collection, data analysis and drafting of the manuscript. SG, PW, AW, JG contributed to the data interpretation. All the authors are responsible for critical revision of the article and gave final approval of the version to be published.

Competing interests
The authors declare that they have no competing interests.

Author details
[1]Division of Rheumatology, Center for Pediatric Clinical Effectiveness, Children's Hospital of Philadelphia, Philadelphia, PA, USA. [2]Department of Biostatistics, Epidemiology and Informatics, Perelman School of Medicine at the University of Pennsylvania, Philadelphia, PA, USA. [3]Division of Neurology, Children's Hospital of Philadelphia, Philadelphia, PA, USA. [4]Division of Infectious Diseases, Center for Pediatric Clinical Effectiveness, Children's Hospital of Philadelphia, Philadelphia, PA, USA.

References
1. Zephir H, Bernard-Valnet R, Lebrun C, Outteryck O, Audoin B, Bourre B, Pittion S, Wiertlewski S, Ouallet JC, Neau JP, et al. Rituximab as first-line therapy in neuromyelitis optica: efficiency and tolerability. J Neurol. 2015; 262:2329–35.
2. Kimbrough DJ, Fujihara K, Jacob A, Lana-Peixoto MA, Leite MI, Levy M, Marignier R, Nakashima I, Palace J, de Seze J, et al. Treatment of neuromyelitis optica: review and recommendations. Mult Scler Relat Disord. 2012;1:180–7.
3. Kim SH, Kim HJ. Rituximab in Neuromyelitis Optica Spectrum disorders: why not as first-line therapy. JAMA Neurol. 2017;74:482.
4. Tenembaum S, Chitnis T, Nakashima I, Collongues N, McKeon A, Levy M, Rostasy K. Neuromyelitis optica spectrum disorders in children and adolescents. Neurology. 2016;87:S59–66.

5. Longoni G, Banwell B, Filippi M, Yeh EA. Rituximab as a first-line preventive treatment in pediatric NMOSDs: preliminary results in 5 children. Neurol Neuroimmunol Neuroinflamm. 2014;1:e46.

6. Torres J, Pruitt A, Balcer L, Galetta S, Markowitz C, Dahodwala N. Analysis of the treatment of neuromyelitis optica. J Neurol Sci. 2015;351:31–5.

7. Evangelopoulos ME, Andreadou E, Koutsis G, Koutoulidis V, Anagnostouli M, Katsika P, Evangelopoulos DS, Evdokimidis I, Kilidireas C. Treatment of neuromyelitis optica and neuromyelitis optica spectrum disorders with rituximab using a maintenance treatment regimen and close CD19 B cell monitoring. A six-year follow-up. J Neurol Sci. 2017;372:92–6.

8. Radaelli M, Moiola L, Sangalli F, Esposito F, Barcella V, Ferre L, Rodegher M, Colombo B, Fazio R, Martinelli V, Comi G. Neuromyelitis optica spectrum disorders: long-term safety and efficacy of rituximab in Caucasian patients. Mult Scler. 2016;22:511–9.

9. Kim SH, Huh SY, Lee SJ, Joung A, Kim HJ. A 5-year follow-up of rituximab treatment in patients with neuromyelitis optica spectrum disorder. JAMA Neurol. 2013;70:1110–7.

10. Kim SH, Jeong IH, Hyun JW, Joung A, Jo HJ, Hwang SH, Yun S, Joo J, Kim HJ. Treatment outcomes with rituximab in 100 patients with neuromyelitis optica: influence of FCGR3A polymorphisms on the therapeutic response to rituximab. JAMA Neurol. 2015;72:989–95.

11. Bienia B, Balabanov R. Immunotherapy of neuromyelitis optica. Autoimmune Dis. 2013;2013:741490.

12. Cree BA, Lamb S, Morgan K, Chen A, Waubant E, Genain C. An open label study of the effects of rituximab in neuromyelitis optica. Neurology. 2005;64:1270–2.

13. Damato V, Evoli A, Iorio R. Efficacy and safety of rituximab therapy in neuromyelitis optica spectrum disorders: a systematic review and meta-analysis. JAMA Neurol. 2016;73:1342–8.

14. Hardin AP, Hackell JM. Age limit of pediatrics. Pediatrics. 2017;140:e20172151.

15. Derle E, Gunes HN, Konuskan B, Tuncer-Kurne A. Neuromyelitis optica in children: a review of the literature. Turk J Pediatr. 2014;56:573–80.

16. Olivieri G, Nociti V, Iorio R, Stefanini MC, Losavio FA, Mirabella M, Mariotti P. Rituximab as a first-line treatment in pediatric neuromyelitis optica spectrum disorder. Neurol Sci. 2015;36:2301–2.

17. Tackley G, O'Brien F, Rocha J, Woodhall M, Waters P, Chandratre S, Halfpenny C, Hemingway C, Wassmer E, Wasiewski W, et al. Neuromyelitis optica relapses: race and rate, immunosuppression and impairment. Mult Scler Relat Disord. 2016;7:21–5.

18. Chalmoukou K, Alexopoulos H, Akrivou S, Stathopoulos P, Reindl M, Dalakas MC. Anti-MOG antibodies are frequently associated with steroid-sensitive recurrent optic neuritis. Neurol Neuroimmunol Neuroinflamm. 2015;2:e131.

19. Kitley J, Woodhall M, Waters P, Leite MI, Devenney E, Craig J, Palace J, Vincent A. Myelin-oligodendrocyte glycoprotein antibodies in adults with a neuromyelitis optica phenotype. Neurology. 2012;79:1273–7.

20. Waters P, Woodhall M, O'Connor KC, Reindl M, Lang B, Sato DK, Jurynczyk M, Tackley G, Rocha J, Takahashi T, et al. MOG cell-based assay detects non-MS patients with inflammatory neurologic disease. Neurol Neuroimmunol Neuroinflamm. 2015;2:e89.

19

The economic profile of peginterferon beta-1a in the treatment of relapsing-remitting multiple sclerosis

Diego Centonze[1,5*], Sergio Iannazzo[2], Laura Santoni[3], Cecilia Saleri[3], Elisa Puma[3], Luigi Giuliani[2] and Pier Luigi Canonico[4]

Abstract

Multiple sclerosis (MS) is a chronic inflammatory disease of the central nervous system with a very high economic impact. Peginterferon beta-1a is the first approved pegylated interferon beta-1a for the treatment of relapsing-remitting multiple sclerosis (RRMS). Its efficacy and safety were demonstrated in the placebo-controlled ADVANCE trial. A complete path to the assessment of a new health technology requires, in addition to a clinical evaluation, also an economic evaluation. In Italy, two economic evaluations were conducted and recently published.

The objective of this article is focused on the two Italian economic analyses in order to describe the methods used, to summarize the main results, and to give a comprehensive picture of the pharmacoeconomic profile of peginterferon beta-1a in Italy in approved indication.

The two analyses were conducted to evaluate such profile; the former was a cost-effectiveness analysis, the latter was a budget impact analysis:

1) The cost-effectiveness analysis – developed through a lifetime Markov model – compared peginterferon beta-1a with injectable first-line treatments for RRMS in Italy from the perspective of the Italian National Healthcare Service (NHS) and from the societal perspective. Efficacy data were derived from a published Network Meta-analysis. Unit costs were based on current prices and tariffs, and the published literature.

From the Italian NHS perspective, peginterferon beta-1a was dominant in one case, while in all others its incremental cost-effectiveness ratio (ICER) was between €10,580/QALY and €22,023/QALY. From the societal perspective, peginterferon beta-1a was dominant versus every comparator.

2) The budget impact analysis estimated – using a simple decision analytic model from the perspective of the Italian NHS – the financial impact due to the introduction of peginterferon beta-1a on the Italian drug market. The cumulative budget impact over 3 years was a cost saving of approximately €3.1 million.

Based on the results of both analyses, the adoption of peginterferon beta-1a for the treatment of RRMS is not only clinically effective, but also economically efficient and financially sustainable from the Italian NHS perspective.

Keywords: Cost-effectiveness, Budget impact, Multiple sclerosis, Disease modifying therapies, Italy

* Correspondence: centonze@uniroma2.it
[1]Dipartimento di Medicina dei Sistemi, Università degli Studi di Roma Tor Vergata, Rome, Italy
[5]IRCCS Istituto Neurologico Mediteranneo Neuromed, Pozzilli, IS, Italy
Full list of author information is available at the end of the article

Background

Multiple sclerosis (MS) is a chronic inflammatory disease of the central nervous system, entailing a progressive disability. In 85% of patients with multiple sclerosis (MS) the onset form is relapsing–remitting MS (RRMS) [1].

MS affects 2.1 to 2.3 million people all over the world, including 600,000 in Europe and 75,000 in Italy (where an incidence is estimated of about 2000 cases/year) [2, 3].

The disease onset in full working age, its chronicity and its progression all heavily impact patients' quality of life and societal costs [4].

The annual societal cost of MS is estimated in Italy at €2.7 billion [3], 29% of which is for direct medical costs (hospitalizations, drugs, diagnostics), 29% for indirect costs (productivity losses), and 42% for direct non-medical costs (informal care, transportation, aids) [5].

The estimated average cost per patient/year from the perspective of the Italian society (i.e., including direct and indirect costs) amounts to €38,000 ca. It varies from €23,000 ca. in patients with mild disability (Expanded Disability Status Scale [6] (EDSS) score: 0–3), to €44,000 ca. in patients with moderate disability (EDSS: 4–6.5), to €63,000 ca. in patients with severe disability (EDSS ≥7) [7].

The correlation between disease severity and cost significance was reported in several sources [3–9]. The Disease Modifying Therapies (DMTs) reduce the frequency of clinical relapses and delay disability progression.

Interferon (IFN) beta-1a, IFN beta-1b and glatiramer acetate (GA) are among the DMTs used in the first line treatment of patients with RRMS in Italy. They are available in injectable formulations (subcutaneous [SC] or intramuscular [IM]), with a variable administration frequency from once a day to once a week.

The European Commission granted marketing authorization to peginterferon beta-1a (Plegridy®) on July 18, 2014. This is the first pegylated formulation for the treatment of RRMS and the only therapy administered with the frequency of one SC injection every 2 weeks.

In the randomized, double-blind, phase 3 clinical trial ADVANCE [10, 11] the efficacy and safety of peginterferon beta-1a were evaluated on a 2-year time horizon. The primary endpoint was the annualized relapse rate (ARR) at 48 weeks.

In the first year patients were treated with peginterferon beta-1a, administered every two (Q2W) or 4 weeks (Q4W) or with placebo; in the second year all patients were treated with peginterferon beta-1a, as placebo patients were re-randomized to be treated with either peginterferon beta-1a Q2W or Q4W. In the first year, patients treated with peginterferon beta-1a reported on average fewer relapses than those taking placebo (0.26 for the Q2W group [p = 0.0007], 0.29 for the Q4W group [p = 0.0114]. The confirmed disability progression 24 weeks decreased significantly (p = 0.0069) in patients

treated with peginterferon beta-1a Q2W compared with placebo.

In the second year peginterferon beta-1a efficacy was maintained, with greater effects for the Q2W vs Q4W dosing.

Moreover, in both administration regimens the ADVANCE study indicated a good safety and tolerability profile of peginterferon beta-1a, similar to the profile of the currently available IFN beta-1a therapies.

A complete path to the assessment of a new health technology requires, in addition to a clinical evaluation, also an economic evaluation.

The economic profile of peginterferon beta-1a versus other injectable first line therapies for the treatment of RRMS was recently evaluated In Italy with two different analyses: cost-effectiveness analysis and budget impact analysis [12, 13].

Both analyses are published in Italian language, on a journal mostly addressed to pharmacoeconomists; a purpose of the present article is to provide with new data a wider area of readers, since it is written in English, on a journal which is read mainly by clinicians.

The primary objective of the present article is focused on the two cited analyses [12, 13], in order to describe the methods used, to summarize the main results, and to give a comprehensive, unified picture of the pharmacoeconomic profile of peginterferon beta-1a in Italy in the approved indication.

Materials and methods

Economic evaluations reflect the need to rationalize the allocation of the available resources (scarce by definition), offering the decision-maker some criteria (on the basis of the information available and their reliability) such as to make justifiable choices [14]. Normally, such evaluations follow two steps.

The first (fundamental) step is aimed at estimating the economic efficiency in the allocation of healthcare resources, assuming they are invested in a given technology instead of another. The technique preferably used is the cost-effectiveness analysis (CEA) [15], with the objective of quantifying (as far as possible, consistent with the specificity of the assessed technology) how much the new technology costs in order to gain one additional benefit (typically, a life year, LY) as compared to a competitor. Such measure, on which many economic evaluations are based in healthcare, is named incremental cost-effectiveness ratio (ICER). In the decision process, the ICER is compared to an acceptability threshold value, an acknowledged (not necessarily official) benchmark to which the meaning may be given of how much the society or the National Healthcare Service (NHS) is willing to pay (willingness to pay, WTP) for one additional benefit gained (for example, as above, a life year). When the new technology is more effective and less expensive than the standard, then it is named dominant.

A LY takes the name of QALY (quality-adjusted life year) when it is weighted with the patient's quality of life. One QALY is a measure unit "equivalent" to the benefit provided by one LY in full health. When QALYs are used, the evaluation technique may be called cost-utility analysis (CUA) – "utility" because the quality of life is converted into a synthetic coefficient which can be related, in economics, to a concept of utility such as "the degree of personal satisfaction", with values varying from 1 (full health) to 0 (death). CEAs/CUAs are preferably conducted on a medium to long term time horizon.

No economic acceptability threshold has been officially defined in Italy to date. Some proposals have been formulated by Italian authors [16–18]. In other countries official thresholds are used [19], or thresholds are proposed by authors or organizations [20, 21]). Based on data from these sources, an ICER value was assumed to be economically acceptable in Italy when it is less or equal to a range from €30,000 to €50,000 per QALY gained.

The second (complementary) step of an economic evaluation is aimed at answering a more immediate and frequent question from the decision-maker, regarding the financial sustainability of a new technology in the short term (1–3 years). Such objective is pursued with the budget impact analysis (BIA), with a view to estimate how and how much a change in the mix of therapies (following the introduction and spread of the new technology) used in the treatment of a given health condition will impact on the trend of the expenditure for such condition [22] from the perspective of the National Healthcare Service.

In the next sections we describe the methods which were followed to perform the two steps (CEA and BIA [12, 13]) to evaluate the economic performance of peginterferon beta-1a for the treatment of RRMS in Italy.

The cost-effectiveness analysis (CEA) of peginterferon beta-1a in Italy

The analysis was conducted using a Markov model (a tool particularly useful when a decision problem involves risk that is continuous over time, when the timing of events is important, and when important events may happen more than once – such as the transitions that a patient performs from one health state to another, often in a recursive way [23]). The model was based on a previously published one [24], reviewed and accepted by – among several agencies – the National Institute for Health and Clinical Excellence (NICE) in the UK [25].

General description of the model

The economic perspective of the Italian National Health Service (NHS) is adopted, with an additional scenario taking into consideration the perspective of the whole Italian society. The time horizon is lifetime; costs and outcomes are discounted at the annual rate of 3.5% (to account for the effect of time on current cost and outcomes values).

Peginterferon beta-1a is compared to other injectable DMTs used in the first line therapy of RRMS:

- IFN beta-1a, 30 μg, intramuscular (IM), once a week (Avonex®)
- IFN beta-1a, 22 μg, subcutaneous (SC), three times a week (Rebif 22®)
- IFN beta-1a, 44 μg SC, three times a week (Rebif 44®)
- IFN beta-1b, 250 μg SC, every other day (Betaferon® and Extavia®)
- GA, 20 mg SC, once a day (Copaxone®).

The model simulates the mortality, the disease progression between EDSS levels, the relapse frequency and the transition to secondary progressive multiple sclerosis (SPMS), estimating the survival (LYs), the survival adjusted for quality of life (QALYs), the overall costs, the incremental cost per QALY gained (ICER).

Twenty-one health states are included in the model (Fig. 1):

- 10 states in the RRMS form (EDSS levels 0; 1–1.5; 2–2.5; ....; 9–9.5)
- 10 states in the SPMS form (EDSS levels 0; 1–1.5; 2–2.5; ....; 9–9.5)
- Death

The simulation starts with a hypothetical cohort distributed in the different EDSS levels of RRMS, according to the initial distribution and demographic characteristics of the patients in the ADVANCE study [10, 11]. At each (annual) simulation cycle the patients can progress/regress between the EDSS levels or remain in the same EDSS level in the RRMS form, progress to the SPMS form, have a relapse according to the specific probability in each level, or die. Patients cannot return from SPMS to RRMS, nor regress to lower EDSS levels in the SPMS form.

The treatments included in the model exert their effect both slowing down the disability progression (compared to the natural history of the disease) and reducing the relapse incidence in the RRMS form. Such effects

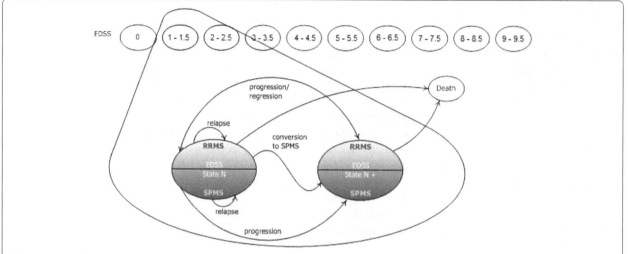

Fig. 1 CEA Model structure. EDSS = Expanded Disability Status Scale; RRMS = relapsing-remitting multiple sclerosis; SPMS = secondary-progressive multiple sclerosis; State N = current EDSS state. Adapted from Gani et al. [23], Iannazzo et al. [12]

persist over the long term [26–30]. No effect is considered on the progression from RRMS to SPMS, on the transition between EDSS levels in the SPMS form and on mortality.

It is assumed that patients stop therapy, with the DMTs included in the analysis, when reaching an EDSS level ≥ 7 in the RRMS form or when passing to the SPMS form.

In respect to each treatment adverse events are simulated.

Clinical data

The annual transition probabilities between EDSS scores of RRMS patients were obtained on the basis of data from the ADVANCE study [10, 11] (for levels 0–5), together with data from the London database, Ontario [31, 32] (for levels 6–9). The annual transition probabilities from RRMS to SPMS, and between EDSS scores of SPMS patients, were derived only from the London database (patients with SPMS were not enrolled in the ADVANCE study).

Annual relapse incidence data were obtained from the ADVANCE study [10, 11], pooled with more data from literature [33–35].

The death probability was estimated for each cycle considering the general mortality of the Italian population broken down by age and gender [36], adjusted for the specific relative risk (RR) in each EDSS score (risk obtained by fitting data reported in the literature [37]).

The treatment efficacy was simulated reducing the disability progression and the relapse incidence, using data derived from the recently published comprehensive Network Meta-analysis [38].

The adverse events (AEs) for all therapies included in the model were those occurred with an incidence ≥5%

for peginterferon beta-1a 125 mcg in the ADVANCE study as well as AEs that occurred at an incidence of ≥3% in the overall peginterferon beta-1a group compared to the placebo group (even if the overall incidence in the peginterferon beta-1a arms was <5%). The serious adverse events were excluded, considering their very low frequency in the ADVANCE study. Annual incidences for comparators were obtained from several sources [39–46].

The utility (related to the quality of life) in the EDSS scores of RRMS patients was assessed by Kobelt et al. [5], together with a disutility (a decrement of utility, due to a health worsening) equal to 0.18 for each relapse (independent from the EDSS score). The utility in the EDSS scores of SPMS patients was estimated subtracting a disutility equal to 0.045 from the utility in the same level in RRMS [32].

The disutilities of the adverse events were obtained from literature or based on expert opinion [47–51].

A zero utility value was assumed when subtracting disutility gave a negative value.

Economic data

The analysis from the Italian NHS perspective identified, measured and quantified the direct medical costs relative to the health management of patients with MS.

The annual treatment cost per patient was calculated based on the ex-factory price per pack, net of temporary low reductions and any negotiated hidden discounts, multiplied by the number of units needed to cover 1 year. For all DMTs included in the model, adherence to treatment was considered equal to 100%.

Administration costs were not considered, since all DMTs in the model can be self-administered subcutaneously or intramuscularly, i.e. at zero cost from the perspective of the Italian NHS.

Annual monitoring costs were calculated based on MS healthcare regional recommendations adopted in Emilia-Romagna [52] and Lazio [53]; resources consumption was valued according to current tariffs [54]. For peginterferon beta-1a, the same consumption was assumed as for non pegylated IFN beta-1a therapies.

The direct medical management cost per relapse was calculated on the basis of an elaboration of the societal cost of one relapse assessed by Kobelt et al. [5], inflated to December 2014 with the Italian consumption price index [36].

The management cost of adverse events was calculated multiplying the annual incidence rates of the adverse events associated to each DMT included in the model by the unit cost of each event. It was assumed that adverse events included in the analysis were managed in the outpatient setting, by a general practitioner [55] or by a specialist [54].

Disease management costs (hospitalizations, outpatient care, visits and lab tests, drugs except DMTs) in the different EDSS scores of RRMS and SPMS patients were estimated processing data reported in the MS cost of illness analysis by Karampampa et al. [56].

In the additional scenario where the Italian society perspective was adopted, indirect costs due to productivity losses (sick leaves, early retirements) caused by MS were also valued, together with direct non-medical costs, e.g. for informal care (from relatives and/or friends) [56].

Sensitivity analysis

The sensitivity analysis was conducted in order to check the robustness of the results and the impact of uncertainties in the data used, considering that the clinical and economic parameters of the model might – in the real life and over time – take values both more or less favorable as compared to those adopted in the basic configuration of the model.

In the one-way sensitivity analysis (OWSA) the value of each parameter was separately varied, and the impact was calculated and registered of such change on the results. For each parameter the low and high value of its uncertainty interval were given. Such interval was defined as the 95% statistical confidence interval (95%CI) when available or as ±10% of the parameter basic value.

The probabilistic sensitivity analysis (PSA) was performed by simultaneously and randomly varying (through 1000 replications) the values of all parameters. To each of them a probability distribution was assigned, centered on the parameter base value and with a variance derived from the 95%CIs reported in the cited Network Meta-analysis [38] (for relapse and progression parameters) or with a standard error assumed equal to 25% of the base value (in all other cases).

The budget impact analysis (BIA) of peginterferon beta-1a in Italy

A simple decision analysis model was used in order to evaluate the potential financial impact of the introduction of peginterferon beta-1a in the Italian drug market for the treatment of RRMS, from the perspective of the Italian NHS, on a 3-year time horizon.

General description of the model

The overall treatment costs were analyzed of a population with RRMS (target population) in Italy, by comparing two different scenarios (Fig. 2):

- A scenario in which the target population is treated with the injectable first line DMTs available in Italy (IFNs beta, GA) excluding peginterferon beta-1a (base scenario)
- A scenario including peginterferon beta-1a among the injectable first line DMTs available in Italy (alternative scenario)

By processing drug consumption data in Italy [57], the number of patients treated with a first line injectable DMT (target population) in the first year of observation was estimated at 35,472. To this number, the number of naïve patients (2000 per year [3]) was added for the following years. The mortality was not taken into account in the budget impact analysis, in view of the short period of observation.

The treatment mix in the base scenario was derived from estimated market shares [57], assuming it remains constant during the three observed years.

In the alternative scenario, the number was initially estimated of the patients that might start the treatment with peginterferon beta-1a in the first 3 years after launch. The number of equivalent patients per year was then calculated (such number allows to consider that every patient is treated for 1 year). Based on the

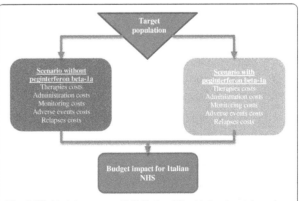

Fig. 2 BIA Model structure. NHS: National Health Service; Adapted from Iannazzo et al. [13]

similarity between active principles, it was assumed that peginterferon beta-1a could compete mainly with IFN beta-1a therapies, and only marginally with IFN beta-1b and GA (considering other characteristics too: ways of use in the clinical practice, action mechanism, etc.).

Clinical data

Efficacy data – in terms of relapse incidence rate without treatment, and of relapse relative risk reduction associated to the drug treatments of the RRMS – were derived from the recently published Network Meta-analysis [38].

With the objective of maintaining a simple cost structure, among the adverse events only those related to the injection site necrosis and flu-like syndrome were considered. The respective incidences were derived from the Prescribing Information of each DMT included in the analysis [58–63].

Economic data

The treatment cost (for which a general adherence of 85% was assumed [64]), the annual monitoring costs and the management cost per relapse were valued with the same criteria adopted in the cost-effectiveness model (see point 2.1.3). The management cost of adverse events was assumed equal to the cost of an outpatient specialist visit [54].

The sensitivity analysis

An OWSA was performed, based on the same criteria adopted in the cost-effectiveness evaluation (see point 2.1.4). The analysis was focused on the maximum budget impact occurring in the third year.

Results

Similarly to the order followed in the Methods section, results are presented sequentially in the two steps of the economic evaluation of peginterferon beta-1a: CEA and BIA respectively.

The cost-effectiveness analysis (CEA) of peginterferon beta-1a in Italy
The comparison of peginterferon beta-1a with IFN beta-1a in the NHS perspective

Results of the analysis indicated that peginterferon beta-1a appeared more effective than IFN beta-1a, in terms both of survival (LYs, discounted) and of survival adjusted for quality of life (QALYs, discounted) (Table 1).

The (discounted) total direct medical cost of a patient treated with peginterferon beta-1a was slightly higher than that of a patient treated with IFN beta-1a 30 μg or with IFN beta-1a 22 μg; in fact, the higher drug and monitoring cost is only partially offset by lower costs for relapses, adverse events and disease management (as compared with the two comparators). On the contrary, the total direct medical cost of peginterferon beta-1a was lower than that of IFN beta-1a 44 μg (Table 1).

Peginterferon beta-1a was dominant vs IFN beta-1a 44 μg because it was more effective and with lower costs. The ICER of peginterferon beta-1a vs IFN beta-1a 30 μg and vs IFN beta-1a 22 μg resulted equal to €11,112 and €12,604 per QALY respectively. In both cases, the ICER is below the acceptability threshold of €30,000–50,000/QALY (Table 1).

Comparing peginterferon beta-1a with IFN beta-1a 30 μg and with IFN beta-1a 22 μg, the OWSA showed that the parameters which most impact on the cost-effectiveness results are the disability progression hazard rates and the outcomes discount rate. However, only the

Table 1 CEA of peginterferon beta-1a vs IFN beta-1a in Italy from the NHS perspective

Outcomes		peginterferon beta-1a 125 μg	IFN beta-1a 30 μg	IFN beta-1a 22 μg	IFN beta-1a 44 μg
Clinical outs.	LYs	19.94	19.71	19.73	19.81
	QALYs	9.07	8.09	8.19	8.55
[a]			0.98	0.87	0.51
Cost outs. (€)	Drugs & mon.	113,095	92,599	93,511	129,261
	Relapses	8789	9331	9078	8768
	Adverse events	102	153	107	150
	Disease manag.	111,107	120,152	119,651	116,368
	Total cost	233,091	222,235	222,077	254,547
[b]			10,856	11,014	−21,456
ICER (€) [c]			11,112	12,532	Dominant

outs. = outcomes
drugs & mon. = treatment acquisition and monitoring
manag. = management
[a] = Incremental benefit (QALYs) (peginterferon beta-1a vs comparators)
[b] = Incremental cost (total) (peginterferon beta-1a vs comparators)
[c] = [b]/[a]

variation in the hazard rates can give rise to ICERs exceeding the €30,000/QALY threshold. Also in the comparison between peginterferon beta-1a and IFN beta-1a 44 μg, where the former was dominant (Table 1), the most impacting parameters are the same – but in no case the ICER exceeds €30,000/QALY.

The PSA primarily showed that the results are robust to variations in the input parameters, in all cases. Moreover, over the 1000 simulations where parameters were varied from the base-case assumptions, in the comparison with IFN beta-1a 22 μg, the probability that peginterferon beta-1a was cost-effective when WTP is assumed to be €30,000/QALY was 74.1% (79.8% if WTP is €50,000/QALY). In the comparison with IFN beta-1a 30 μg, the analogous probability was 79.7% for peginterferon beta-1a when WTP is assumed to be €30,000/QALY (85.1% when WTP is €50,000/QALY).

Finally, in the comparison with IFN beta-1a 44 μg, the PSA showed that peginterferon beta-1a is dominant in 76.2% of cases and cost-effective in 97.6% when WTP is €30,000/QALY.

The comparison of peginterferon beta-1a with other injectable first line DMTs in the NHS perspective

Peginterferon beta-1a was more effective than IFN beta-1b and GA (in terms both of LYs and of QALYs), with a total medical direct cost per patient slightly higher (Table 2).

The ICER of peginterferon beta-1a was €10,580, €16,702, and €22,023 per QALY vs IFN beta-1b 250 μg (Betaferon), IFN beta-1a 250 μg (Extavia), and GA

20 mg, respectively – below the acceptability threshold of €30,000–50,000/QALY in all comparisons (Table 2).

The results of the OWSA are in line with those relative to the comparisons between peginterferon beta-1a with IFN beta-1a (reported above).

In the PSA, the comparisons show trends analogous to those described for IFN beta-1a. In particular, the probability for peginterferon beta-1a to be cost-effective is 74.7% vs GA, 81.4% vs IFN beta-1b 250 μg (Extavia) and 87.0% vs IFN beta-1b 250 μg (Betaferon) when WTP is €50,000/QALY.

The analysis in the societal perspective

The total societal cost of a patient treated with peginterferon beta-1a was lower than those of all the comparators included in the analysis (Table 3).

Peginterferon beta-1a was dominant vs all injectable first line DMTs (IFN beta-1a, IFNβ-1b, GA) because it is more effective, in terms both of survival (LYs) and of survival adjusted for quality of life (QALYs) and with a lower total societal cost (Table 3).

The PSA showed peginterferon beta-1a dominant vs all comparators, with probabilities between 76.3% (vs IFN beta-1a 44 μg) and 85.8% (vs IFN beta-1b 250 μg).

The budget impact analysis (BIA) of peginterferon beta-1a in Italy

In the base scenario (without peginterferon beta-1a), the total medical cost of the target population was equal to €321,530,021, €339,658,686, and €357,787,352 in the first, second, third year of the observation period, respectively (Table 4). In the alternative scenario (with

Table 2 CEA of peginterferon beta-1a vs IFN beta-1b and GA in Italy from the NHS perspective

Outcomes		peginterferon beta-1a 125 μg	IFN beta-1b 250 μg[a]	IFN beta-1a 250 μg[b]	GA 20 mg
Clinical outs.	LYs	19.94	19.68	19.68	19.68
	QALYs	9.07	8.06	8.06	8.15
[a]			1.01	1.01	0.92
Cost outs. (€)	Drugs & mon.	113,095	92,105	86,019	82,887
	Relapses	8789	8808	8808	8502
	Adverse events	102	110	110	94
	Disease manag.	111,107	121,277	121,277	121,424
	Total cost	233,091	222,399	216,213	212,908
[b]			10,691	16,877	20,183
ICER (€) [c]			10,580	16,702	22,023

outs. = outcomes
drugs & mon. = treatment acquisition and monitoring
manag. = management
[a] = Incremental benefit (QALYs) (peginterferon beta-1a vs comparators)
[b] = Incremental cost (total) (peginterferon beta-1a vs comparators)
[c] = [b]/[a]
[a]Betaferon
[b]Extavia

Table 3 CEA of peginterferon beta-1a vs the other injectable first line DMTs in Italy from the societal perspective

Outcomes		peg-IFN β-1a 125 μg	IFN β-1a 30 μg	IFN β-1a 22 μg	IFN β-1a 44 μg	IFN β-1b 250 μg[a]	IFN β-1b 250 μg[b]	GA 20 mg
Clinical outcomes								
	LYs	19.94	19.71	19.73	19.81	19.68	19.68	19.68
	QALYs	9.07	8.09	8.19	8.55	8.06	8.06	8.15
[a]			0.98	0.87	0.51	1.01	1.01	0.92
Direct medical costs (€)								
	Drugs & mon.	113,095	92,599	93,511	129,261	92,105	86,019	82,887
	Relapses	8789	9331	9078	8768	8808	8808	8502
	Adverse evts.	102	153	107	150	110	110	94
	Disease man.	111,107	120,152	119,651	116,368	121,277	121,277	121,424
Indirect and non-medical costs (€)								
	Relapses	8901	9453	9196	8882	8922	8922	8613
	Other costs	528,222	586,700	583,313	561,586	594,367	594,357	595,374
Total cost		770,213	818,388	814,585	825,015	825,689	819,503	816,894
[b]			−48,175	−44,372	−54,801	−55,475	−49,289	−46,681
ICER (€) [c]			dominant	dominant	dominant	dominant	dominant	dominant

Peg-IFNβ-1a = peginterferon beta-1a
IFNβ = IFN beta
adrugs & mon. = treatment acquisition and monitoring
evts. = events
man. = management
[a] = Incremental benefit (QALYs) (peginterferon beta-1a vs comparators)
[b] = Incremental cost (total) (peginterferon beta-1a vs comparators)
[c] = [b]/[a]
[a]Betaferon
[b]Extavia

peginterferon beta-1a) the analogous costs were lower: €321,118,561, €338,559,367, and €356,201,191, respectively. Therefore, from the perspective of the Italian NHS, the introduction of peginterferon beta-1a to the Italian market of first line injectable therapies for the treatment of RRMS resulted in a 3-year cumulative impact of about €3.1 million savings (−0.3% of the expenditure).

The comparison of the detailed cost items in the two scenarios showed that the reduction of the total expenditure in the alternative scenario was mainly due to the reduction of the overall acquisition cost for the pharmacological therapy and to the lower costs for the relapse management thanks to the reduction of the total number of relapses.

The OWSA, focused on the cumulative impact of the 3 years, showed that the acquisition cost of peginterferon beta-1a is the most relevant parameter, the variation (±10%) of which can result in an impact with a positive value (i.e. in a cost to the Italian NHS). The result is influenced, albeit to a lesser extent, also by the efficacy parameters of the treatments (in terms of relapse increase or reduction) and by the cost per relapse; the variation of these parameters, however, can never give rise to a sign change in the result, which remains consistently favourable in the alternative scenario (with peginterferon beta-1a).

Table 4 BIA of peginterferon beta-1a in Italy from the NHS perspective

Costs	Year 1	Year 2	Year 3	Cumulative
Base scenario (without peg-IFNβ-1a) (€)	321,530,021	339,658,686	357,787,352	1,018,976,059
Alternative scenario (with peg-IFNβ-1a) (€)	321,118,561	338,559,367	356,201,191	1,015,879,119
Absolute impact(€)	−411,460	−1,099,319	−1,586,161	−3,096,940
Relative impact (%)	−0.13%	−0.32%	−0.44%	−0.30%

Peg-IFNβ-1a = peginterferon beta-1°
Adapted from Iannazzo et al. [13]

Discussion

The economic profile of peginterferon beta-1a in the treatment of RRMS in Italy was assessed with two analyses.

In the cost-effectiveness analysis (CEA), peginterferon beta-1a was compared with other injectable first line DMTs on a lifetime horizon, and was found to be the most effective. From the NHS perspective, peginterferon beta-1a was dominant versus IFN beta-1a 44 µg. The ICER of peginterferon beta-1a versus IFN beta-1a, IFN beta-1b and GA was consistently below the acceptability threshold adopted (€30,000–50,000/QALY [16–21]) – or, from another point of view, well below the level considered acceptable in another jurisdiction like UK [19]. From the societal perspective, peginterferon beta-1a was always dominant versus all the alternatives included in the cost-effectiveness model.

The analysis of the budget impact (BIA) from the NHS perspective showed that the introduction of peginterferon beta-1a results in a health expenditure reduction over the three analysed years, starting from the first year.

In both the CEA and the BIA, the sensitivity analysis confirmed the reliability of the base case results.

On the other hand, it is worth highlighting the major limitations associated to these assessments, starting from those which are common to both the CEA and the BIA of peginterferon beta-1a.

The first limitation is due to the unavailability of a head-to-head study comparing peginterferon beta-1a with the alternatives included in the analysis. As a consequence, for clinical data about the efficacy of the treatments the Network Meta-analysis [38] was used, which provides indirect comparisons. This is likely acceptable, however, considering that such analyses are numerically grown very much in the last years [65] and that their use in pharmacoeconomic evaluations is now well established [66, 67].

The second limitation lies in not having captured, in the design of the models, all the features that might be differentiating for peginterferon beta-1a, such as the administration frequency and the degree of immunogenicity.

In fact, peginterferon beta-1a is administered subcutaneously once every 2 weeks. Considering that the number of administrations per month of comparator first line injectable DMTs currently available in Italy is between 4 and 28, a reduction in administration frequency between 50% and 94% can be achieved with peginterferon beta-1a. Such a reduction might result in better adherence to treatment, with clinical and economic benefits for both patients and NHS. The adherence to therapies for MS has proved inversely correlated to the relapse incidence and to the total direct and indirect costs; in particular, the comparison between adherent and non-adherent patients showed that in the former the incidence of serious relapses is significantly lower (12.4% vs 19.9%, $p < 0.013$), and the average total direct and indirect costs are also significantly lower ($14,095 vs $16,638, $p < 0.048$) too [68].

In the pivotal study peginterferon beta-1a showed a low immunogenicity. This results in a low risk of producing neutralizing antibodies (NAbs), which reduce treatment efficacy. Patients with NAbs show a significant increase of the relapse incidence rate ratio (IRR = 1.38; $p = 0.0247$) and a significant decrease of the time to the first relapse (IRR = 1.51; $p = 0.0111$) [69]. This means that a low immunogenicity results in a low economic impact from the perspective of both the NHS and the society: the annual increment of the management cost of a patient who develops NAbs is equal to €1111 from the perspective of the Italian NHS and to €3100 from the perspective of the Italian society [70].

In any case, it should be noted that assuming an equal adherence to treatment (100% in the CEA and 85% in the BIA) in all the DMTs included in the analysis, and not considering a different immunogenicity degree among the IFNs, is a conservative approach in assessing peginterferon beta-1a.

Another limitation is represented by the value used for the relapse cost from the perspective of the Italian NHS: not having found ad hoc data in the literature, such value was calculated processing the societal cost estimated by Kobelt et al. [5]. Moreover, this source is not recent and the relapse management mode has meantime changed in the clinical practice, with a reduction of the number of relapses associated to a hospitalization. To keep into consideration the potential weakness of the adopted value, its variation interval was extended to −30% of the basic value in the OWSA.

Among the limitations specific to peginterferon beta-1a CEA only, the first one regards the model configuration, which is limited to the first line of treatment and cannot simulate possible further treatments. This is due to the fact that no therapeutic algorithm is reported in the Italian guidelines for the MS treatment.

Finally, the analysis does not capture the patient's satisfaction/dissatisfaction effects nor the effects of increment/decrement of the quality of life associated to a MS therapy as compared with another. Due to the unavailability of data in the literature to this purpose, the utilities adopted to assess the quality of life do not keep into account the possible preferences of patients for the individual drugs.

As to the budget impact analysis, not including costs due to disability progression is a specific limitation. On the other hand, this choice was made because a three-year time horizon looked too short to appreciate the possible economic consequences of a slowing in the disability progression.

Some evidence and confirmations could be given in addition to the results of this study.

The first one regards the cost-effectiveness analysis where the average proportion between the total lifetime per patient cost from the NHS perspective (direct medical costs) and the society perspective (direct and indirect costs) is about 28% (Tables 1–3). This percentage is in line with the estimated proportion of direct medical costs in the Kobelt study [5]. The second one regards the budget impact analysis where the cost per patient per year which can be derived from Table 4 (about € 9200) looks comparable with the mean direct medical cost per patient per year reported in the Kobelt study [5] (€ 11,100) considering also that in the BIA were not considered all costs included in the Kobelt study (such as: physical visits, over the counter drugs, rehabilitation).

Further supports are available for CEA only. They show how the results from the Italian analysis are in line with those reported for US, Scotland, and Ireland.

A study was conducted in the US assessing the cost-effectiveness of peginterferon beta-1a vs IFN beta-1a (44 μg SC three times per week) and GA (20 mg SC once daily) in the treatment of RRMS from the perspective of a US payer [71].

The Markov model used for the analysis is the same (both in structure and in assumptions) as that above described in Section 2, only differing in some options (e.g., time horizon: 10 years in the base case instead of lifetime; annual discount rate: 3% instead 3.5%) and in the data concerning the US demographic and economic environment (mortality, medical costs) instead of the Italian one.

Compared with IFN beta-1a 44 μg and GA 20 mg, peginterferon beta-1a was associated with a slower rate of disability progression during RRMS and of progression to SPMS. This resulted in peginterferon beta-1a being dominant over both competitors, with cost savings of $ 22,070 (€ 19,424) and $ 19,163 (€ 16,865) respectively and additional 0.06 and 0.07 QALYs gained respectively (original monetary values were converted from $ to € @0.88 [72]).

A comparison of results from Italian and USA analyses – specific data are not reported here – shows that LYS and QALYs are fewer in the former, due to the shorter time horizon adopted in the US model. However, all (but one) cost items are higher (in particular, the cost for drugs and monitoring) than in Italy, which might be explained by a positive difference between the unit prices in the respective health systems.

The only cost item which appears higher in Italy is the cost for disease management: a kind of cost particularly increasing with the worsening of the disease, which can be better assessed in a longer time horizon.

The probabilistic sensitivity analysis showed that peginterferon beta-1a was dominant over both competitors in >90% of 5000 replications and was cost-effective in 95% of the replications when using a WTP threshold equal to $50.000 (€ 44,000) per QALY gained.

The study [67] showed that peginterferon beta-1a has a favorable cost-efficacy profile relative to its comparators, confirming the results from the Italian CEA [12].

In Scotland, the cost-effectiveness evaluation of peginterferon beta-1a vs IFNs beta and GA from the NHS perspective showed peginterferon beta-1a dominant vs IFN beta-1a 30 μg, IFN beta-1a 22 μg and IFN beta-1b and cost-effective (assuming a WTP equal to £20,000) vs IFN beta-1a 44 μg and GA 20 mg [73].

Also in Ireland, in the cost-effectiveness evaluation of peginterferon beta-1a vs IFNs beta and GA from the perspective of a third payer, peginterferon beta-1a resulted dominant vs all comparators [74].

Conclusions

In conclusion, the results from the cost-effectiveness analysis show that peginterferon beta-1a in the treatment of RRMS in Italy is a cost-effective alternative, vs both IFN beta-1a and other injectable first line treatments (IFN beta-1b and GA) from the perspective both of the Italian NHS and of the Italian society. In the light of the budget impact analysis, the introduction of peginterferon beta-1a among the first line injectable available alternatives does not result in additional costs but, on the contrary, it generates savings for the NHS.

Overall, reading together the results from two analyses (CEA and BIA), peginterferon beta-1a is a cost-effective and financially sustainable alternative from the NHS perspective and a valid option in the treatment of patients with RRMS in Italy.

Acknowledgments
The authors thank Doctor Carlo Lucioni and Doctor Silvio Mazzi, professional pharmacoeconomists contracted to HPS (Health Publishing & Services Srl, Milan), for assistance in the preparation of the manuscript.

Funding
This manuscript was financially supported by Biogen Italia (Milan, Italy).

Authors' contributions
All the authors are the same who published the two economic analyses [12, 13] which the present article is focused on. All authors read and approved the final manuscript.

Competing interests
• SI is a consultant that received fees by Biogen Italia for other projects
• DC is an Advisory Board member of Bayer Schering, Biogen, Merck-Serono, Teva and received honoraria for speaking or consultation fees from Almirall, Bayer Schering, Biogen, Genzyme, GW Pharmaceuticals, Merck Serono,

Novartis, Sanofi-Aventis, Teva. He is also principal investigator in clinical trials for Bayer Schering, Biogen, Novartis, Merck Serono, Sanofi-Aventis, Teva
• PLC has received research grants, contributions and fees by the following pharmaceutical companies: Abbvie, Almirall, Amgen, A.C.R.A.F. – Angelini, Astellas, Astra Zeneca, Baxter, Bayer, Biogen, BioMarine, Bristol Mayers Squibb, Celgene, Chiesi, Daiichi Sankyo, Eli Lilly, Grunenthal, GSK, Hospira, Lundbeck, LeoPharma, Merck Serono, MSD, Menarini, Mundipharma, Novartis Consumer Health, Novartis Pharma, Otsuka, Pfizer, Roche, Sandoz, Sanofi, Sigma Tau, Takeda, Zambon
• LG received fee by Biogen Italia for other projects
• LS, CS, EP are employees of Biogen Italia

Author details
[1]Dipartimento di Medicina dei Sistemi, Università degli Studi di Roma Tor Vergata, Rome, Italy. [2]SIHS srl, Health Economics Consulting, Torino, Italy. [3]Biogen Italia, Milan, Italy. [4]Dipartimento di Scienze del Farmaco, Università del Piemonte Orientale, Novara, Italy. [5]IRCCS Istituto Neurologico Mediteranneo Neuromed, Pozzilli, IS, Italy.

References
1. Compston A, Coles A. Multiple Sclerosis. Lancet. 2008;372:1502–17.
2. MSIF - Multiple Sclerosis International Federation. Atlas of MS 2013. http://www.msif.org/wp-content/uploads/2014/09/Atlas-of-MS.pdf. Accessed 29 Feb 2016.
3. AISM – Associazione Italiana Sclerosi Multipla. Bilancio Sociale 2014. http://bilanciosociale.aism.it/wp-content/uploads/2014/05/AISM-Bilancio-2014.pdf. Accessed 29 Feb 2016.
4. Kobelt G, Pugliatti M. Cost of multiple sclerosis in Europe. Eur J Neurol. 2005;12(Suppl 1):63–7.
5. Kobelt G, Berg J, Lindgren P, Battaglia M, Lucioni C, Uccelli A. Costs and quality of life of multiple sclerosis in Italy. Eur J Health Econ. 2006;7(Suppl 2): S45–54.
6. Kurtzke JF. A new scale for evaluating disability in multiple sclerosis. Neurology. 1955;5(8):580–3.
7. Ponzio M, Gerzeli S, Brichetto G, Bezzini D, Mancardi GL, Zaratin P, et al. Economic impact of multiple sclerosis in Italy: focus on rehabilitation costs. Neurol Sci. 2015;36(2):227–34.
8. Amato MP, Battaglia MA, Caputo D, Fattore G, Gerzeli S, Pitaro M, et al., Mu. S. I. C. Study Group. The costs of multiple sclerosis: a cross-sectional, multicenter cost-of-illness study in Italy. J Neurol. 2002;249(2):152–63.
9. Berto P, Amato MP, Bellantonio P, Bortolon F, Cavalla P, Florio C, et al. Multiple sclerosis in Italy: cost-of-illness study. Neurol Sci. 2011;32(5):787–94.
10. Calabresi PA, Deykin A, Arnold DL, Balcer L, Boyko A, Pelletier J, Hung S, Sheikh S, Seddighzadeh A, Zhu Y, Liu S, Kieseier BC - analysis of 2-year clinical efficacy and safety of Peginterferon Beta-1a in patients with relapsing-remitting multiple sclerosis: data from the pivotal phase 3 ADVANCE study - American Academy of Neurology, 66th annual meeting 2014.
11. Calabresi PA, Kieseier BC, Arnold DL, Balcer LJ, Boyko A, Pelletier J, et al., ADVANCE Study Investigators. Pegylated interferon beta-1a for relapsing-remitting multiple sclerosis (ADVANCE): a randomised, phase 3, double-blind study. Lancet Neurol. 2014;13(7):657–65.
12. Iannazzo S, Santoni L, Saleri C, Puma E, Vestri G, Giuliani L, et al. Analisi di costo-efficacia dell'utilizzo di peginterferone β-1a nel trattamento della sclerosi multipla recidivante remittente in Italia. Farmeconomia. Health Econ Therapeut Pathways. 2016;17(Suppl 2):13–36.
13. Iannazzo S, Santoni L, Saleri C, Puma E, Vestri G, Giuliani L, et al. Valutazione dell'impatto economico di peginterferone beta-1a nel trattamento della sclerosi multipla recidivante remittente in Italia. Farmeconomia. Health Econ Therapeut Pathways. 2016;17(Suppl 2):37–48.
14. Fantelli V, van de Vooren K, Garattini L, Budget Impact Analysis: stato dell'arte in letteratura e proposta per una definizione in Italia. QF 2011;15.
15. Drummond MF, Sculpher MJ, Torrance GW, O'Brien BJ, Stoddart GL. Methods for the Economic Evaluation of Health Care Programmes. Third edition. Oxford University Press 2005, pp. 379.
16. Gruppo di lavoro AIES coordinato da Fattore G. Proposta di linee guida per la valutazione economica degli investimenti sanitari in Italia. Pharmaco Economics Italian Res Articles. 2009;11(2):83–93.
17. Lucioni C, Ravasio R. Come valutare i risultati di uno studio farmacoeconomico? Pharmaco Economics Italian Res Articles. 2004;6(3):121–30.
18. Messori A, Santarlasci B, Trippoli S, Vaiani M. Controvalore economico del farmaco e beneficio clinico: stato dell'arte della metodologia e applicazione di un algoritmo farmacoeconomico. Pharmaco Economics Italian Res Articles. 2003;5(2):53–67.
19. National Institute for Clinical Excellence (NICE). Guide to the Methods of Technology Appraisal 2013. https://www.nice.org.uk/process/pmg9/resources/guide-to-the-methods-of-technology-appraisal-2013-pdf-2007975843781 Accessed 15 Mar 2016.
20. Jönsson B. Changing health environment: the challenge to demonstrate cost-effectiveness of new compounds. PharmacoEconomics. 2004;22(Suppl 4):5–10.
21. World Health Oranisation. Cost effectiveness and strategic planning (WHO-CHOICE). http://www.who.int/choice/costs/CER_levels/en/. Accessed 14 Mar 2016.
22. Tarricone R. Valutazione economica: definizioni, principali tecniche di valutazione e ruolo della Budget Impact Analysis. Giornale Italiano di Farmacoeconomia e Farmacoutilizzazione. 2012;4(2):5–24.
23. Sonnenberg FA, Beck JR. Markov models in medical decision making: a practical guide. Med Decis Mak. 1993;13(4):322–38.
24. Gani R, Giovannoni G, Bates D, Kemball B, Hughes S, Kerrigan J. Cost-effectiveness analyses of Natalizumab (Tysabri®) compared with other disease-modifying therapies for people with highly active relapsing-remitting multiple sclerosis in the UK. PharmacoEconomics. 2008;26(7):617–27.
25. Peninsula Technology Assessment Group (PenTAG). The effectiveness and cost-effectiveness of natalizumab for multiple sclerosis: an evidence review of the submission from Biogen. Evidence Review Group Report commissioned by NHS R&D HTA Programme on behalf of: NICE. 2007. https://www.nice.org.uk/guidance/ta127/documents/multiple-sclerosis-natalizumab-evaluation-report-evidence-review-group-report2. Accessed 20 Apr 2016.
26. Fiore D, Hung TW, Cui Y, You X, Shang S, Scott T. ADVANCE phase 3 extension study (ATTAIN): Peginterferon Beta-a 125 mcg every 2 weeks demonstrated sustained efficacy in RRMS patients treated up to 5 years. AAN Annual Meeting. 2016;P4:010.
27. Kappos L, Kuhle J, Multanen J, Kremenchutzky M. Verdun di Cantogno E, Cornelisse P, Lehr L, Casset-Semanaz F, Issard D, Uitdehaag BM. Factors influencing long-term outcomes in relapsing-remitting multiple sclerosis: PRISMS-15. J Neurol Neurosurg Psychiatry. 2015;86(11):1202–7.
28. Ford C, Goodman AD, Johnson K, Kachuck N, Lindsey JW, Lisak R, et al. Continuous long-term immunomodulatory therapy in relapsing multiple sclerosis: results from the 15-year analysis of the US prospective open-label study of glatiramer acetate. Mult Scler. 2010;16(3):342–50.
29. Goodin DS, Reder AT, Ebers GC, Cutter G, Kremenchutzky M, Oger J, et al. Survival in MS: a randomized cohort study 21 years after the start of the pivotal IFNβ-1b trial. Neurology. 2012;78(17):1315–22.
30. Bermel RA, Weinstock-Guttman B, Bourdette D, Foulds P, You X, Rudick RA. Intramuscular interferon beta-1a therapy in patients with relapsing-remitting multiple sclerosis: a 15-year follow-up study. Mult Scler. 2010;16(5):588–96.
31. Weinshenker BG, Bass B, Rice GP, et al. The natural history of multiple sclerosis: a geographically based study. 2.Predictive value of the early clinical course. Brain 1989;112:1419–1428.
32. Weinshenker BG, Bass B, Rice GP, et al. The natural history of multiple sclerosis: a geographically based study. I. Clinical course and disability. Brain. 1989;112:133–46. http://dx.doi.org/10.1093/brain/112.1.133
33. Orme M, Kerrigan J, Tyas D, Russell N, Nixon R. The effect of disease, functional status, and relapses on the utility of people with multiple sclerosis in the UK. Value Health. 2007;10(1):54–60.
34. Tyas D, Kerrigan J, Russell N, Nixon R. The distribution of the cost of multiple sclerosis in the UK: how do costs vary by illness severity? Value Health. 2007;10(5):386–9.
35. Patzold U, Pocklington PR. Course of multiple sclerosis. First results of a prospective study carried out of 102 MS patients from 1976–1980. Acta Neurol Scand. 1982;65(4):248–66.
36. ISTAT. Annuario statistico italiano 2015. http://www.istat.it/it/archivio/171864. Accessed 4 Mar 2016.
37. Pokorski RJ. Long-term survival experience of patients with multiple sclerosis. J Insur Med. 1997;29(2):101–6.
38. Tolley K, Hutchinson M, You X, Wang P, Sperling B, Taneja A, et al. A network meta-analysis of efficacy and evaluation of safety of subcutaneous Pegylated interferon Beta-1a versus other Injectable therapies for the

treatment of relapsing-remitting multiple sclerosis. PLoS One. 2015:1–21. doi:10.1371/journal.pone.0127960.

39. Lublin FD, Cofield SS, Cutter GR, Conwit R, Narayana PA, Nelson F, et al. Wolinsky JS; CombiRx investigators. Randomized study combining interferon and glatiramer acetate in multiple sclerosis. Ann Neurol. 2013;73(3):327–40.

40. Schwid SR, Panitch HS. Full results of the evidence of interferon dose-response-European north American comparative efficacy (EVIDENCE) study: a multicenter, randomized, assessor-blinded comparison of low-dose weekly versus high-dose, high-frequency interferon beta-1a for relapsing multiple sclerosis. Clin Ther. 2007;29(9):2031–48.

41. Durelli L, Verdun E, Barbero P, Bergui M, Versino E, Ghezzi A, et al. Zaffaroni M; independent comparison of interferon (INCOMIN) trial study group. Every-other-day interferon beta-1b versus once-weekly interferon beta-1a for multiple sclerosis: results of a 2-year prospective randomised multicentre study (INCOMIN). Lancet. 2002;359(9316):1453–60.

42. Calabrese M, Bernardi V, Atzori M, Mattisi I, Favaretto A, Rinaldi F, et al. Effect of disease-modifying drugs on cortical lesions and atrophy in relapsing-remitting multiple sclerosis. Mult Scler. 2012;18(4):418–24.

43. Etemadifar M, Janghorbani M, Shaygannejad V. Comparison of Betaferon, Avonex, and Rebif in treatment of relapsing-remitting multiple sclerosis. Acta Neurol Scand. 2006;113(5):283–7.

44. Ebers GCR, Lesaux G, Paty J, Oger D, Li J, Beall DKB, et al. Randomised double-blind placebo-controlled study of interferon (beta)-1a in relapsing/remitting multiple sclerosis. Lancet. 1998;352(9139):1498–504.

45. Cadavid D, Wolansky LJ, Skurnick J, Lincoln J, Cheriyan J, Szczepanowski K, et al. Efficacy of treatment of MS with IFNbeta-1b or glatiramer acetate by monthly brain MRI in the BECOME study. Neurology. 2009;72(23):1976–83.

46. O'Connor P, Filippi M, Arnason B, Comi G, Cook S, Goodin D, et al., BEYOND Study Group. 250 microg or 500 microg interferon beta-1b versus 20 mg glatiramer acetate in relapsing-remitting multiple sclerosis: a prospective, randomised, multicentre study. Lancet Neurol. 2009;8(10):889–97.

47. National Institute for Clinical Excellence (NICE). Natalizumab for the treatment of adults with highly active relapsing-remitting multiple sclerosis. NICE technology appraisal guidance [TA127], 2007. https://www.nice.org.uk/guidance/TA127. Accessed 25 May 2016.

48. Parsons S, Carnes D, Pincus T, Foster N, Breen A, Vogel S, et al. Measuring troublesomeness of chronic pain by location. BMC Musculoskelet Disord. 2006;7:34.

49. National Institute for Clinical Excellence (NICE). Depression in adults: recognition and management. NICE guidelines [CG90]. 2009. http://www.nice.org.uk/guidance/cg90. Accessed 11 May 2015.

50. National Institute for Clinical Excellence (NICE). Irritable bowel syndrome in adults: diagnosis and management. NICE guidelines [CG61]. 2008. http://www.nice.org.uk/guidance/cg61. Accessed 11 May 2015.

51. van Hoek AJ, Underwood A, Jit M, Miller E, Edmunds WJ. The impact of pandemic influenza H1N1 on health-related quality of life: a prospective population-based study. PLoS One. 2011;6:e17030. http://dx.doi.org/10.1371/journal.pone.0017030

52. R Emilia-Romagna. Assessorato Politiche per la Salute. Percorso regionale (Emilia-Romagna) di diagnosi e terapia della sclerosi multipla. Versione 1.1, maggio 2011. http://salute.regione.emilia-romagna.it/documentazione/ptr/elaborati/128_sclerosi_multipla.pdf. Accessed 17 Mar 2016.

53. Regione Lazio. Decreto del Commissario ad acta (delibera del Consiglio dei Ministri del 21 marzo 2013) N. U00386 del 13/11/2014. Percorso Diagnostico Terapeutico Assistenziale Sclerosi Multipla. http://www.teresapetrangolini.it/wordpress-4/wp-content/uploads/2014/11/Decreto_sclerosi-multipla_13112014.pdf. Accessed 17 Mar 2016.

54. MINISTERO DELLA SALUTE Remunerazione delle prestazioni di assistenza ospedaliera per acuti, assistenza ospedaliera di riabilitazione e di lungodegenza post acuzie e di assistenza specialistica ambulatoriale. DECRETO 18 ottobre 2012. Supplemento ordinario alla "Gazzetta Ufficiale" n. 23 del 28 gennaio 2013 - Serie generale.

55. Garattini L, Castelnuovo E, Lanzeni D, Viscarra C. Durata e costo delle visite in medicina generale: il progetto DYSCO. Farmeconomia e Percorsi terapeutici. 2003;4(2):109–14.

56. Karampampa K, Gustavsson A, Miltenburger C, Teruzzi C, Fattore G. Treatment experience, burden and unmet needs (TRIBUNE) in MS study: results from Italy. Mult Scler. 2012;18(Suppl 2):29–34.

57. IMS Health. Aprile 2014 - Marzo 2015. Dati IMFO. ©IMS Health S.p.A. Tutti i diritti riservati.

58. Avonex Prescribing Information. http://www.accessdata.fda.gov/drugsatfda_docs/label/2014/103628s5129s5177s5194s5224lbl.pdf. Accessed May 2016.

59. Plegridy Prescribing Information. http://www.accessdata.fda.gov/drugsatfda_docs/label/2014/125499s000lbl.pdf. Accessed May 2016.

60. Rebif Prescribing Information. http://www.accessdata.fda.gov/drugsatfda_docs/label/2014/103780s5178s5179lbl.pdf. Accessed May 2016.

61. Extavia Prescribing Information. http://www.accessdata.fda.gov/drugsatfda_docs/label/2009/125290s0000lbl.pdf. Accessed May 2016.

62. Copaxone_Prescribing Information. http://www.accessdata.fda.gov/drugsatfda_docs/label/2009/020622s057lbl.pdf. Accessed May 2016.

63. Betaferon_Prescribing Information. http://www.accessdata.fda.gov/drugsatfda_docs/label/2015/103471s5186lbl.pdf. Accessed May 2016.

64. Furneri G, Scalone L, Ciampichini R, Cortesi PA, Fornari C, Madotto F, Chiodini V, Cesana G, Mantovani LG. Utilization of disease modifying agents in multiple sclerosis: analysis from an Italian administrative database. ISPOR 15th Annual European Congress. 2012.

65. Lee AW. Review of mixed treatment comparisons in published systematic reviews shows marked increase since 2009. J Clin Epidemiol. 2014;67(2):138–43.

66. Jansen JP, Fleurence R, Devine B, Itzler R, Barrett A, Hawkins N, et al. Interpreting indirect treatment comparisons and network meta-analysis for health-care decision making: report of the ISPOR task force on indirect treatment comparisons good research practices: part 1. Value Health. 2011;14(4):417–28.

67. Hoaglin DC, Hawkins N, Jansen JP, Scott DA, Itzler R, Cappelleri JC, et al. Conducting indirect-treatment-comparison and network-meta-analysis studies: report of the ISPOR task force on indirect treatment comparisons good research practices: part 2. Value Health. 2011;14(4):429–37.

68. Ivanova JI, Bergman RE, Birnbaum HG, Phillips AL, Stewart M, Meletiche DM. Impact of medication adherence to disease-modifying drugs on severe relapse, and direct and indirect costs among employees with multiple sclerosis in the US. J Med Econ. 2012;15(3):601–9.

69. Paolicelli D, D'Onghia M, Pellegrini F, Direnzo V, Iaffaldano P, Lavolpe V, et al. The impact of neutralizing antibodies on the risk of disease worsening in interferon b–treated relapsing multiple sclerosis: a 5 year post-marketing study. J Neurol. 2013;260(6):1562–8.

70. Paolicelli D, Iannazzo S, Santoni L, D'Onghia M, Direnzo V, Iaffaldano A, et al. The cost of patients with relapsing-remitting multiple sclerosis who develop Neutralising antibodies while treated with interferon Beta. Milano: ISPOR 2015. p. 2015.

71. Hernandez L, Guo S, Kinter E, Fay M. Cost-effectiveness analysis of peginterferon beta-1a compared with interferon beta-1a and glatiramer acetate in the treatment of relapsing-remitting multiple sclerosis in the United States. J Med Econ. Published online: 07 Mar 2016. Journal homepage: http://www.tandfonline.com/loi/ijme20

72. Data source: https://currency-conter.net/?gclid=CN2h_LnZmswCFRUTGwodEIUEBg. Accessed 19 Apr 2016.

73. Hernandez L, Guo S, Toro-Diaz H, Carroll S, SFS F. Cost-effectiveness analysis of Peginterferon Beta-1a in the treatment of relapsing-remitting multiple sclerosis in Scotland. Milano: ISPOR 2015; 2015.

74. Hernandez L, Guo S, Toro-Diaz H, Carroll S, SFS F. Cost-effectiveness analysis of Peginterferon Beta-1a in the treatment of relapsing-remitting multiple sclerosis in Ireland. Milano: ISPOR 2015; 2015.

20

The role of puberty and adolescence in the pathobiology of pediatric multiple sclerosis

Vincenzo Salpietro[1], Agata Polizzi[2,3], Gaia Recca[3] and Martino Ruggieri[4*]

Abstract

Multiple sclerosis (**MS**) is increasingly recognized in the paediatric age. In a smaller, but well-established, proportion of paediatric MS patients [20% of total paediatric MS cases: 0.2% to 0.7% of the total MS patients] the onset of disease is before 10 years of age [pre-pubescent (*childhood*) MS]; in the majority [80%] of paediatric MS patients, however [1.7% to 5.6% of the total MS population], the onset of disease is between 10 and 18 years [post-pubertal (*juvenile*) MS]. Notably, while pre-pubertal MS occurs almost equally in both genders (female/male ratio = 0.9:1; reverting to 0.4–0.6/1 in pre-school MS children) the female/male ratio rises to 2.2/3:1 in the post-pubertal age. Interestingly, precocious puberty has been associated to: (**a**) a higher risk of developing MS; and (**b**) a more severe disease course. In addition to that, males are more susceptible to MS (and manifest more neurodegeneration) than females the latter being however more inflammatory than males; pregnancy however reduces MS relapses. All the above findings led to the suggestion of an underlying female sex hormonal involvement in the pathophysiology of MS vs. a protective role of male sex hormones. Epigenetic perspectives indicate that the interplay between genetic background, environmental triggers and neuroendocrine changes, typically occurring around the time of *adolescence*, could all play a combined role in initiating and/or promoting MS with onset in the paediatric age including many of the most frequent disease-associated risk factors (e.g., overweight/obesity, low vitamin D levels, reduced sunlight exposure, Epstein-Barr virus infection). According to this proposed *complex multifactorial model*, susceptibility to MS may be thus acquired during pre-pubertal age and children have probably to wait until the adolescence to manifest their first clinical signs/symptoms.

Keywords: *Paediatric multiple sclerosis, Childhood multiple sclerosis, Early-onset multiple sclerosis, Puberty, Hormones, Pathophysiology, Leptin, PI3K, Demyelination*

Background

The *World Health Organisation* (**WHO**) - *Multiple Sclerosis International Federation* reported that the interquartile range for signs/symptom onset in MS is between 25.3 and 31.8 years, placing the average age of MS onset at 29.2 years [1]. However, *late-onset* cases have been well documented [2] and the occurrence of MS at the other end of the spectrum of life (i.e., < age 18 years: *childhood MS*) is now well established (1.7% to 10% of total MS patients) [3–19]. A small, but well-established subgroup of paediatric MS cases is younger than (or had the onset of symptoms before) 10 years of age (pre-pubescent MS: 0.2% to 0.7% of total MS cases) [7, 18] including children with onset of disease in pre-school years [17] and (exceptionally) during early infancy (i.e., < age 2 years) [17, 19]. The mean annual incidence rates for childhood/paediatric MS is at 0.1/100,000–0.9/100,000 [3–16] whilst annual incidence figures for *pre-pubescent* onset MS are at 0.09/100,000] [7, 17–19]. While pre-pubescent MS occurs almost equally in both genders (female/male ratio = 0.9:1; reverting to 0.4/0.6/1 in pre-school MS children, as it occurs in acute disseminated encephalomyelitis - ADEM) [20] the female/male ratio rises to 2.2/3:1 in the post-pubertal age ("*juvenile* MS": i.e., MS with onset between age 10–18 years) [7, 12, 17–19, 21, 22].

* Correspondence: m.ruggieri@unict.it
[4]Unit of Rare Diseases of the Nervous System in Childhood, Department of Clinical and Experimental Medicine, Section of Pediatrics and Child Neuropsychiatry, University of Catania, AOU "Policlinico-Vittorio Emanuele", Via S. Sofia, 78, 95124 Catania, Italy
Full list of author information is available at the end of the article

In the present review, we summarize the gender effects on inflammatory and neurodegenerative processes in MS and the relationship between pubertal hormonal and/or neuroendocrine changes and the risk of paediatric MS.

Pathophysiology of MS and the rationale for disease-modifying therapies

The hallmark of MS is the demyelinated *"MS plaque"* that is unique and different from that seen in other inflammatory diseases and consists of a well-demarcated hypocellular area characterised by the loss of myelin, the formation of astrocytic scars, and the presence of inflammatory mononuclear cell infiltrates, typically concentrated in perivascular, particularly perivenular, cuffs [23–25]. These infiltrates, which are mainly composed of a mixture of innate (CNS-resident) and adaptive (CNS-infiltrating) components of the immune system [24], include [among the *innate* effectors] monocytes/macrophages, dendritic cells, reactive microglial cells, astrocytes, and mast cells, and [among the *adaptive* effectors] autoreactive lymphocyte T cells, B lymphocytes, and plasma cells plus minor additional components (e.g., ependymal cells), which after their migration into the central nervous system (**CNS**), incite a pro-inflammatory reaction, resulting in local tissue injury, which consists in blood brain barrier (**BBB**: another innate immune component) leakage, destruction of myelin sheaths, oligodendrocytes damage, and cell death, as well as axonal damage and loss, leading in turn to the glial scar (i.e., to the "MS plaque", as seen at imaging and histopathology) [23].

Thus, the migration and/or activation of (innate and adaptive) pro-inflammatory cells into the CNS represent a key stage in the natural history of MS (but what initiates this event still remains unclear) [23]. From a pathophysiologic viewpoint MS appears to be caused by a contact in early childhood with a pathogen coupled with other individual susceptibility factors (e.g., genetic, racial and demographic background), which can elicit their reactivation, triggering innate mechanisms of defence as *toll-like receptors* (**TLRs**: membrane-spanning, non-catalytic receptors expressed on sentinel cells - e.g., macrophages or dendritic cells - recognizing structurally conserved molecules derived from microbes), that signalizes downstream through its adapter protein *MyD88* (myeloid differentiation primary response 88), and the phosphorylated/degraded protein *IKB* which permits translocation of *NF-KB* (nuclear factor kappa-light-chain enhancer of activated B cells: a protein complex, which controls DNA transcription, cytokine production and cell survival) and the transcription of pro-inflammatory cytokines such as IL-6, TNF, IL-1, IL-12, E-selectin, MCP-1, and IL-8. TLR through IRF7 (Interferon regulatory factor 7) gives the signal to the transcription of IFN α/β (i.e., the cytokines used for communication between cells to trigger the protective

defences of the immune system). Another important signal is given by NOD receptors (nucleotide-binding oligomerization domain: i.e., a cytoplasmic pattern recognition receptor, which regulates the innate system and cooperates with TLRs) activated also by potassium efflux-inducing agents such as ATP and TLR stimulation. Additional signalling is provided by PAMS/PAMP (pathogen-associated molecule patterns), toxins, danger or stress, whose triggering induce the *inflammasome* (i.e., a cytoplasmic multiprotein oligomer) via NLRP (NOD-like receptor protein) that form a complex with ASC (apoptosis-associated speck-like protein containing a CARD: caspase recruitment domain) and caspase-1 (i.e., the interleukin-1 converting enzyme, which converts the IL precursors into mature active IL proteins), activating IL-1b, a major factor inducing inflammation, autophagy and cell death, particularly necrosis [23].

All the above pro-inflammatory soluble factors activate microglia and endothelial cells [i.e., innate effectors], up-regulating expression of adhesion molecules (e.g., E-selectin), facilitating the migration of T cells into the CNS. Matrix metalloproteinases (**MMP**) degrades BBB enhancing further migration of autoreactive T cells and macrophages via chemokines (CX3CL-1). The Th1 response evocated via IL-12 and IFN-γ further activates macrophages that in turn do so to T cells CD8+. Th2 response via IL-6 mainly stimulates maturation of B cells and production of autoantibodies. Cytotoxic damage to the oligodendrocyte mediates myelin loss and exposure of the axon to reactive oxygen species, slowing or blocking action potentials and the production of neurological manifestations.

There are intents to remyelinate these lesions via OPCs (oligodendrocyte precursor cells), but neuronal factors such as LINGO-1 (Leucine rich repeat and immunoglobulin-like domain-containing protein 1: a protein important for protein-protein interactions, which regulates/modulates neuronal differentiation and growth, regulation of axon guidance and regeneration processes) or TLR2 inhibit their migration [23–25].

Based on these premises, over the last two decades a dozen different preparations of immunomodulatory/immunosuppressive agents, targeting the above CNS autoimmune mechanisms, have been developed, showing beneficial effects in patients with MS and have been approved as first- or second-line disease-modifying therapies (**DMTs**), including [24, 26]: (**a**) [*first-line DMTs*] interferon-β (IFN-β1a and 1b), glatiramer acetate (GA), dimethyl fumarate (DMF), and teriflunomide; and (**b**) [*second-line DMTs*] mitoxantrone, fingolimod (a small molecule antagonist against SIP and SIP-receptors inhibiting immune cell trafficking), natalizumab (an alpha-4 integrin blocker of immune cell trafficking/migration), alemtuzumab (an anti-CD52 cell-depleting monoclonal antibody), daclizumab (a blocker of the interleukin 2Rα chain), and ocrelizumab (an anti-CD20 cell-depleting monoclonal antibody) [23, 26].

Although these therapies are able to modulate the immune adaptive response, they do not inhibit innate immune cells (e.g., microglial cells, macrophages, and dendritic cells) that participate in the progression of MS. In addition to that, some of these strategies, with their indiscriminate targeting of both pathogenic and protective immune cells, might have side effects. Several new drugs are imminently emerging including strategies targeting the innate immune system [e.g., inhibition of tyrosine kinase, inhibition of NFkB, scavengers for active oxygen species and nitric oxide, or pharmacological interference with their production], or targeting the inflammasome [23].

Disease-modifying therapies in pediatric MS

No medication currently approved for adults with (relapsing-remitting) MS has completed testing for pediatric MS in randomized placebo-controlled trials, although several pediatric MS trials have recently been launched [27]. Use of DMTs in pediatric MS remains off-label in many countries, especially in patients younger than 12 years; nevertheless, these medications are widely used. At present, IFN-b and GA continue to be the standard first-line treatments for pediatric patients with MS, as supported by observational studies and experts' consensus guidelines [26, 27]. Trials are on-going evaluating the clinical outcome of pediatric patients with MS treated with fingolimod, dimethyl fumarate, and teriflunomide [27].

Ages at presentation of MS in childhood and the "*true*" pre-*pubertal* threshold

Currently, MS in the paediatric age group is divided into two main groups according to the age at presentation of first signs/symptoms [3–19]:

(1) *Childhood MS* (when the first acute demyelinating event occurs prior to age 12 years);
(2) *Juvenile MS* (when onset of disease ranges from 12 to 18 years);

A separate group defines (**3**) *adult MS*, when disease onset is after age of 18 years [1, 2].

The cut-off period up to 12 years to define childhood MS was chosen by most Authors in their studies because this period was (and still is) considered as the pre- or early pubertal period [Tanner stages (i.e., Breast, Genitalia, Pubic hair) I or II]. A restricted number of Authors have proposed, in their studies, a lower cut-off for defining "*true*" childhood MS at 10 years of age [12, 17, 19]; this (lowered) period better reflects the biological pre-

pubertal period irrespective to gender [Tanner stages (i.e., Breast, Genitalia, Pubic hair) I vs. I or II: Tanner stage I represents the *true* pre-pubertal stage]. By lowering the cut-off period down to 10 years one could be surer: (**a**) to exclude early pubertal children in analysis of paediatric MS cases, thus avoiding inclusion of MS patients already targeted by the postulated effects of pubertal sex hormones on predisposed tissues [e.g., bone marrow, thymus, central nervous system]; and (**b**) to limit multiple viral exposures as by age 10 years most children (e.g., in Italy) have usually completed their vaccination schedule of mandatory and recommended vaccines [17, 19].

Pre-pubescent onset MS is characterised by peculiar clinical, laboratory and imaging features and outcome [17, 19, 28], including inversion of sex ratios, low to null family history for MS, preponderance of atypical manifestations at onset (e.g., hemiparesis, seizures, lethargy, brainstem signs/symptoms or cerebellar ataxia), polyfocal presentation, highest relapse number/year and fastest recovery time, more severe neurological deficits at relapses with more completely or near-completely recovery, ADEM/leukodystrophy-like MRI patterns at onset vs. typical MS MRI patterns attained years after the first attacks, a worse outcome in the earliest onsets (i.e., < 2 years of age) vs. a better outcome (as compared to post-pubertal MS) in onsets at toddler ages.

Age- and *gender*-related peculiarities of pediatric MS vs. similar disorders

A peculiar female responsiveness to environmental triggers is noted across many disease models and is usually attributed to the need, in the female gender, to make repeated, rapid and consistent physiologic accommodations to pregnancy. In female adolescents with MS, a number of genetic, non-genetic and lifestyle factors have possibly sexually dimorphic effects on MS disease predisposition and on its clinical course [29, 30].

Similarly to what occurs in MS, the so-called *pseudotumour cerebri syndrome* (**PTCS**) is a neurological disorder, which, within childhood, mostly affects post-pubertal females, who often are overweight. PTCS is a condition of unclear aetiology, characterised by increased intracranial pressure (**ICP**) without any radiographic evidence of brain tissue abnormalities, and with normal chemical and cytological cerebrospinal fluid (**CSF**) composition [31–33]. Multiple causes have been taken into consideration in the pathophysiology and aetiology of PTCS [32, 33] including obesity, endocrine abnormalities (e.g., hyperaldosteronism, Cushing syndrome, hyperandrogenism, Addison disease), kidney disease (e.g., nephrotic syndrome), systemic disease (e.g., systemic lupus erythematous, Guillain-Barrè syndrome, antiphospholipid antibody syndrome, polycystic ovary syndrome - PCOS, Behcet disease, familial

Mediterranean fever), medications (e.g., recombinant growth hormone therapy, tetracycline, steroids, mycophenolate mofetil, vitamins A and D, cytarabine, and cyclosporine A), viral infections (e.g., chickenpox, measles, reactivation of varicella infection) and changes in CSF volume and in cerebral CSF hemodynamic (increased cerebral blood volume, increased cerebrospinal fluid production, decreased cerebrospinal fluid resorption or venous flow abnormalities); PTCS has been also observed in members of the same family presenting in either an autosomal dominant or recessive manner. A recently proposed *unifying (neuroendocrine) hypothesis* inferred that [32] multiple neuroendocrine interactions (e.g., cortisol, aldosterone, progesteron) could influence the activation of the mineralocorticoid receptor (**MR**) in the choroid plexus epithelial cells, which in turn stimulates (via a nuclear pathway) the ATPase/Na$^+$/K$^+$ pump leading to raised intracranial CSF production [25]. Even though it typically affects both genders and all age groups, the post-pubertal PTCS typically occurs in overweight girls/women during their reproductive age [34]. Notably, the overall incidence of PTCS is estimated to be 0,9/100,000 rising to 19/100,000 in overweight women [34, 35].

Paediatric PTCS is known to occur in association with a broad variety of conditions, especially obesity and endocrine derangements (e.g., cortisol deficiency or excess, hyperandrogenism, hyperaldosteronism) [32, 36]. Although pre-pubertal PTCS can occur in both genders and ages, post-pubertal PTCS is usually recorded in women during their reproductive age [34, 35]: in this respect, it has been previously proposed that the proneness of some women to develop PTCS could be linked to an estrogenic gynecoid (pear-shaped) fat distribution [34]. Adipose tissue contains aromatase, which may be a link between obesity and PTCS. Aromatase, which catalyses the production of oestrogens from plasma androstenedione, is more prevalent in the fat of the buttock regions (reflecting the typical female fat distribution) vs. the abdominal (visceral) regions [34–36]. Of note, the reports of the onset of PTCS in postmenopausal women following the initiation of hormone replacement therapy further support the notion of an oestrogen involvement in the pathophysiology of this condition [31–33, 37, 38].

The PTCS neuroendocrine pathophysiology [32] cannot be applied to MS, as the mechanism underlying the rise of CSF pressure cannot be compared to the process of demyelination and unlikely involves an autoimmune aetiology [39]. Nonetheless, higher values of ICP have been recently documented in the paediatric MS population [31, 32], thus reflecting the fact that both these conditions (PTCS and MS) could share similar precipitating factors (e.g., obesity, female sex hormones) on a background of alike clinical and anthropometric features. A tenable hypothesis of common possible trigger(s) underlying both diseases could be represented by the putative involvement of *Leptin*, which seem to be centrally involved either in PTCS and in MS pathophysiology [7, 32] (Fig. 1).

The role of *gender* factors in paediatric MS

The sex discrepancy (with a female preponderance) in MS is evident only in individuals who manifest disease symptoms after puberty [1, 7, 17, 19], implicating a likely role of female sex hormones in initiating and/or promoting the disease [7] and of post-pubertal male (high) levels of testosterone in protecting from the disease [40]. The above notion is supported by a number of clinical and laboratory evidences: (**a**) men with MS present at an older age, concurrent with the start of the age-related decline in testosterone levels; (**b**) a decrease of androgen levels in MS adult males is associated with a more severe disease course and a faster progression to disability; and (**c**) testosterone administration may ameliorate the clinical course of MS in males [41, 42].

Oestrogens (17β-estradiol-E2- and estriol-E3), progesterone and testosterone may provide anti-inflammatory and neuroprotective effects on induction and effector phases of experimental allergic encephalomyelitis (**EAE**) [29, 30]. Anti-inflammatory effects appear mainly mediated by oestrogen nuclear receptors alpha (ERα) and beta (ERβ) expressed by regulatory CD4 + CD25+ T cells (Treg), regulatory B (Breg) cells and dendritic cells and may be abrogated in the absence of B cells and the co-inhibitory receptor, Programmed Death-1 (PD-1) on CD4+ Foxp3+ Treg cells. E2 protective effects on EAE seem to be mediated by binding to the membrane G-protein-coupled receptor 30(GPR30). Testosterone may work through androgen receptors or after its conversion to oestrogen through ERs, or GPR30. Androgens may induce remyelination in cuprizone-induced CNS demyelination by acting on neural androgen receptors. Experimental studies also showed that androgens exert a protective role against the development of EAE, the animal model of MS [30]. Additionally, therapeutic trials with dihydrotestosterone (**DHT**) in castrated animals ameliorate both symptoms and inflammation [29, 30, 40].

Some neuroprotective effects of oestrogens in EAE are mediated by ERα expressed on astrocytes: ERβ ligands can prevent demyelination and stimulate remyelination and ERβ treatment can affect microglia with protective effects in CNS inflammation. Progesterone appears to affect axonal protection and remyelination, and testosterone can restore synaptic transmission deficits in the hippocampus.

Sex hormones play a pivotal role in the human *immune system*, regulating antigen presentation, cytokine gene expression, lymphocyte activation and autoimmune

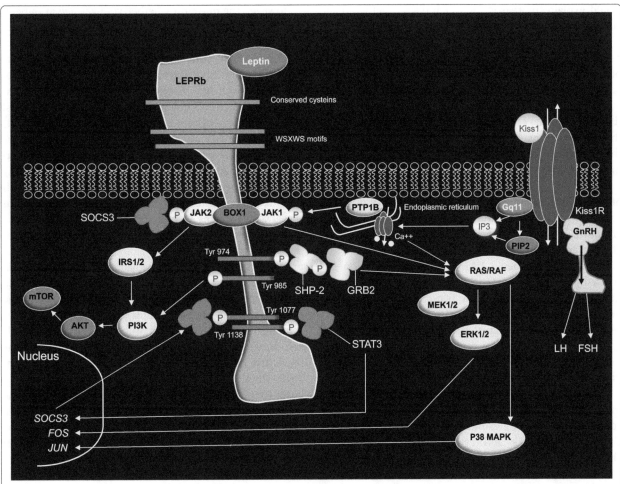

Fig. 1 Mechanisms of Leptin signalling in immune and neuroendocrine cells. Leptin binds to one of its receptors, LEPRb, activating JAK2 by auto-phosphorylation or cross-phosphorylation, and phosphorylates tyrosine residues in the receptor's cytoplasmic domain. Four of the phosphorylated residues [974, 985, 1077, 1138] function as docking sites for cytoplasmic adaptors for STAT factors, particularly STAT3, which dimerizes translocating into the nucleus, where it induces expression of *SOCS3*, *FOS* and *JUN* genes. SOCS3 participates in a feedback loop that inhibits Leptin signalling by binding to phosphorylated tyrosines. SHP-2 is recruited to Tyr985 and Tyr974 and activates ERK1/2 and p38 MAPK pathways through the adaptor protein GRB2, ultimately inducing *FOS* and *JUN* gene expression [*FOS* and *JUN* encode for fos and jun proto-oncogene proteins, which form heterodimers (C-fos:c-jun) resulting in the formation of AP-1 (Activator Protein-1) complex, which binds DNA at AP-1 specific sites at the promoter and enhancer regions of target genes and converts extracellular signals into changes of gene expression]. PTP-1B is localized on the surface of the *endoplasmic reticulum*, and is involved in negative regulation of LEPRb signalling through dephosphorylation of JAK2 after internalization of the LEPRb complex; the endoplasmic reticulum is also the site of action (via Ca++) of the IP3-PIP2-mediated pathway of the Kissprotein1, which in turn modulates GnRH secretion and ultimately LH and FSH secretion [neuroendocrine cells are hereby represented as if they were inside the membrane for practical purposes: in the real pathways the Kiss1 protein binds to the Kiss1 receptor (R), which is expressed on the membrane surface of both immune and neuroendocrine cells: the latter cells promote secretion of GnRH, which in turn stimulate secretion of LH and FSH]. JAK2 can also induce phosphorylation of the IRS1 and 2 proteins, which are responsible for PI3K/AKT and mTOR pathway activation

processes [30, 41]. Also, immune central tolerance at the thymus level is strictly dependent on the hormonal status [29, 30, 42]. Elevation of sex steroids during puberty has been, de facto, linked to the typical decline of the thymus, which starts around adolescence; the thymus rejuvenation after ablation of sex steroids further supports this notion [29, 30, 43]. It is unsure whether puberty and its related hormonal changes affect the susceptibility to environmental factors such as infections.

There are gender-related differences in immune response and women have higher levels of immunoglobulin and more vigorous T-cell activation when compared to males [44]. Oestrogens appear to have a controversial role on inflammation in EAE. At lower levels, oestrogens - such as estradiol - may promote inflammation; but at higher levels, oestrogens - such as the pregnancy hormone estriol - may induce a shift in the immune response from a T helper 1 (**TH1**) response to a T helper 2 (**TH2**) response, muting inflammation [45]. This would explain the reason for which disease activity usually decreases during late pregnancy, which is typically characterized by high levels of estriol and also the beneficial effects of estriol administration to non-pregnant MS females in improving the disease manifestations [46–48].

Studies in EAE also show that low dose oestrogen therapy may have also profound effects in inhibiting the development of autoimmunity, likely influencing the immune reaction towards a protective anti-inflammatory cytokine response [29, 30]. However, in one of these studies, oestrogen treatment at the onset of active EAE failed to reduce disease severity, a result that is consistent with the hypothesis that naive cells are more sensitive to sex hormones than differentiated effector cells [49].

Of note, post-pubertal EAE female mice develop increased myelin reactive T-cell responses compared to age-matched mice that had been prevented from entering puberty via pre-pubertal ovariectomy surgery [49, 50]. Together, these studies suggest that puberty in females enhances central nervous system (CNS) autoimmune mechanisms, further explaining the female preponderance of MS, at the post-pubertal ages.

Lastly, the role of the female chromosome X on immunity and MS should be also regarded as crucial. This could involve hormones-independent mechanisms, including microRNAs and cytokine genes present on chromosome X [51].

Precocious puberty and the risk of MS

Recent MS studies, further deepened, the (causal) relationship between puberty and the disease: initially, only the peri-pubertal period was regarded as typically associated to a dramatic, female-specific, rise in disease incidence; later studies, however, demonstrated that an earlier occurrence of puberty and menarche was also associated to higher risks of disease onset and a more severe clinical course. One study demonstrated that the age at first symptoms increased by 1.16 years as the age of menarche increased by one year [52]. A further MS collaborative Canadian study showed that females with MS were younger at menarche (i.e., 12.4/12 years vs. 12.6/12 years) compared to controls [53]. An association between earlier age at menarche in females and a more severe disease course has been also recorded [54].

A potential effect of age of puberty and menarche on MS, further strengthens the putative involvement of female sex hormones in disease pathophysiology, due to oestrogen-related changes in CNS and immune system (as outlined above). Thus, an earlier menarche may possibly upset a delicate oestrogen balance, making some susceptible girls prone to develop MS.

However, the question whether younger age at puberty is a real trigger for the disease or a mere trigger factor on a background of multiple genetic and environmental determinants remains unsolved. Additionally, it has also been speculated that earlier menarche is a surrogate for the effect of an MS disease causative factor that influences the risk of MS independently by oestrogens, whilst affecting the age of menarche as a by-product [53].

Of note, puberty onset requires specific changes in the secretion of the pituitary gonadotropins, luteinizing hormone (LH) and follicle-stimulating hormone (FSH), which are dependent on the release of Gonadotropin [LH/FSH] releasing hormone (GnRH) from the hypothalamus (Fig. 1); thus, timing of puberty is strictly dependent on a specific genetic susceptibility and on environmental conditions that can influence physiological and pathological processes acting on the hypothalamic-pituitary axis, including nutrition, adiposity, bone mass, emotional and psychological factors, light-darkness cycles/melatonin and endocrine disrupting compounds [55].

Interestingly, also low vitamin D levels are usually associated with an earlier age of pubertal onset in the paediatric population [56]. In this context, it is still unclear whether environmental exposures affecting puberty timing also affect the risk of developing MS in an independent manner. Thus, the correlation between precocious timing of puberty and menarche and the risk of onset and/or worsening of MS and the higher prevalence of obesity within the paediatric MS population are overall factors, which reflect a possible underlying endocrinology/metabolic involvement in the pathophysiology of MS.

Some important MS-associated risk factors (i.e., low vitamin D level, obesity) are also known to be causes of early puberty per se, further supporting the possibility that earlier puberty is a surrogate for the effect of an MS disease causative factor that influences both the risk of MS and an earlier menarche.

Obesity and Leptin: Correlations between metabolism and paediatric MS

Pediatric obesity has been demonstrated in one study to be a risk factor for later development of adult-onset MS in women whilst obesity occurring in adulthood carried out a null risk of developing MS [57]. Another study found that paediatric obesity was independently associated with an increased risk of paediatric onset MS in girls but not in boys: the association between body mass index (BMI) and paediatric MS was strikingly pronounced in extremely obese adolescent girls [7].

Despite these findings, still there are many underexplored and/or not yet fully understood aspects on these relationships. The relative percentages of body fat during the paediatric age are known to be associated with accelerated sexual maturation and precocious puberty: it is unclear if overweight and obesity may predispose independently to both earlier puberty and MS, or if it happens in a consecutive manner [58, 59]. Obesity is characterized by a low-grade inflammation state and it is known to be associated with a T helper 17 (**Th17**) bias predisposing to autoimmune reactions [60]. Additionally, interactions between obesity and vitamin D status remains unexplored [47].

Adipose tissue is not an inert tissue implied only in energy storage, but can be regarded as a part of an *endocrine organ*, which releases many mediators that in turn may predispose to both puberty and MS; additionally, some of these mediators and/or adipokines released by adipocytes are involved in several inflammatory processes, including tumor necrosis factor alpha (**TNF-a**), interleukin 6 (**IL-6**) and Leptin. The adipokine hormone **Leptin** is an amino-acid cytokine-like protein, which is known to play a crucial role in regulating puberty, especially in females. At central (hypothalamic) level, Leptin facilitates puberty onset likely stimulating the Kisspeptin1 (**Kiss1**) pathways, the upstream regulators of GnRH neurons [55] (Fig. 1).

Besides its metabolic role in promoting puberty onset, Leptin has many additional central and/or peripheral actions, including regulation of both innate and adaptive immunity. In fact Leptin stimulates the secretion of pro-inflammatory cytokines (e.g., Il-6, IL-18) and at the adaptive immune system level, Leptin promotes switch towards pro-inflammatory Th1 immunological responses [61].

Leptin mediates its effects by binding to Leptin receptors (**LepRs**) expressed in the brain and a in wide array of peripheral tissues. Various alternatively spliced isoforms of LepRs have been described, but the long isoform of Leptin receptor (**LepRb**) is primarily responsible for Leptin signalling (Fig. 1). The binding of Leptin to LepRb activates a number of signalling pathways, including AK2/STAT 3 and STAT5, SHP2/MAPK and PI3K/AKT/mTOR [59–61]. Notably, the activation of the phosphatidylinositol-3 kinase (**PI3K**) pathway by Leptin is one of the most studied effects of Leptin signalling in the brain and it has been demonstrated to play crucial roles in several metabolic and energetic processes [61]. A number of studies have demonstrated the relevance of PI3K as an underlying mechanism of Leptin actions in vivo [52]. In rats, peripheral Leptin administration was found to activate PI3K in the brain and pre-treatment with inhibitors of PI3K abolished the anorectic response induced by Leptin [61–63].

Interestingly, the balance of PI3K/AKT pathway is essential for oligodendrocytes survival and axon myelination and *gain of functions* mutations of genes enclosed in this pathway (especially mutations in *PIK3CA* gene) have been linked to various types of overgrowth

syndromes [known as *PIK3-related overgrowth syndromes*, or **PROS**] [64, 65], which are also characterized by diffuse white matter abnormalities and increased signal on T2-weighted images on MRI [66, 67]. Studies that investigate potential interactions between Leptin and the PI3K signalling in MS patients are needed.

One of the principal observations, which indicate that Leptin could represent a key mediator in the pathogenesis of MS, is due to its female-specific rise during the peri-pubertal age. In fact, numerous studies showed that during pubertal age Leptin levels continue to increase in girls but not in boys due to the testosterone-related inhibition on Leptin secretion [63]. Besides its interaction with the PIK/AKT pathway, possibly implicated in early cytodegenerative processes of myelin, the actions of Leptin include a strong influence in both the innate and the adaptive immune system. In the innate system, Leptin stimulate the activation of the monocyte-macrophage lineage and the secretion of pro-inflammatory cytokines; in the adaptive immune system Leptin induces pro-inflammatory Th1 responses [61, 62]. Interestingly, the Leptin deficient mice are resistant to the induction of EAE, and administration of Leptin in this animal model shifts the Th2-type response, characteristic of this animal model, to a Th1-type response [68].

Moreover, it has been observed that Leptin is able to maintain environmental conditions that promote loss of immune self-tolerance [69, 70]; in particular, both in vitro and in vivo, leptin can affect the generation, proliferation and responsiveness of t_{reG} cells, a key type of t cells that is involved in the control of immunological tolerance [71].

Thus, the crucial involvement of leptin in initiating and promoting puberty, the observation that it continues to rise in female but not in male adolescents, the increased levels of leptin in the pediatric obese population, the central role of this hormone in regulating inflammatory and autoimmune processes, the demonstration of its necessary role for the induction of the animal model of MS (i.e., EAE), are all convincing evidences of the involvement of leptin in pathogenesis of MS, especially in the post-pubertal pediatric age group.

Conclusions and future directions

In conclusion, within the post-pubertal MS group both the disease prevalence and the female-male ratio are much higher if compared to the pre-pubertal MS group. Furthermore, a more precocious onset of puberty has been associated to both a higher risk of developing MS and an even more severe disease course. Additional support linking puberty with the pathogenesis of MS may be driven from the observations of remarkable similarities between the neuroendocrine mechanisms underlying the onset of puberty and those associated with the postpartum period [72]. In fact, the hypogonadotrophic state of the postpartum phase resembles the pre-pubertal (hypogonadotrophic) state [73, 74].

Interestingly, the postpartum recovery of gonadotropin release follows a predictable sequence of a preferential rise of FSH followed by LH secretion, a pattern identical to that of the peri-pubertal state [72]. For these reasons, the neuroendocrine changes in the postpartum period have been also known as *"puberty in miniature"* and have been frequently associated to the significantly increased risk of onset and relapse of MS after partum. Thus, it is possible that the biological mechanisms, which are responsible for the development of the clinical manifestations of MS in the pubertal or post-pubertal periods, are also involved in the onset or the reactivation of the disease in the post-partum period.

Thus, recent researches in the field suggest that the neuroendocrine changes, typically occurring around the time of puberty, could play a role in initiating and/or promoting pediatric MS associated with additional genetic/non-genetic (e.g., environmental) factors.

According to this multifactorial model, susceptibility to MS may be thus acquired during a wide window of risk through childhood and most pre-pubertal children acquiring susceptibility to the disease have probably to wait until the *"pubertal switch"* to manifest the clinical symptoms. Further experimental studies are required in future to fully understand the gene-neuroendocrine-immune-environment-lifestyle interactions underlying the molecular pathobiology of pediatric-onset MS.

Abbreviations
AKT: AK (Akr mouse) strain transforming; FOS: Finkel osteogenic sarcoma [Finkel-Biskis-Jinkins murine osteogenic sarcoma virus]; FSH: Follicle stimulating hormone; GnRH: Gonadotropin [LH/FSH] releasing hormone; Gq11: Guanine nucleotide binding protein q 11; GRB2: Growth factor receptor-bound protein 2; IRS: Insulin receptor substrate; JAK2: Janus kinase 2; JUN: Jinkins avian sarcoma virus oncogene; Kiss1: Kissprotein 1; Kiss1R: Kissprotein receptor; LEPRb: Leptin receptor, long form b; LH: Luteinizing hormone; MAPK: Mitogen-activated protein kinase; MEK2: MAPK-extracellular kinase 2; mTOR: Mammalian target of rapamycin; PI3K: Phosphatidylinositol-3-kinase; PIP3: Phosphatidylinositol tri-phosphate; PTP-1B: Tyrosine-protein phosphatase non-receptor type 1; RAF: Rapidly accelerated fibrosarcoma protein; RAS: *Rat sarcoma* viral (V-ras) oncogene homolog; SHP-2: SHP protein tyrosine phosphatase-2; SOCS3: suppressor of cytokine signalling 3; STAT3: transducer and activator of transcription 3; IP3: Inositol 1,4,5-trisphosphate receptor, type 3; ERK1/2: Extracellular-signal regulated kinases 1 and 2

Acknowledgements
We wish to thank Dr. G.H. Tutino (Catania) for his valuable comments and support.

Funding
None

Authors' contributions
VS and MR conceived the review, participated in its design and coordination and wrote the initial draft. VS and GR reviewed the existing literature. VS and AP drafted the final version. AP along with MR designed and drew Fig. 1. All authors read and approved the final manuscript.

Competing interests
The authors declare that they have no competing interests.

Author details
[1]Department of Molecular Neuroscience, University College of London, London, UK. [2]National Centre for Rare Diseases, Istituto Superiore di Sanità, Rome, Italy. [3]Institute of Neurological Sciences, National Research Council, Catania, Italy. [4]Unit of Rare Diseases of the Nervous System in Childhood, Department of Clinical and Experimental Medicine, Section of Pediatrics and Child Neuropsychiatry, University of Catania, AOU "Policlinico-Vittorio Emanuele", Via S. Sofia, 78, 95124 Catania, Italy.

References
1. Compston A, Coles A. Multiple sclerosis. Lancet. 2008;372:1502–17.
2. Kis B, Rumberg B, Berlit P. Clinical characteristics of patients with late-onset multiple sclerosis. J Neurol. 2008;255:697–02.
3. Duquette P, Murray TJ, Pleines J, Ebers GC, Sadovnick D, Weldon P, Warren S, Paty DW, Upton A, Hader W, et al. Multiple sclerosis in childhood: clinical profile in 125 patients. J Pediatr. 1987;111:359–63.
4. Ghezzi A, Deplano V, Faroni J, Grasso MG, Liguori M, Marrosu G, Pozzilli C, Simone IL, Zaffaroni M. Multiple sclerosis in childhood: clinical features of 149 cases. Mult Scler. 1997;3:43–6.
5. Mikaeloff Y, Caridade G, Assi S, Suissa S, Tardieu M. Prognostic factors for early severity in a childhood multiple sclerosis cohort. Pediatrics. 2006;118:1133–9.
6. Renoux C, Vukusic S, Mikaeloff Y, Edan G, Clanet M, Dubois B, Debouverie M, Brochet B, Lebrun-Frenay C, Pelletier J, Moreau T, Lubetzki C, Vermersch P, Roullet E, Magy L, Tardieu M, Suissa S, Confavreux C, Adult Neurology Departments KIDMUS Study Group. Natural history of multiple sclerosis with childhood onset. N Engl J Med. 2007;356:2603–13.
7. Banwell B, Ghezzi A, Bar-Or A, Mikaeloff Y, Tardieu M. Multiple sclerosis in children: clinical diagnosis, therapeutic strategies, and future directions. Lancet Neurol. 2007;6:887–902.
8. Krupp LB, Tardieu M, Amato MP, Banwell B, Chitnis T, Dale RC, Ghezzi A, Hintzen R, Kornberg A, Pohl D, Rostasy K, Tenembaum S, Wassmer E, International Pediatric Multiple Sclerosis Study Group. International pediatric multiple sclerosis study group criteria for pediatric multiple sclerosis and immune-mediated central nervous system demyelinating disorders: revisions to the 2007 definitions. Mult Scler. 2013;19:1261–7.
9. Pohl D, Hennemuth I, von Kries R, Hanefeld F. Paediatric multiple sclerosis and acute disseminated encephalomyelitis in Germany: results of a nationwide survey. Eur J Pediatr. 2007;166:405–12.
10. Chitnis T, Glanz B, Jaffin S, Healy B. Demographics of pediatric-onset multiple sclerosis in an MS center population from the northeastern United States. Mult Scler. 2009;15:627–31.
11. Simone IL, Carrara D, Tortorella C, Liguori M, Lepore V, Pellegrini F, Bellacosa A, Ceccarelli A, Pavone I, Livrea P. Course and prognosis in early-onset MS: comparison with adult-onset forms. Neurology. 2002;59:1922–8.
12. Achiron A, Garty BZ, Menascu S, Magalashvili D, Dolev M, Ben-Zeev B, Pinhas-Hamiel O. Multiple sclerosis in Israeli children: incidence, an clinical, cerebrospinal fluid and magnetic resonance imaging findings. Isr Med Assoc J. 2012;14:234–9.
13. Reinhardt K, Weiss S, Rosenbauer J, Gartner J, von Kries R. Multiple sclerosis in children and adolescents: incidence and clinical picture - new insights

from the nationwide german surveillance (2009-2011). Eur J Neurol. 2014;21:654–9.

14. Ghezzi A, Ruggieri M, Trojano M, Filippi M, ITEMS Study Group. Italian studies on early onset multiple sclerosis: the present and the future. Neurol Sci. 2004;25(suppl4):S346–9.

15. Van Haren K, Waubant E. Therapeutic advances in paediatric multiple sclerosis. J Pediatr. 2013;163:631–7.

16. Chitnis T, Tardieu M, Amato MP, Banwell B, Bar-Or A, Ghezzi A, Kornberg A, Krupp LB, Pohl D, Rostasy K, Tenembaum S, Waubant E, Wassmer E. International pediatric MS study group clinical trials summit: meeting report. Neurology. 2013;80:1161–8.

17. Ruggieri M, Polizzi A, Pavone L, Grimaldi LME. Multiple sclerosis in children under 6 years of age. Neurology. 1999;53:478–84.

18. Huppke B, Ellenberger D, Rosewich H, Friede T, Gärtner J, Huppke P. Clinical presentation of pediatric multiple sclerosis before puberty. Eur J Neurol. 2014;21:441–6.

19. Ruggieri M, Iannetti P, Polizzi A, Pavone L, Grimaldi LM, Italian Society of Paediatric Neurology Study Group on Childhood Multiple Sclerosis. Multiple sclerosis in children under 10 years of age. Neurol Sci. 2004;25(Suppl 4):S326–35.

20. Pavone P, Pettoello-Mantovano M, Le Pira A, Polizzi A, Giardino I, Parano E, Pulvirenti A, Giugno R, Ferro A, Pavone L, Ruggieri M. Acute disseminated encephalomyelitis. A long-term prospective study and meta-analysis of the literature. Neuropediatrics. 2010;41:246–55.

21. Orton SM, Herrera BM, Yee IM, Valdar W, Ramagopalan SV, Sadovnick AD, Ebers GC, Canadian Collaborative Study Group. Sex ratio of multiple sclerosis in Canada: a longitudinal study. Lancet Neurol. 2006;5:932–6.

22. O'Connor KC, Lopez-Amaya C, Gagne D, Lovato L, Moore-Odom NH, Kennedy J, Krupp L, Tenembaum S, Ness J, Belman A, Boyko A, Bykova O, Mah JK, Stoian CA, Waubant E, Kremenchutzky M, Ruggieri M, Bardini MR, Rensel M, Hahn J, Weinstock-Guttman B, Yeh EA, Farrell K, Freedman MS, Iivanainen M, Bhan V, Dilenge M, Hancock MA, Gano D, Fattahie R, Kopel L, Fournier AE, Moscarello M, Banwell B, Bar-Or A. Anti-myelin antibodies modulate clinical expression of childhood multiple sclerosis. J Neuroimmunol. 2010;223:92–9.

23. Hernández-Pedro NY, Espinosa-Ramirez G, de la Cruz VP, Pineda B, Sotelo J. Initial immunopathogenesis of multiple sclerosis: innate immune response. Clin Dev Immunol. 2013;2013:413465.

24. Waisman A, Liblau RS, Becher B. Innate and adaptive immune response in the CNS. Lancet Neurol. 2015;14:945–55.

25. Koudriavtseva T, Mainero C. Neuroinflammation, neurodegeneration and regeneration in multiple sclerosis: intercorrelated manifestations of the immune response. Neural Regen Res. 2016;11:1727–30.

26. Ingwersen J, Aktas O, Hartung HP. Advances in and algorithms for the treatment of relapsing-remitting multiple sclerosis. Neurotherapeutics. 2016;13:47–57.

27. Ghezzi A, Amato MP, Makhani N, Shreiner T, Gärtner J, Tenembaum S. Pediatric multiple sclerosis: conventional first-line treatment and general management. Neurology. 2016;87(9 Suppl 2):S97–S102.

28. Waldman A, Ness J, Pohl D, Simone IL, Anlar B, Amato MP, Ghezzi A. Pediatric multiple sclerosis: clinical features and outcome. Neurology. 2016;87(9 Suppl 2):S74–81.

29. Miller DH, Fazekas F, Montalban X, Reingold SC, Trojano M. Pregnancy, sex and hormonal factors in multiple sclerosis. Mult Scler. 2014;20:527–36.

30. Ramien C, Taenzer A, Lupu A, Heckmann N, Engler JB, Patas K, Friese MA, Gold SM. Sex effects on inflammatory and neurodegenerative processes in multiple sclerosis. Neurosci Biobehav Rev. 2016;67:137–46.

31. Soiberman U, Stolovitch C, Balcer LJ, Regenbogen M, Constantini S, Kesler A. Idiopathic intracranial hypertension in children: visual outcome and risk of recurrence. Childs Nerv Syst. 2011;27:1913–8.

32. Salpietro V, Polizzi A, Bertè LF, Chimenz R, Chirico V, Manti S, Ferraù V, Salpietro A, Arrigo T, Ruggieri M. Idiopathic intracranial hypertension: a unifying neuroendocrine hypothesis through the adrenal-brain axis. Neuro Endocrinol Lett. 2012;33:569–73.

33. Salpietro V, Mankad K, Kinali M, Adams A, Valenzise M, Tortorella G, Gitto E, Polizzi A, Chirico V, Nicita F, David E, Romeo AC, Squeri CA, Savasta S, Marseglia GL, Arrigo T, Johanson CE, Ruggieri M. Pediatric idiopathic intracranial hypertension and the underlying endocrine-metabolic dysfunction: a pilot study. J Pediatr Endocrinol Metab. 2014;27:107–15.

34. Andrews LE, Liu GT, Ko MW. Idiopathic intracranial hypertension and obesity. Horm Res Paediatr. 2014;81:217–25.

35. Radhakrishnan K, Ahlskog JE, Cross SA, Kurland LT, O'Fallon WM. Idiopathic intracranial hypertension (pseudotumor cerebri). Descriptive epidemiology in Rochester, Minn, 1976 to 1990. Arch Neurol. 1993;50:78–80.

36. Sheldon CA, Kwon YJ, Liu GT, McCormack SE. An integrated mechanism of pediatric pseudotumor cerebri syndrome: evidence of bioenergetic and hormonal regulation of cerebrospinal fluid dynamics. Pediatr Res. 2015;77:282–9.

37. Salpietro V, Ruggieri M. Pseudotumor cerebri pathophysiology: the likely role of aldosterone. Headache. 2014;54:1229.

38. Khan MU, Khalid H, Salpietro V, Weber KT. Idiopathic intracranial hypertension associated with either primary or secondary aldosteronism. Am J Med Sci. 2013;346:194–8.

39. Narula S, Liu GT, Avery RA, Banwell B, Waldman AT. Elevated cerebrospinal fluid opening pressure in a pediatric demyelinating disease cohort. Pediatr Neurol. 2015 Apr;52:446–9.

40. Voskuhl RR, Palaszynski K. Sex hormones in experimental autoimmune encephalomyelitis: implications for multiple sclerosis. Neuroscientist. 2001;7:258–70.

41. Cossburn M, Ingram G, Hirst C, Ben-Shlomo Y, Pickersgill TP, Robertson NP. Age at onset as a determinant of presenting phenotype and initial relapse recovery in multiple sclerosis. Mult Scler. 2012;18:45–54.

42. Morley JE, Kaiser FE, Perry HMIII, Patrick P, Morley PM, Stauber PM, Vellas B, Baumgartner RN, Garry PJ. Longitudinal changes in testosterone, luteinizing hormone, and follicle-stimulating hormone in healthy older men. Metabolism. 1997;46:410–3.

43. Gold SM, Voskuhl RR. Estrogen and testosterone therapies in multiple sclerosis. Progr Brain Res. 2009;175:239–51.

44. Whitacre CC. Sex differences in autoimmune disease. Nat Immunol. 2001;2:777–80.

45. Walker LS, Abbas AK. The enemy within: keeping selfreactive T cells at bay in the periphery. Nat Rev Immunol. 2002;2:11–9.

46. Hince M, Sakkal S, Vlahos K, Dudakov J, Boyd R, Chidgey A. The role of sex steroids and gonadectomy in the control of thymic involution. Cell Immunol. 2008;252:122–38.

47. Bove R, Chitnis T. The role of gender and sex hormones in determining the onset and outcome of multiple sclerosis. Mult Scler. 2014 Apr;20:520–6.

48. Coyle PK. Pregnancy and multiple sclerosis. Neurol Clin. 2012;30:877–88.

49. Sicotte NL, Liva SM, Klutch R, Pfeiffer P, Bouvier S, Odesa S, TC W, Voskuhl RR. Treatment of multiple sclerosis with the pregnancy hormone estriol. Ann Neurol. 2002;52:421–8.

50. Bebo BF Jr, Fyfe-Johnson A, Adlard K, Beam AG, Vandenbark AA, Offner H. Low dose estrogen therapy ameliorates experimental autoimmune encephalomyelitis in two different inbred mouse strains. J Immunol. 2001;166:2080–9.

51. Rubtsova K, Marrack P, Rubtsov AV. Sexual dimorphism in autoimmunity. J Clin Invest. 2015;125:2187–93.

52. Sloka JS, Pryse-Phillips WE, Stefanelli M. The relation between menarche and the age of first symptoms in a multiple sclerosis cohort. Mult Scler. 2006;12:333–9.

53. Ramagopalan SV, Valdar W, Criscuoli M, DeLuca GC, Dyment DA, Orton SM, Yee IM, Ebers GC, Sadovnick AD. Age of puberty and the risk of multiple sclerosis: a population based study. Eur J Neurol. 2009;16:342–7.

54. D'Hooghe B, Haentjens MP, Nagels G, D'Hooghe T, De Keyser J. Menarche, oral contraceptives, pregnancy and progression of disability in relapsing onset and progressive onset multiple sclerosis. J Neurol. 2012;259:855–61.

55. Chirico V, Lacquaniti A, Salpietro V, Buemi M, Salpietro C, Arrigo T. Central precocious puberty: from physiopathological mechanisms to treatment. J Biol Regul Homeost Agents. 2014;28:367–75.

56. Villamor E, Marin C, Mora-Plazas M, Baylin A. Vitamin D deficiency and age at menarche: a prospective study. Am J Clin Nutr. 2011;94:1020–5.

57. Munger KL, Chitnis T, Ascherio A. Body size and risk of MS in two cohorts of US women. Neurology. 2009;73:1543–50.

58. Lee JM, Appugliese D, Kaciroti N, Corwyn RF, Bradley RH, Lumeng JC. Weight status in young girls and the onset of puberty. Pediatrics. 2007;119:e624–30.

59. Davison KK, Susman EJ, Birch LL. Percent body fat at age 5 predicts earlier pubertal development among girls at age 9. Pediatrics. 2003;111:815–21.

60. Winer S, Paltser G, Chan Y, Tsui H, Engleman E, Winer D, Dosch HM. Obesity predisposes to Th17 bias. Eur J Immunol. 2009;39:2629–35.

61. Demerath EW, Towne B, Wisemandle W, Blangero J, Chumlea WC, Siervogel RM. Serum leptin concentration, body composition, and gonadal hormones during puberty. Int J Obes Relat Metab Disord. 1999;23:678–85.

62. Harlan SM, Rahmouni K. PI3K signaling: a key pathway in the control of sympathetic traffic and arterial pressure by leptin. Mol Metab. 2013;2:69–73.

63. Beretta M, Bauer M, Hirsch E. PI3K signaling in the pathogenesis of obesity: the cause and the cure. Adv Biol Regul. 2015;58:1–15.
64. Ruggieri M, Praticò AD. Mosaic neurocutaneous disorders and their causes. Semin Pediatr Neurol. 2015;22:207–33.
65. Vahidnezhad H, Youssefian L, Uitto J. Molecular genetics of the PI3K-AKT-mTOR pathway in Genodermatoses: diagnostic implications and treatment opportunities. J Invest Dermatol. 2015 Sep 24; https://doi.org/10.1038/jid.2015.331.
66. Lebrun-Julien F, Bachmann L, Norrmén C, Trötzmüller M, Köfeler H, Rüegg MA, Hall MN, Suter U. Balanced mTORC1 activity in oligodendrocytes is required for accurate CNS myelination. J Neurosci. 2014;34:8432–48.
67. Conway RL, Pressman BD, Dobyns WB, Danielpour M, Lee J, Sanchez-Lara PA, Butler MG, Zackai E, Campbell L, Saitta SC, Clericuzio CL, Milunsky JM, Hoyme HE, Shieh J, Moeschler JB, Crandall B, Lauzon JL, Viskochil DH, Harding B, Graham JM Jr. Neuroimaging findings in macrocephaly-capillary malformation: a longitudinal study of 17 patients. Am J Med Genet A. 2007;143A:2981–08.
68. Matarese G, La Cava A, Sanna V, Lord GM, Lechler RI, Fontana S, Zappacosta S. Balancing susceptibility to infection and autoimmunity: a role for leptin? Trends Immunol. 2002;23:182–7.
69. Matarese G, Carrieri PB, Montella S, De Rosa V, La Cava A. Leptin as a metabolic link to multiple sclerosis. Nat Rev Neurol. 2010;6:455–61.
70. Procaccini C, Pucino V, Mantzoros CS, Matarese G. Leptin in autoimmune diseases. Metabolism. 2015;64:92–104.
71. De Rosa V, Procaccini C, Calì G, Pirozzi G, Fontana S, Zappacosta S, La Cava A, Matarese G. A key role of leptin in the control of regulatory T cell proliferation. Immunity. 2007;26:241–55.
72. Sandyk R, Awerbuch GI. Multiple sclerosis: the role of the pineal gland in its timing of onset and risk of psychiatric illness. Int J Neurosci. 1993;72:95–106.
73. Lage M, Garcia-Mayor RV, Tomé MA, Cordido F, Valle-Inclan F, Considine RV, Caro JF, Dieguez C, Casanueva FF. Serum leptin levels in women throughout pregnancy and the postpartum period and in women suffering spontaneous abortion. Clin Endocrinol. 1999;50:211–6.
74. Chehab FF. 20 years of leptin: leptin and reproduction: past milestones, present undertakings, and future endeavors. J Endocrinol. 2014;223:T37–48.

21

Differentiating Vogt-Koyanagi-Harada syndrome from recurrent optic neuritis

Marta Scarioni[1*†] ⓘ, Anna M. Pietroboni[1†], Alessandro Invernizzi[2,3], Francesco Viola[2], Laura Ghezzi[1], Alberto Calvi[1], Tiziana Carandini[1], Milena De Riz[1], Daniela Galimberti[1] and Elio Scarpini[1]

Abstract

Background: First recognized at the beginning of twentieth century and named after three authors who independently described some affected patients, Vogt-Koyanagi-Harada syndrome is a rare multisystemic autoimmune disease targeting melanin-containing tissues of the eye, meninges, inner ear and skin. It predominantly affects Asian people, but also people with darker skin pigmentation such as Native Americans and Hispanics (Mestizos), whose ancestors moved from Asia across the Bering strait to North America and further down to Central and South America. Heterogenous presentation is observed, especially among different ethnic groups. Here we describe the case of an Hispanic South American patient presenting with multiple visual relapses and thus mimicking recurrent optic neuritis; we provide insights into the differential diagnosis and a brief review of the literature concerning the epidemiology of Vogt-Koyanagi-Harada syndrome in Hispanic patients compared with other ethnic groups.

Case presentation: A 34-year-old Ecuadorian woman presented over years with multiple relapses involving the visual system. She was investigated in both neurologic and ophthalmic clinical settings. Brain Magnetic Resonance Imaging, cerebrospinal fluid examination, Spectral Domain Optical Coherence Tomography and Fluorescein Angiography were performed. She was misdiagnosed first as an optic neuritis pointing to a demyelinating disorder, then as a posterior scleritis. Due to the protean manifestations of Vogt-Koyanagi-Harada syndrome and the incomplete clinical presentation at the beginning, the right diagnosis was made only at a later disease stage using retrospective criteria.

Conclusions: Hispanic patients often present without extraocular symptoms in early phases of the disease and they have globally lower rates of integumentary signs compared to Asian patients. The diagnosis of a multisystemic disease such as Vogt-Koyanagi-Harada syndrome is a challenge involving specialists operating in different medical fields; especially in urban multiethnic populations, rare etiologies of common symptoms have to be taken into account when performing a differential diagnosis.

Keywords: Vogt-Koyanagi-Harada syndrome, Epidemiology, Case report, South America, Hispanic, Differential diagnosis, Optic neuritis, Uveitis, Multiple sclerosis

* Correspondence: marta.scarioni@gmail.com
†Equal contributors
[1]Department of Pathophysiology and Transplantation, Neurology Unit, Dino Ferrari Center, University of Milan, Fondazione IRCCS Ca' Granda, Ospedale Maggiore Policlinico, Milan, Italy
Full list of author information is available at the end of the article

Background

First recognized at the beginning of twentieth century and named after three authors who independently described some affected patients [1], Vogt-Koyanagi-Harada (VKH) is a rare multisystemic autoimmune disease targeting melanin-containing tissues of the eye, meninges, inner ear and skin [2]. It predominantly affects Asian people, but also people with darker skin pigmentation such as Native Americans and Hispanics (Mestizos), whose ancestors moved from Asia across the Bering strait to North America and further down to Central and South America [3, 4]. Genetic susceptibility is linked to certain HLA alleles, the most relevant being HLA-DRB1*0405, which has been reported as the predominant allele across different ethnic groups [5]. The typical age of incidence is between 20 and 50 years, and women are affected twice than men. The most prominent feature of VKH is bilateral uveitis, accompanied by various combinations of neurological, auditory and cutaneous signs and symptoms. The typical disease course includes four phases (prodromic, uveitic, convalescent and recurrent/chronic), with very protean clinical manifestations [6]. New diagnostic criteria take into account such clinical variability [7].

Case presentation

A 34-year-old Ecuadorian women was referred to our hospital for sudden loss of vision and pain in her right eye, immediately followed by the same symptoms in the left eye. At presentation bilateral visual impairment with a best corrected visual acuity (BCVA) of 20/200 in the right eye and 20/60 in the left eye was detected. Ophthalmoscopic examination revealed optic nerve head edema without any other sign of inflammation. The patient was hence referred to the neurological ward with a diagnose of "bilateral papilledema – suspected optic neuritis (ON)". Here, she underwent neurological examination, brain and spinal cord Magnetic Resonance Imaging (MRI), lumbar puncture (LP) and autoantibodies testing (anti AQP4 and anti-MOG) to rule out a demyelinating disease of the Central Nervous System (CNS). Neurological examination and MRI resulted within normal limits. Autoantibodies testing was negative. Cerebrospinal fluid (CSF) examination showed a mild pleocytosis in the absence of oligoclonal bands (OCBs). She was treated with a short-term steroid therapy and discharged with the diagnosis of "bilateral ON with liquor pleocytosis".

Six years later, another episode of sudden loss of vision and pain in the left eye occurred, and the patient was admitted to the ophthalmology ward for worsening symptoms. She underwent a complete ophthalmological examination, including Spectral Domain Optical Coherence Tomography (SD-OCT) and Fluorescein Angiography

(FA). SD-OCT revealed a large exudative retinal detachment (ERD) at the posterior pole in the left eye and bilateral choroidal folds (Fig. 1). FA showed optic disc hyperfluorescence during late phases of the angiogram as well as multiple areas of leakage in the left eye (Fig. 2). A work-up for posterior uveitis was hence performed. Blood tests for infectious diseases commonly causing uveitis (herpetic viruses, syphilis, borreliosis, tuberculosis) were negative as well as autoantibodies (ANA, ASMA, ANCA, anti-dsDNA, ENA) screening. A complete neurological evaluation was then repeated; this time CSF examination was normal, with neither pleocytosis nor OCBs, while MRI of the eyes and orbits revealed a scleroretinal thickening with enhancement in the posterior chamber of the left eye. According to these findings the disease was labelled as "probable posterior scleritis (PS)". A three-days high-dose intravenous steroid treatment was started, followed by slow oral taper in the following months. The patient improved both clinically and instrumentally.

A year and a half later, the patient came to our attention complaining of loss of vision in the right eye, accompanied by headache, neck stiffness, slight subjective left hearing loss and tinnitus. At fundoscopic examination, optic nerve head edema was detected in the right eye (Fig. 3). The relapsing nature of the condition along with the protean clinical manifestations of the disease through the years raised the suspect of VKH disease. The medical history of the patient was hence retrospectively investigated and the CSF pleocytosis identified at the first presentation was finally correctly reinterpreted. In addition to those described, the patient reported other preceding episodes of visual loss diagnosed elsewhere as ONs and treated with intravenous steroid therapy followed by slow oral taper. There was no laboratory evidence suggestive of other autoimmune or infective ocular disease entities, nor a previous history of penetrating ocular trauma or surgery. According to revised diagnostic criteria for VKH disease (Read et al., 2001), a diagnosis of incomplete VKH was finally made. She was treated with oral steroid therapy, with partial edema resolution on a 3-months eye examination. A long-term treatment with Azathioprine was then started.

In order to support our diagnosis, a HLA haplotype typization was performed. However, HLA-DRB1*0405 allele was absent.

Discussion and conclusions

Here, we describe a case of VKH, whose diagnosis was done retrospectively due to the protean manifestations of this condition. The first presentations, including loss of vision accompanied by pain in the eye, suggested in fact ON [8] or posterior scleritis (PS) [9].

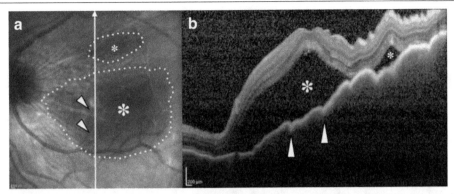

Fig. 1 Combined Near Infrared Reflectance (NIR) (**a**) and Spectral Domain Optical Coherence Tomography (SD-OCT) (**b**) of the left eye performed during a disease recurrence occurred six years after the first presentation. The white arrow crossing NIR image corresponds to the position of the SD-OCT scan. Multiple pockets of fluid accumulation (white asterisk) detaching the neuroretina are visible as dark gray areas (encircled by white dotted lines) on NIR and as empty spaces on SD-OCT. Choroidal folds are also clearly visible in both the images (white arrowheads)

The first clinical episode was investigated in a neurological setting, with optic nerve head edema as solely clinical finding leading to high suspicion of ON as a Clinically Isolated Syndrome (CIS) pointing to a demyelinating disorder such as Multiple Sclerosis (MS) or, given the bilateral and exclusive involvement of the visual system, a Neuromyelitis Optica Spectrum Disorder (NMOSD) [10]; little attention was hence given to liquoral pleocytosis in the absence of OCBs, since both these findings were still compatible with a CNS demyelinating disease. According to the misdiagnosis, a suboptimal dose of steroid was administered at that time, which can at least partially explain the subsequent propensity for recurrence [11].

The second clinical episode was investigated by ophthalmologists. On that occasion clinical and instrumental findings (OCT, FA) could rise the suspicion of both a PS and a VKH [12, 13], but the absence of CSF pleocytosis (probably due to prior long-term steroid administration) did not support the latter hypothesis, which seemed also the less likely from a purely epidemiological point of view.

The third clinical episode manifested with polymorphic symptoms suggesting a VKH syndrome and the patient was evaluated in a multidisciplinary setting, so that the right diagnosis was made at a later disease stage using retrospective criteria.

The lack of communication between specialists operating in different medical fields can lead to a significant diagnostic delay, especially with rare multisystemic diseases. Crossing knowledge boundaries, which are often not clearly defined in such disorders, is essential to reach

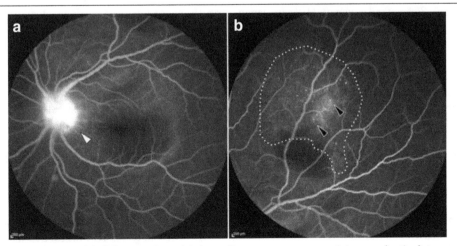

Fig. 2 Fluorescein angiography (FA) of the left eye performed during a disease recurrence occurred six years after the first presentation. Images of the posterior pole (**a**) during the late phases of the angiogram reveal leakage of dye from the optic nerve head (white arrowhead) demonstrating the inflammatory status. Multiple leaking points (black arrowheads) feeding a pocket of subretinal fluid (encircled by white dotted lines) are visible along the supero-temporal vascular arcade (**b**)

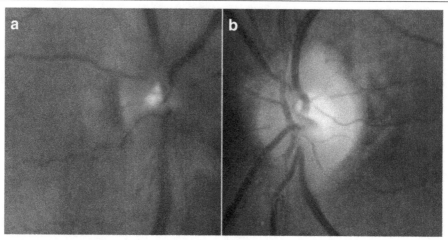

Fig. 3 Fundus photography of both eyes (optic nerve head field) performed during the last disease recurrence. Optic nerve head appears hyperemic and swollen in the right eye (**a**) as compared to the left eye (**b**) where the disc looks within normal limits

the goal of early diagnosis and treatment which, in turn, significantly affects prognosis, avoiding long-term complications such as severe iris depigmentation and persistent ocular hypotony, which have been described in South American patients [14].

VKH is a rare disease in Europe. In Switzerland, where the first patient was described by Vogt [5], VKH represents 0.7% of all uveitis [15]. Two studies from the North of Italy, where our hospital is located, report VKH as accounting for 1,37–4,1% of all uveitis (the former being a percentage even lower then the rest of Europe) [16, 17]. VKH is mostly seen (and thus, suspected) among patients of Asian origin. In China the highest percentage of panuveitis is reported [18], due to the high incidence of both VKH and Bechet disease (accounting respectively for 29–30% of all uveitis) [19]. In Japan VKH was considered the first cause of uveitis [18, 20], but differences in etiology of uveitis are being observed over time [21], and in most recent studies it is reported as the second cause of uveitis (7% of all uveitis) after sarcoidosis [22, 23]. On the other hand, higher VKH rates than expected are being recorded in South America: in Chile [24] VKH has been reported as the most frequent cause of uveitis, accounting for 17,2% of all uveitis, and in Argentina as the second cause after toxoplasmosis, accounting for 16.7% of all uveitis [18]. An epidemiologic study on uveitis conducted in Barcelona and highlighting the challenge of globalization in urban multiethnic populations reported a South American ethnicity in 47% of cases of VKH [25].

Ethnic groups do not only differ with respect to incidence and prevalence of the disease, but also for the frequency of clinical manifestations: Hispanic patients often present without extraocular symptoms in early

phases of the disease [26], as we observed in this case, and they have globally lower rates of integumentary signs (between 11 and 16%) and hearing impairment (9%) compared to Asian patients [27]. On the other hand, neurological signs and dysacousia are quite common (74–76%) among Japanese patients [23, 28], while integumentary signs are more often seen in Chinese patients (39–41%) [29]. When looking at ocular manifestations, studies conducted on South American patients are concordant in rating a optic disc swelling occurrence significantly lower than in Asian patients (8,6% - 9% versus 50–73%, respectively) [26–30], but they differ in rating ERD (91% according to Sutavachtarin et al.... and 45,7% according to Giordano et al..) and anterior uveitis (100% according to Sutavachtarin et al. and 45,1% according to Giordano et al) [26, 30]. Response to therapy and complication rates are reported to be similar among ethnic groups [26].

Such epidemiological considerations have to be taken into account when performing a differential diagnosis. In our case, also the hypothesis of a NMOSD was considered, due the history of bilateral and recurrent ONs, but diagnostic criteria where not fulfilled [10]. Also NMOSDs have higher occurrence rates in Asian patients [31]. In South America NMOSDs have been reported to have a higher prevalence in non-white populations, while MS (which is another possible misdiagnosis in VKH patients, as recently described by Algathani et al) [32] has a higher prevalence in white South Americans [33].

The present case reinforces the notion that also in Western European countries, especially in urban multiethnic populations, rare etiologies of common symptoms have to be taken into account when performing a differential diagnosis.

Abbreviations

BCVA: best corrected visual acuity; CIS: Clinically Isolated Syndrome; CNS: Central Nervous System; CSF: cerebrospinal fluid; ERD: exudative retinal detachment; FA: Fluorescein Angiography; LP: lumbar puncture; MRI: Magnetic Resonance Imaging; MS: Multiple sclerosis; NMOSD: Neuromyelitis Optica Spectrum Disorder; OCB: oligoclonal bands; ON: optic neuritis; PS: posterior scleritis; SD-OCT: Spectral Domain Optical Coherence Tomography; VKH: Vogt-Koyanagi-Harada

Funding

The authors declare that they didn't receive any funding for this publication.

Authors' contributions

MS contributed to conception, design and draft of the manuscript for intellectual content. AP contributed to conception, design and draft of the manuscript for intellectual content. AI contributed to conception, design and draft of the manuscript for intellectual content. FV contributed to conception, design and revision of the manuscript for intellectual content. LG contributed to revision of the manuscript for intellectual content. AC contributed to revision of the manuscript for intellectual content. TC contributed to revision of the manuscript for intellectual content. MD contributed to revision of the manuscript for intellectual content. DG contributed to revision of the manuscript for intellectual content. ES contributed to revision of the manuscript for intellectual content. All authors read and approved the final manuscript.

Competing interests

The authors declare that they have no competing interests.

Author details

[1]Department of Pathophysiology and Transplantation, Neurology Unit, Dino Ferrari Center, University of Milan, Fondazione IRCCS Ca' Granda, Ospedale Maggiore Policlinico, Milan, Italy. [2]Department of Clinical Sciences and Community Health, Ophtalmological Unit, University of Milan, Fondazione IRCCS Ca' Granda, Ospedale Maggiore Policlinico, Milan, Italy. [3]Department of Biomedical and Clinical Science "Luigi Sacco", Eye Clinic, Luigi Sacco Hospital, University of Milan, Milan, Italy.

References

1. Sakata VM, da Silva FT, Hirata CE, de Carvalho JF, Yamamoto JH. Diagnosis and classification of VKH disease. Autoimmun Rev 2014;13:550–550.
2. Silpa-archa S, Silpa-archa N, Preble JM, Foster CS. Vogt-Koyanagi-Harada syndrome: perspectives for immunogenetics, multimodal imaging, and therapeutic options. Autoimmun Rev. 2016;15:809–19.
3. Moorthy RS, Inomata H, Rao NA. Vogt-Koyanagi-Harada syndrome. Surv Ophthalmol. 1995;39(4):265–92.
4. Abad S, Monnet D, Caillat-Zucman S, Mrejen S, Blanche P, Chalumeau M, Mouthon L, Dhote R, Brézin AP. Characteristics of Vogt-Koyanagi-Harada disease in a French cohort: ethnicity, systemic manifestations, and HLA genotype data. Ocul Immunol Inflamm. 2008;16(1–2):3–8.
5. Lavezzo MM, et al. Vogt-Koyanagi-Harada disease: review of a rare autoimmune disease targeting antigens of melanocytes. Orphanet Journal of Rare Diseases. 2016;11:29.
6. Greco A, Fusconi M, Gallo A, Turchetta R, Marinelli C, Macri GF, De Virgilio A, de Vincentiis M. Vogt-Koyanagi-Harada syndrome. Autoimmun Rev. 2013;12:1033–8.
7. Read RW, Holland GN, Rao NA, Tabbara KF, Ohno S, Arellanes-Garcia L, Pivetti-Pezzi P, Tessler HH, Usui M. Revised diagnostic criteria for VKH disease: report of an international committee on nomenclature. American Journal of Ophthalmology. 2001;131(5):647–52.
8. Toosy AT, Mason DF, Miller DH. Optic neuritis. Lancet Neurol. 2014; 13(1):83–99.
9. Gonzalez-Gonzalez LA, Molina-Prat N, Doctor P, Tauber J, Sainz de la Maza M, Foster CS. Clinical features and presentation of posterior scleritis: a report of 31 cases. Ocul Immunol Inflamm. 2014;22(3):203–7.
10. Wingerchuk DM, Banwell B, Bennett JL, et al. International consensus diagnostic criteria for neuromyelitis optica spectrum disorders. Neurology. 2015;85:177–89.
11. Kawaguchi T, Horie S, Bouchenaki N, Ohno-Matsui K, Mochizuki M, Herbort CP. Suboptimal therapy controls clinically apparent disease but not subclinical progression of Vogt-Koyanagi-Harada disease. International Ophtalmology. 2010;30:41–50.
12. Fardeau C, Tran TH, Gharbi B, Cassoux N, Bodaghi B, LeHoang P. Retinal fluorescein and indocyanine green angiography and optical coherence tomography in successive stages of Vogt-Koyanagi-Harada disease. International Ophtalmology. 2007;27(2–3):163–72.
13. Nakai K, Gomi F, Ikuno Y, Yasuno Y, Nouchi T, Ohguro N, Nishida K. Choroidal observations in Vogt-koyanagi-Harada disease using high-penetration optical coherence tomography. Graefes Arch Clin Exp Ophthalmol. 2012;250(7):1089–95.
14. Cuevas M, De-la-Torre A, Córdoba A. Bilateral iris depigmentation and ocular Hypotony as end-stage manifestations of untreated Vogt-Koyanagi-Harada disease. Ocul Immunol Inflamm. 2017:1–6.
15. Rathinam SR, Namperumalsamy P. Global variation and pattern changes in epidemiology of uveitis. Indian J Ophthalmol. 2007;55(3):173–83.
16. Mercanti A, Parolini B, Bonora A, Lequaglie Q, Tomazzoli L. Epidemiology of endogenous uveitis in north-eastern Italy. Analysis of 655 new cases. Acta Ophtalmologica. Scandinavica. 2001;79(1):64–8.
17. Cimino L, Aldigeri R, Salvarani C, Zotti CA, Boiardi L, Parmeggiani M, Casali B, Cappuccini L. The causes of uveitis in a referral centre of northern Italy. Int Ophthalmol. 2010;30(5):521–9.
18. Chams H, et al. Epidemiology and prevalence of uveitis: review of literature. Iranian. J Ophthalmol. 2009;21(4):4–16.
19. Yang P, Zhang Z, Zhou H, Li B, Huang X, Gao Y, Zhu L, Ren Y, Klooster J, Kijlstra A. Clinical patterns and characteristics of uveitis in a tertiary center for uveitis in China. Curr Eye Res. 2005;30(11):943–8.
20. Wakabayashi T, Morimura Y, Miyamoto Y, Okada AA. Changing patterns of intraocular inflammatory disease in Japan. Ocul Immunol Inflamm. 2003; 11(4):277–86.
21. Iwata D, Mizuuchi K, Aoki K, Horie Y, Kase S, Namba K, Ohno S, Ishida S, Kitaichi N. Serial frequencies and clinical features of uveitis in Hokkaido, Japan. Ocul Immunol Inflamm. 2016:1–4.
22. Ohguro N, Sonoda KH, Takeuchi M, Matsumura M, Mochizuki M. The 2009 prospective multi-center epidemiologic survey of uveitis in Japan. Jpn J Ophthalmol. 2012 Sep;56(5):432–5.
23. Takahashi R, et al. Uveitis incidence in Jichi Medical University hospital, Japan, during 2011–2015. Clin Ophthalmol. 2017;11:1151–6.
24. Liberman P, Gauro F, Berger O, Urzua CA. Causes of uveitis in a tertiary Center in Chile: a cross-sectional retrospective review. Ocul Immunol Inflamm. 2014:1–7.
25. Llorenç V, et al. Epidemiology of uveitis in a western urban multiethnic population. The challenge of globalization. Acta Ophthalmol. 2015;93(6): 561–7.
26. Sukavatcharin S, et al. Vogt-Koyanagi–Harada disease in Hispanic patients. Int Ophthalmol. 2007;27:143–8.
27. Hedayaftar et al. The spectrum of Vogt-Koyanagi-Harada disease in Iran. Int Ophtalmol. 2017.
28. Sasamoto Y, Ohno S, Matsuda H. Studies on corticosteroid therapy in Vogt-Koyanagi-Harada disease. Ophthalmologica. 1990;201(3):162–7.
29. Chee SP, Jap A, Bacsal K. Spectrum of Vogt-Koyanagi-Harada disease in Singapore. Int Ophthalmol. 2007;27(2–3):137–42.
30. Giordano VE, Schlaen A, Couto C, et al. Spectrum and visual outcomes of Vogt-Koyanagi-Harada disease in Argentina. Int J Ophthalmol. 2017; 10(1):98–102.
31. Jacob A, et al. Current concept of neuromyelitis optica (NMO) and NMO spectrum disorders. J Neurol Neurosurg Psychiatry. 2013;84(8):922–30.
32. Algathani H, et al. Vogt Koyanagi Harada syndrome mimicking multiple sclerosis: a case report and review of the literature. Mult Scler Relat Disord. 2017;12:44–8.
33. Papais-Alvarenga RM, et al. Central nervous system idiopathic inflammatory demyelinating disorders in south Americans: a descriptive, multicenter, cross-sectional study. PLoS One. 2015;10(7):e0127757.

22

Baseline characteristics associated with NEDA-3 status in fingolimod-treated patients with relapsing-remitting multiple sclerosis

Manuela Giuliani, Alessandra Logoteta, Luca Prosperini[*] ⓘ, Maria Neve Hirsch and Carlo Pozzilli

Abstract

Background: Fingolimod is an efficacious treatment for relapsing-remitting multiple sclerosis (RRMS) and there is class I evidence that it is superior to standard care in reducing relapse rate. However, real-world data investigating its effectiveness and potential predictors of response are still scarce.

Objective: To estimate (i) the proportion of fingolimod-treated patients who achieved the no evidence of disease activity (NEDA-3) status; and (ii) to determine which baseline (i.e. at treatment start) clinical and magnetic resonance imaging (MRI) variables were associated with better outcomes.

Methods: We collected clinical and MRI data of RRMS patients treated with fingolimod and followed-up for 24 months. The proportion of patients who had NEDA-3 - i.e. absence of relapses, sustained Expanded Disability Status Scale (EDSS) worsening and radiological activity on MRI - was estimated. A Cox proportional hazard model was carried out to investigate which baseline characteristics were associated with the NEDA status at follow-up.

Results: We collected data of 201 patients who started fingolimod. Of them, 24 (12%) were treatment-naïve, 115 (58%) were switched after failing a self-injectable drug, and 60 (30%) switching from natalizumab. Five patients who discontinued fingolimod early (within 3 months) (bradycardia, $n = 2$; leukopaenia, $n = 2$; macular oedema, $n = 1$) were removed from the analysis. At follow-up, 118 (60%) patients achieved the NEDA-3 status, while 78 experienced clinical and/or MRI activity. The risk of not achieving the NEDA-3 status was associated with higher baseline EDSS score (hazard ratio [HR] = 1.18, $p = 0.024$) and more relapses in the 12 months prior to fingolimod start (HR = 1.61, $p = 0.014$).

Conclusion: Our findings suggest that fingolimod may lead to a better control of the disease if started in patients with a less aggressive disease (i.e. fewer pre-treatment relapses and milder disability level), thus supporting its possible role as an early treatment for MS.

Keywords: Multiple sclerosis [190], Clinical outcome measures [40], Therapeutics [360], Fingolimod

Background

Multiple Sclerosis (MS) is a chronic, inflammatory, demyelinating, immune mediate disease of the central nervous system (CNS) that affects almost 2.1 million people worldwide. At least 70–75% of these patients are suffering from the relapsing-remitting type of MS (RRMS) that is characterized by acute inflammatory episodes of CNS demyelination [1]. Relapses may be also

---
* Correspondence: luca.prosperini@uniroma1.it
Department of Neurology and Psychiatry, S. Andrea Hospital Sapienza University, Viale dell'Università 30, 00185 Rome, Italy

associated with disability worsening [2], therefore the main therapeutic aim in RRMS is to control disease activity by reducing the number of relapses and preventing disability progression [3]. Relapses and disability worsening assessed by the Expanded Disability Status Scale (EDSS) [4] are indeed currently accepted as main endpoints in large, phase III, randomized clinical trials [5]. More recently, the No Evidence of Disease Activity (NEDA-3) has been proposed as a new outcome measure for RRMS based on (i) absence of relapses; (ii) absence of sustained disability worsening, defined as ≥1-point increase in EDSS score confirmed 3-6 months apart; (iii) absence of radiological activity, seen on magnetic resonance imaging (MRI) as gadolinium-enhancing lesions or new/enlarged T2-hyperintense lesions [6].

Fingolimod 0.5 mg (Gilenya®, FTY720, Novartis Pharma AG, Basel Switzerland) is a sphingosine-1-phosphate receptor modulator which has been approved as once daily orally administered therapy for RRMS [7]. As evidenced by the phase III trials FREEDOMS, FREEDOMS II and TRANSFORMS, fingolimod significantly reduces relapses rate compared with both placebo and intramuscular Interferon beta (IFNB)-1a [8–10]. Moreover, fingolimod is superior to both placebo and IFNB-1a with regard to MRI-related measures, namely the number of new or enlarged lesions on T2-weighted images, gadolinium-enhancing lesions, and brain-volume loss [7–9]. A post-hoc analysis of the FREEDOMS trial also demonstrated a higher proportion of patients treated with fingolimod achieving the NEDA-3 status than those treated with placebo (33 vs. 13%) [11].

However, real world data on the effectiveness of fingolimod are still scarce and post-marketing studies were mainly designed to either compare fingolimod with other DMTs (self-injectable drugs, natalizumab, dimethyl fumarate) [12–20] or investigate the role of fingolimod as an exit strategy after natalizumab discontinuation [21–27]. Therefore, here we aimed at estimating the proportion of patients achieving the NEDA-3 status in a real-world population. Baseline characteristics associated with a better chance to achieve the NEDA-3 status were also investigated.

Methods

Study design and participants

This was a 24-month, retrospective, independent, single-centre, post-marketing, study. Given its retrospective design, this study in no way interfered in the care received by patients. The present study was conducted in accordance with specific national laws, the International Conference on Harmonization Guidelines of Good Clinical Practice and the ethical standards laid down in the 1964 Declaration of Helsinki and its later amendments.

We collected clinical and MRI data of patients with RRMS according to revised McDonald criteria [28] and starting treatment with fingolimod at the MS Centre of S. Andrea Hospital in Rome according to the Italian regulatory criteria. Only patients having a regular follow-up for at least 24 months from fingolimod start were included in the present study.

Demographic and clinical information were collected at baseline visit (i.e. at fingolimod start) and included sex, time since first symptom, number of exacerbations in the previous year, EDSS score, treatment history,

presence of contrast-enhancing lesions at MRI scan of brain and spinal cord.

Ethical standard

This study was conducted in accordance with the International Conference on Harmonization Guidelines of Good Clinical Practice and the Declaration of Helsinki. In no way did this study interfere in the Care received by patients. The Ethical Committee of Sapienza University provided exemption of approval for post-authorisation observational studies. Each patient involved in this study signed an informed consent before collecting, storing and analysing individual data.

Follow-up assessments

Clinical relapses and changes in EDSS score during treatment, as well as any other medical event occurred as a result of fingolimod treatment, were recorded.

We collected also MRI data after approximately 6, 12, and 24 months of fingolimod treatment, focusing on the presence of gadolinium-enhancing lesions on post-contrast T1-weighted scans and the appearance of new hyperintense lesions on T2-weighted sequences (when compared to the previous scan). Unscheduled MRI scans were also performed, if necessary, to confirm suspect relapses.

To ensure a more reliable comparison between each scan, images were acquired in the same outpatient centre using a superconducting 1.5 T magnet (GE Excite), according to published guidelines [29]. Reproducible slice positioning was maintained throughout the follow-up using the same anatomical landmarks for each patient. All MRI scans were interpreted by experienced radiologists unaware of clinical data.

Outcome measures

As primary outcome, we estimated the proportions of patients who achieved the NEDA-3 status at the end of the 24-month follow-up. As mentioned, NEDA-3 is a combined measure defined as absence of either a clinical relapse, or disability worsening, or radiological activity [6]. The NEDA-3 has been recently proposed as a principal aim in management of relapsing MS because it leads to better long-term outcomes [6–30].

We also analyzed individually the subcomponents of disease activity as secondary outcomes (time to relapse, disability worsening, radiological activity).

A relapse was defined as the appearance or reappearance of one or more symptoms attributable to MS, accompanied by objective deterioration on neurological examination lasting at least 24 h, in the absence of fever and preceded by neurological stability for at least 30 days [28].

Disability worsening was defined as ≥1.5-point increase (if baseline EDSS score was 0), ≥1.0-point increase (if baseline EDSS score was <5.5), or ≥0.5-point increase (if baseline EDSS score was ≥5.5) confirmed 6 months apart [31].

Radiological activity was defined as the occurrence of ≥1 GD-enhancing lesion or ≥1 new T2-hyperintense lesion. We decided to not consider enlarged T2-hyperintense lesions since a previous study demonstrated a poor between-rater agreement for this metric under routine clinical setting [32].

Statistical Analyses

All values are expressed as mean (standard deviation, SD), median (range), or proportion, as appropriate.

We considered the following baseline (i.e. at fingolimod start) characteristics: sex, age, time since first symptom, EDSS score, number of relapses in the previous 12 months, presence of gadolinium-enhancing lesions at brain MRI scan. The multiple sclerosis severity score (MSSS) was also estimated for each participant to obtain a variable accounting for the disease severity [33].

Patients were also divided according to their treatment history as 'treatment-naïve', 'switchers for failure', i.e. switching from self-injectable DMTs, 'switchers for safety', i.e. switching from natalizumab. Between-subgroup differences were tested using the Kruskall-Wallis test and the Chi-squared test for continuous and dichotomous variables, respectively.

A time-to-event multivariable model was performed to investigate which baseline characteristics were associated with NEDA-3 status and its subcomponents at the end of the 24-month follow-up. Specifically, we inserted the counterpart of NEDA-3 (i.e. the occurrence of any evidence of disease activity, such as relapses, disability worsening and/or radiological activity) as dependent variable in a Cox proportional hazards regressions. The aforementioned baseline patients' characteristics and interaction terms were added in the model as independent variables in a stepwise fashion (for predictor inclusion: $F \geq 1$ and $p \leq 0.05$; for exclusion: $F < 1$ and $p > 0.10$). As main time variable we used the length of the observation (in months), between the baseline and the last visit over the 24-months period, or outcome reach, whichever came first.

Patients lost to follow-up and those who discontinued fingolimod within the first three months of treatment were excluded from the main analysis. A post-estimation sensitivity analysis was also done by applying the best-case scenario (i.e. the NEDA-3 status) and worst-case scenario (i.e. any evidence of disease activity due to relapses, and disability worsening and/or radiological activity) to patients who were excluded from the case-base analysis.

All p-values less than 0.05 in either directions were considered as significant. Analyses were carried out using a PC version of Statistical Package for Social Sciences 16.0 (IBM SPSS, Chicago, IL, USA).

Results

Participants

The Table 1 shows the baseline characteristics of patients. We analysed data of 201 patients (141 females, 60 males) with mean (SD) age of 37.9 (9.4), mean time since first symptom of 8.8 (5.9) years, and median EDSS score of 2.0 (range 0–6.5). Twenty-four (12%) patients were treatment-naïve, 117 (58%) were switched after failing a first-line DMT, and 60 (30%) were switched from natalizumab treatment due to safety reasons (i.e. they were tested positive for the John Cunningham virus and then were considered at high risk for developing Progressive Multifocal Leukoencephalopathy). There were significant between-subgroup differences across patients with different treatment history. The time since first symptom was shorter in treatment-naïve patients than in both switchers for failure ($p < 0.05$) and switchers for safety ($p < 0.001$).

The disability level, assessed by EDSS score, was higher in switchers for safety than in both switchers for failure ($p < 0.001$) and treatment-naïve ($p < 0.05$). The number of relapses in previous year was lower in switchers for safety than in both switchers for failure ($p < 0.05$) and treatment-naïve ($p < 0.05$). Sex, age, presence of gadolinium-enhancement at baseline MRI scan did not differ between subgroups defined by treatment history.

Five (2.5%) patients who discontinued fingolimod within 3 months from treatment start were removed from subsequent analyses. They were discontinued early for the following reasons: bradycardia, $n = 2$; leukopaenia, $n = 2$; macular oedema, $n = 1$. There was no patient lost to follow-up.

Study outcomes

The Fig. 1 shows the proportion of patients who achieved the NEDA-3 status at the end of the 24-month follow-up. At follow-up, 118 (60%) patients achieved the NEDA-3 status; 149 (76%) were free from relapses; 168 (86%) were free from disability worsening; 135 (69%) were free from radiological activity.

Among the 78 patients who had any evidence of disease activity, 15 experienced relapses, disability worsening and radiological activity; 23 relapsed with concomitant radiological activity, but without disability worsening; three relapsed with subsequent disability worsening, but without evidence of radiological activity; 1 had MRI activity and subsequent disability worsening, but without any evident clinical exacerbation; the remaining 36 patients had only either relapses ($n = 8$), disability worsening ($n = 8$), or radiological activity ($n = 20$).

Table 1 Baseline characteristics of patients (n = 201)

	Whole sample	Tretament-naive	Switchers for failure	Switchers for safety
N	201	24	117	60
Gender, n (%)				
Female	141 (70)	17 (71)	88 (75)	36 (60)
Male	60 (30)	7 (29)	29 (25)	24 (40)
Age, years				
mean (SD)	37.9 (9.3)	37.2 (8.0)	37.5 (9.9)	39.0 (8.5)
median [range]	38 [18–60]	37 [20–53]	38 [18–60]	39 [18–60]
Time since first symptom, years				*
mean (SD)	8.8 (6.0)	5.1 (5.8)	8.2 (5.8)	11.3 (5.6)
median [range]	8 [<1–23]	2 [<1–18]	7 [1–21]	11 [2–23]
EDSS score				*
mean (SD)	2.7 (1.4)	2.5 (1.0)	2.4 (1.3)	3.4 (1.5)
median [range]	2.0 [0–6.5]	2.0 [0–5.0]	2.0 [1.0–5.5]	3.5 [1.0–6.5]
No. of relapses in previous year				*
mean (SD)	1.1 (0.6)	1.3 (0.5)	1.2 (0.4)	0.9 (0.8)
median [range]	1 [0–3]	1 [1, 2]	1 [1–3]	1 [0-3]
Presence of gadolinium-enhancing lesions, n (%)	125 (62)	17 (71)	78 (67)	30 (50)

*$p < 0.01$ by the Kruskal-Wallis test

Baseline variables associated with NEDA-3 status

Previous treatment history affected the chance of NEDA-3 at follow-up. We found indeed that the proportions of patients reaching the NEDA-3 status were 81% (17/21), 61% (70/115) and 52% (29/60) in treatment-naïves, switchers for failure and switchers for safety, respectively (see Fig. 2). However, only the comparison between treatment-naïve and switchers for safety reached the statistical significance ($p = 0.02$ by the Chi-squared

test), while there was a trend towards statistical significance by comparing treatment-naives and switchers for failure ($p = 0.08$). There was no difference between switchers for failure and switchers for safety ($p = 0.24$).

The Table 2 shows the findings of the Cox proportional hazard model for the NEDA-3 status in the case-

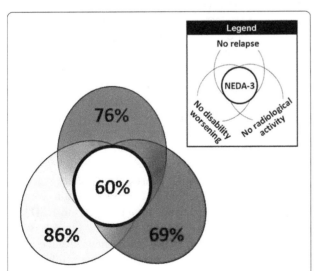

Fig. 1 Description of different components of no evidence of disease activity (NEDA-3) at the end of the 24-month follow-up in 196 patients with relapsing-remitting multiple sclerosis treated with fingolimod

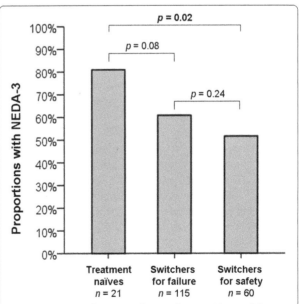

Fig. 2 Proportions of patients achieving the no evidence of disease activity (NEDA-3) at the end of the 24-month follow-up according to previous treatment history (n = 196); statistical comparisons were done by the Chi-squared test

Table 2 Stepwise Cox proportional hazard regression model showing baseline variables associated with evidence of disease activity (NEDA-3) at 24 months after fingolimod start (n = 196)

Independent variables	Hazard Ratio	95% confidence intervals	P-value
Expanded Disability Status Scale (EDSS) score (each step)	1.18	1.02–1.37	0.024
Relapses (each unit)	1.61	1.10–2.35	0.014

Inserted variables that did not contribute to fit the model were as follows: sex, age, time since first symptom, multiple sclerosis severity score (MSSS), presence of gadolinium–enhancing lesions at brain MRI scan.

Hazard ratios >1.0 indicates an increased risk of occurrence of any evidence of disease activity, i.e. relapses, disability worsening and/or radiological activity

base scenario (n = 196). We found an increased risk of not achieving the NEDA-3 status in patients who were more disabled (HR = 1.18, p = 0.024) and in those who experienced more relapses in the 12 months prior to fingolimod start (HR = 1.61, p = 0.014). Previous treatment history did not contribute to fit the model.

The post-estimation sensitivity analysis showed that all these estimates were not altered in the best-case and worst-case scenarios (data not shown).

Discussion

The aim of the present study was two-fold: estimating the proportion of patients achieving the NEDA status in a real-world population taking fingolimod and identifying baseline characteristics associated with a better outcome after 24 months of follow-up.

We found 60% of patients achieving the NEDA-3 status, an almost double proportion with respect to post-hoc analysis (33%) from the FREEDOMS trial [11]. This confirms data from other post-marketing studies showing that the effectiveness of DMTs for MS is often better than their efficacy [34]. A very similar proportion (60%) of patients achieving NEDA-3 was instead reported in a 4.5-year extension phase of TRANSFORMS trial after switching from IFNB-1a to fingolimod [35].

The discrepancy in proportions with NEDA-3 between experimental and real world setting might be explained by the different way to assess relapses, change in disability and radiological activity [5]. Most relapses were assessed retrospectively in our study, while new symptoms must have been coupled with an increase in EDSS score or functional systems to be defined as a qualified relapses in FREDOMS and TRANSFORMS trials [8, 9]. The time required to confirm disability worsening was 6 months in our study versus 3 months in RCTs. Another difference is that we did not consider enlarged T2 lesions in the assessment of MRI activity, since a previous study demonstrated a poor between-rater agreement for this metric under routine clinical setting [32].

As expected, patients switching from natalizumab (switchers for safety) were at higher risk of not achieving the NEDA-3 status [23]. We also found a trend (p = 0.08) towards a worse outcome in patients who switched from self-injectable DMTs (switchers for failure) with respect to treatment-naïve patients, supporting previous suggestions about the role of fingolimod as first treatment option [11, 20].

However, there were relevant baseline differences across subgroups of patients defined by previous treatment history that are known to act as treatment effect modifiers [36]. We found indeed that fingolimod may lead to a better control of the disease if started in patients with a less aggressive disease, i.e. fewer pre-treatment relapses and milder disability level, regardless of previous treatment history.

Our findings are partially in contrast with the subgroup analyses of the FREEDOMS and TRANSFORMS trials, where the pre-treatment number of relapses did not affect the on-treatment annualised relapse rate [37, 38] and patients with EDSS score ≤3.5 did not have a significant reduction in risk of disability progression compared to placebo [37]. Moreover, subgroup analysis of pivotal trials did not reveal any clear advantage for treatment-naïves with respect to previously treated patients, except for a higher relative reduction in relapse rate for treatment-naive rapidly evolving severe RRMS patients (i.e. patients who had ≥2 relapses within the year before baseline and ≥1 gadolinium-enhancing lesion at baseline) [37].

However, these contradictions are attributable to the intrinsic differences between the NEDA-3 status, based on the absolute absence of clinical and radiological activity, and outcomes considered in RCTs, based on quantitative differences in outcomes with respect to placebo or an active comparator [5, 6, 34]. Lastly, we have also to bear in mind that the potential predictors of response to therapy are indeed strictly dependent on the outcome measure considered as criterion of response [39].

Our study suffers from some limitations, mainly due its retrospective design and lack of control group. Despite the adoption of a very stringent outcome such as NEDA-3, we were not able to estimate brain volume loss, thus missing the chance to obtain data on NEDA-4; therefore our data are mainly weighted towards focal inflammatory activity rather than neurodegeneration processes [40]. Another drawback of our study is the short follow-up (24 months); in this regard, further effort is required to determine whether the NEDA-3 status achieved after 24 months of fingolimod may be sustained even in a longer-term follow-up. Long-term data suggest indeed that the NEDA-3 status is difficult to maintain after 7–10 years from starting self-injectable DMTs, while a longer-term disease remission has been described with natalizumab, but with a greater burden in terms of health cost, surveillance, and averse events [30, 41, 42].

Conclusions

Our study suggests that patients with fewer pre-therapy relapses and milder disability level are the best candidates for a more effective treatment with fingolimod. We hope that these findings might contribute to a more accurate identification of patients likely to have the maximum benefit from the fingolimod treatment in real world practice, despite several biases due to the retrospective study design.

Acknowledgements
none.

Funding
This research was carried out using information collected during normal patient care, and extra time spent in data analysis and interpretation was part of educational programmes within the University; no external source of funding was required.

Authors' contributions
MG: acquisition of the data, analysis and interpretation of the clinical data; AL: acquisition of the data, analysis and interpretation of the clinical data; LP: conception and design of the study, analysis and interpretation of the data; drafting a significant portion of the manuscript/figures; MNH: analysis and interpretation of the MRI data; CP: conception and design of the study, drafting a significant portion of the manuscript/figures. All authors read and approved the final manuscript.

Competing interests
The authors declare that they have no competing interests.

Disclosures
LP has received consulting and/or lecture fees and travel grant from Biogen, Genzyme, Novartis and Teva. CP has received consulting and/or lecture fees and/or research funding and travel grant from Almirall, Bayer Schering, Biogen Idec, Genzyme, Merck Serono, Novartis, Roche and Teva. The other Authors have nothing to disclose.

References
1. Pugliatti M. The epidemiology of multiple sclerosis in Europe. Eur J Neurol. 2006;13:700–22.
2. Lublin FD, Baier M, Cutter G. Effect of relapses on development of residual deficit in multiple sclerosis. Neurology. 2003;61:1528–32.
3. Ransohoff RM, Hafler DA, Lucchinetti CF. Multiple sclerosis-a quiet revolution. Nat Rev Neurol. 2015;11(3):134–42.
4. Kurtzke JF. Rating neurological impairment in multiple sclerosis: an expanded disability status scale (EDSS). Neurology. 1983;33:1444–52.
5. Montalban X. Review of methodological issues of clinical trials in multiple sclerosis. J Neurol Sci. 2011;311 Suppl 1:S35–42.
6. Giovannoni G, Turner B, Gnanapavan S, et al. Is it time to target no evident disease activity (NEDA) in multiple sclerosis? Mult Scler Relat Disord. 2015;4:329–33.
7. http://www.ema.europa.eu/docs/en_GB/document_library/EPAR_-_Summary_for_the_public/human/002202/WC500104530.pdf. Accessed 28 Feb 2017.
8. Kappos L, Radue EW, O'Connor P, FREEDOMS Study Group, et al. A placebo-controlled trial of oral fingolimod in relapsing multiple sclerosis. N Engl J Med. 2010;362:387 401.
9. Cohen JA, Barkhof F, Comi G, TRANSFORMS Study Group, et al. Oral fingolimod or intramuscular interferon for relapsing multiple sclerosis. N Engl J Med. 2010;362:402–15.
10. Calabresi PA, Radue EW, Goodin D, et al. Safety and efficacy of fingolimod in patients with relapsing-remitting multiple sclerosis (FREEDOMS II): a double-blind, randomised, placebo-controlled, phase 3 trial. Lancet Neurol. 2014;13:545–56.
11. Nixon R, Bergvall N, Tomic D, et al. No evidence of disease activity: indirect comparisons of oral therapies for the treatment of relapsing– remitting multiple sclerosis. Adv Ther. 2014;31:1134–54.
12. Braune S, Lang M, Bergmann A, NTC Study Group. Second line use of fingolimod is as effective as natalizumab in a German out-patient RRMS-cohort. J Neurol. 2013;260:2981–5.
13. He A, Spelman T, Jokubaitis V, et al. Comparison of switch to fingolimod or interferon beta/glatiramer acetate in active multiple sclerosis. JAMA Neurol. 2015;72:405–13.
14. Kalincik T, Horakova D, Spelman T, et al. Switch to natalizumab versus fingolimod in active relapsing-remitting multiple sclerosis. Ann Neurol. 2015;77:425–35.
15. Barbin L, Rousseau C, Jousset N, et al. Comparative efficacy of fingolimod vs natalizumab: a French multicenter observational study. Neurology. 2016;86:771–8.
16. Baroncini D, Ghezzi A, Annovazzi PO, et al. Natalizumab versus fingolimod in patients with relapsing-remitting multiple sclerosis non-responding to first-line injectable therapies. Mult Scler. 2016;22:1315–26.
17. Braune S, Lang M, Bergmann A, NTC Study Group. Efficacy of fingolimod is superior to injectable disease modifying therapies in second-line therapy of relapsing remitting multiple sclerosis. J Neurol. 2016;263:327–33.
18. Hersh CM, Love TE, Cohn S, Hara-Cleaver C, Bermel RA, Fox RJ, Cohen JA, Ontaneda D. Comparative efficacy and discontinuation of dimethyl fumarate and fingolimod in clinical practice at 12-month follow-up. Mult Scler Relat Disord. 2016;10:44–52.
19. Kalincik T, Brown JW, Robertson N, MSBase Study Group, et al. Treatment effectiveness of alemtuzumab compared with natalizumab, fingolimod, and interferon beta in relapsing-remitting multiple sclerosis: a cohort study. Lancet Neurol. 2017;4422(17):30007–8.
20. Prosperini L, Saccà F, Cordioli C, et al. Real-world effectiveness of natalizumab and fingolimod compared with self-injectable drugs in non-responders and in treatment-naïve patients with multiple sclerosis. J Neurol. 2017;264(2):284–94.
21. Cohen M, Maillart E, Tourbah A, Club Francophone de la Sclérose en Plaques Investigators, et al. Switching from natalizumab to fingolimod in multiple sclerosis: a French prospective study. JAMA Neurol. 2014;71(4):436–41. doi:10.1001/jamaneurol.2013.6240.
22. Jokubaitis VG, Li V, Kalincik T, MSBase Study Group, et al. Fingolimod after natalizumab and the risk of short-term relapse. Neurology. 2014; 82(14):1204–11.
23. Comi G, Gold R, Dahlke F, et al. Relapses in patients treated with fingolimod after previous exposure to natalizumab. Mult Scler. 2015;21(6):786–90.
24. Iaffaldano P, Lucisano G, Pozzilli C, Italian iMed-Web database, et al. Fingolimod versus interferon beta/glatiramer acetate after natalizumab suspension in multiple sclerosis. Brain. 2015;138(Pt11):3275–86.
25. Kappos L, Radue EW, Comi G, TOFINGO study group, et al. Switching from natalizumab to fingolimod: a randomized, placebo-controlled study in RRMS. Neurology. 2015;85(1):29–39.
26. Alping P, Frisell T, Novakova L, Islam-Jakobsson P, Salzer J, Björck A, Axelsson M, Malmeström C, Fink K, Lycke J, Svenningsson A, Piehl F. Rituximab versus fingolimod after natalizumab in multiple sclerosis patients. Ann Neurol. 2016;79(6):950–8. doi:10.1002/ana.24651.
27. Fragoso YD, Alves-Leon SV, Becker J, et al. Safety of switching from natalizumab straight into fingolimod in a group of JCV-positive patients with multiple sclerosis. Arq Neuropsiquiatr. 2016;74:650–52.
28. Polman CH, Reingold SC, Banwell B, et al. Diagnostic criteria for multiple sclerosis: 2010 revisions to the McDonald criteria. Ann Neurol. 2011;69(2):292–302.
29. Filippi M, Rocca MA, Bastianello S, et al. Guidelines from the Italian neurological and Neuroradiological societies for the use of magnetic

resonance imaging in daily life clinical practice of multiple sclerosis patients. Neurol Sci. 2013;34:2085–93.

30. Rotstein DL, Healy BC, Malik MT, et al. Evaluation of no evidence of disease activity in a 7-year longitudinal multiple sclerosis cohort. JAMA Neurol. 2015;72:152–8.

31. Rio J, Nos C, Tintoré M, et al. Defining the response to interferon beta in relapsing-remitting multiple sclerosis patients. Ann Neurol. 2006;59:344–52.

32. Altay EE, Fisher E, Jones SE, et al. Reliability of classifying multiple sclerosis disease activity using magnetic resonance imaging in a multiple sclerosis clinic. JAMA Neurol. 2013;70:338–44.

33. Roxburgh RH, Seaman SR, Masterman T, et al. Multiple sclerosis severity score: using disability and disease duration to rate disease severity. Neurology. 2005;64:1144–51.

34. Trojano M, Tintore M, Montalban X, et al. Treatment decisions in multiple sclerosis - insights from real-world observational studies. Nat Rev Neurol. 2017;13(2):105–18.

35. Cohen JA, Khatri B, Barkhof F, TRANSFORMS Study Group. Long-term (up to 4.5 years) treatment with fingolimod in multiple sclerosis: results from the extension of the randomised TRANSFORMS study. J Neurol Neurosurg Psychiatry. 2016;87(5):468–75.

36. Signori A, Schiavetti I, Gallo F, Sormani MP. Subgroups of multiple sclerosis patients with larger treatment benefits: a meta-analysis of randomized trials. Eur J Neurol. 2015;22:960–6.

37. Devonshire V, Havrdova E, Radue EW, FREEDOMS study group, et al. Relapse and disability outcomes in patients with multiple sclerosis treated with fingolimod: subgroup analyses of the double-blind, randomised, placebo-controlled FREEDOMS study. Lancet Neurol. 2012;11(5):420–8.

38. Cohen JA, Barkhof F, Comi G, et al. Fingolimod versus intramuscular interferon in patient subgroups from TRANSFORMS. J Neurol. 2013;260(8):2023–32.

39. Portaccio E, Zipoli V, Siracusa G, Sorbi S, Amato MP. Response to interferon beta therapy in relapsing-remitting multiple sclerosis: a comparison of different clinical criteria. Mult Scler. 2006;12:281–6.

40. Kappos L, De Stefano N, Freedman MS et al. Inclusion of brain volume loss in a revised measure of 'no evidence of disease activity' (NEDA-4) in relapsing-remitting multiple sclerosis. Mult Scler. 2016;22:1297–05.

41. De Stefano N, Stromillo ML, Giorgio A, et al. Long-term assessment of no evidence of disease activity in relapsing-remitting MS. Neurology. 2015;85:1722–3.

42. Prosperini L, Fanelli F, Pozzilli C. Long-term assessment of No evidence of disease activity with natalizumab in relapsing multiple sclerosis. J Neurol Sci. 2016;364:145–7.

23

Insights on diagnosis and therapeutic decision-making patterns for multiple sclerosis treatment

Katsutoshi Hiramatsu[1*], Masakazu Hase[1] and Hirofumi Ochi[2]

Abstract

Background: There are few reports about the actual state of diagnosis for multiple sclerosis (MS) in Japan. In addition, in late years multiple disease-modifying drugs (DMDs) were released in Japan, but there are few reports of the actual treatment situation including the choice of DMD as well. Therefore, we conducted a questionnaire survey involving neurologists across Japan to investigate the current practices of diagnosing and determining the treatment strategy for MS.

Methods: A case-based survey was conducted among Japanese neurologists currently treating MS patients with DMD to understand the current situation of MS diagnosis and treatment policy determination in Japan. Respondents were divided into tertiles, group 1 (one to three), group 2 (four to nine) and group 3 ($\geq$ ten) by the number of MS patients under management. Results were evaluated as the whole and in each group. Consensus opinion was defined a priori as at least 75% agreement.

Results: Effective responses were obtained from 205 neurologists by web-based survey. 86.3% of the respondents answered that they are able to diagnose MS in accordance with the 2010 revised McDonald criteria for MS. This proportion increased in accordance with the abundance of experience gained treating MS patients (trend test: $p < 0.014$). All the respondents answered that magnetic resonance imaging (MRI) was to be used for all suspected clinical relapse regardless of the presence or absence of new signs on any neurological examinations, and even when no neurological exams were performed, suggesting that they value MRI testing as a key criterion for diagnosing MS regardless of treatment experience. While no consensus was achieved on DMD selection to treat naïve patients with different disease activities, most of the respondents answered to choose either IFNβ products or fingolimod. The neurologists with abundant treatment experience (group 3) would change DMD as the disease activity increased, whereas the less experienced groups (group 1 and 2) replied that they would choose the same DMDs regardless of disease activity level.

Conclusions: The present study shed light on diagnosis and treatment decision-making patterns for MS in Japan.

Keywords: Diagnosis, Disease-modifying drug, Multiple sclerosis, Relapsing-remitting multiple sclerosis, Therapeutic measures

* Correspondence: katsutoshi.hiramatsu@biogen.com
[1]Biogen Japan Ltd., Nihonbashi 1-chome Mistui Building 14F, 4-1, Nihonbashi 1-chome, Chuo-ku, Tokyo 103-0027, Japan
Full list of author information is available at the end of the article

Background

Multiple sclerosis (MS) is an inflammatory demyelinating disease that affects the white matter of the central nervous system. MS is known to be classified into Relapsing-Remitting MS (RRMS) and Primary Progressive MS (PRMS). RRMS is defined as a type of MS in which patients experience relapse and remission over time whereas PRMS is defined as a type of MS in which patients experience gradual and chronic progression of their symptoms from the onset of the disease, which often results in severe disability in patients [1]. In Japan, compared to Western countries, the prevalence of MS is significantly lower, and the current estimated prevalence is 10/100,000 [2, 3]. The advent of disease-modifying drugs (DMDs) has made it possible to prevent relapse and suppress the progression of physical disabilities [4]. The DMDs that have been approved in Japan include subcutaneous interferon beta-1b (IFNβ-1b; approved in 2000), intramuscular interferon beta-1a (IFNβ-1a; 2006), fingolimod (FTY; 2011), natalizumab (NTZ; 2014), glatiramer acetate (GA; 2015), and dimethyl fumarate (DMF; 2016). For diagnosis of MS, the globally accepted diagnostic criteria proposed by McDonald has been widely used [5]. This criteria set, featured by the use of MRI findings for demonstrating the temporal and spacial multiplicity of inflammatory demyelinating lesions in the central nervous system, was first reported in 2001 and subsequently revised, mainly in MRI criteria, in 2005 and 2010 [5–9]. In Japan, an original criteria set is available for diagnosing MS as a designated intractable disease, which includes MRI criteria developed based on the 2010 revised McDonald criteria [10]. Healthcare system of Japan exempts a major financial burden of patients treated with DMDs if they satisfy both diagnostic criteria for MS as a designated intractable disease and other certain conditions. This requires precise understanding of MS diagnostic criteria and diagnosing of MS in accordance with these in physicians treating MS, suggesting a wide acknowledgement of the McDonald criteria. In terms of the selection of DMDs, since few head-to-head clinical trials assessing a prognosis as an endpoint have been conducted, the Treatment Guidelines for Multiple Sclerosis 2010 [9], as well as treatment response, safety, disease severity, and history of DMD use are used as the basis for drug selection.

In this study, we conducted a questionnaire survey involving neurologists across Japan to investigate the current practices of diagnosing and determining the treatment strategy for MS in Japan.

Methods

This was a cross-sectional survey, conducted through the Internet from April 11 to 18, 2016 by M3 Inc. (Tokyo, Japan). M3 Inc. (Tokyo, Japan) conducted the survey using their healthcare professional panel. A total of 3743 registered neurologists were screened in a preliminary survey and 376 (10.0%) of them fully responded, and 269 (7.2%) neurologists who were treating MS patients with DMDs at the time of survey were included in the questionnaire survey. The questionnaire used was basically the Japanese-translated version of the one used in previous studies conducted in the U.S. [11, 12], and it consisted mostly of the same questions as the English version. After responses were collected, de-identified data were provided by M3, Inc. for the analysis, so that no individual responses were known to us or anyone else involved in data analysis or manuscript development.

Consent to the use and publication of survey results was obtained from all respondents along with the completed questionnaires.

Data analysis

Respondents with valid responses to the questionnaire were included in the analysis. The survey results were summarized descriptively, and a response concordance rate of ≥75% was considered to indicate consensus [11, 12]. Respondents were stratified by tertiles of the number of MS patients under care at the time of survey as a measure of recent experience with MS treatment. This measurement was employed because the treatment paradigm of MS in a clinical setting could have been shifted during 2 years before the survey due to the launch of 2 DMDs in Japan; therefore, the current number of MS patients under care could capture an up-to-date MS treatment experience of the respondents. Respondents were classified into groups 1 (1–3 patients); $n = 69$, 2 (4–9); $n = 58$ and 3 (≥10); $n = 78$, and treatment experience with MS was assessed in relation to survey results. Intergroup comparison was performed using the one-way analysis of variance (ANOVA) for continuous variables and the chi-square test for categorical variables. For the intergroup comparison of trend with increasing treatment experience, the Cochran-Armitage test was used for binary variables and the Cochrane-Mantel-Haenszel test for other variables [13]. All tests were exploratory and not adjusted for differences in demographic factors between groups or multiplicity of analysis. All tests were performed at a two-sided significance level of 5% using SAS Release 9.3 (SAS Institute).

Results
Demographics of respondents

Valid responses were obtained from 205 of the 269 neurologists to whom the questionnaire was sent, yielding a response rate of 76.2%. The demographics of the 205 respondents are summarized in Table 1. The mean number of MS patients under care was 8.78, with 70.3% of the respondents having more than 10 years of

Table 1 Respondent characteristics

Characteristics	Overall (n = 205)	Sub-group by number of MS patients under care			P value[‡]
		Group 1: 1–3 patients (n = 69)	Group 2: 4–9 patients (n = 58)	Group 3: ≥10 patients (n = 78)	
Age, n (%)					
20s	4 (2.0)	3 (4.3)	0 (0.0)	1 (1.3)	0.197
30s	65 (31.7)	25 (36.2)	17 (29.3)	23 (29.5)	
40s	80 (39.0)	25 (36.2)	24 (41.4)	31 (39.7)	
50s	45 (22.0)	13 (18.8)	13 (22.4)	19 (24.4)	
≥ 60s	11 (5.4)	3 (4.3)	4 (6.9)	4 (5.1)	
Number of MS patients under care, mean ± SD, (min–max)	8.78 ± 8.92 (1–50)	2.35 ± 0.78	5.14 ± 1.03	17.17 ± 9.54	< 0.001[*]
Approximate percentages of patients with MS under care, mean ± SD, (min–max)	6.56 ± 7.64 (1–60)	3.14 ± 2.63 (1–10)	5.41 ± 7.41 (1–50)	10.44 ± 9.01 (1–60)	< 0.001[*]
Years of post-residency treatment experience with MS, n (%)					
< 3 years	8 (3.9)	4 (5.8)	2 (3.4)	2 (2.6)	0.009
3–5 years	16 (7.8)	9 (13.0)	2 (3.4)	5 (6.4)	
6–10 years	37 (18.0)	14 (20.3)	12 (20.7)	11 (14.1)	
11–15 years	51 (24.9)	18 (26.1)	14 (24.1)	19 (24.4)	
16–20 years	40 (19.5)	11 (15.9)	14 (24.1)	15 (19.2)	
> 20 years	53 (25.9)	13 (18.8)	14 (24.1)	26 (33.3)	
Affiliation, n (%)					
University hospitals	60 (29.3)	19 (27.5)	8 (13.8)	33 (42.3)	0.019
National/public hospitals	58 (28.3)	18 (26.1)	20 (34.5)	20 (25.6)	
Hospitals in general	79 (38.5)	28 (40.6)	27 (46.6)	24 (30.8)	
Private practice	8 (3.9)	4 (5.8)	3 (5.2)	1 (1.3)	
Membership in professional association[†], n (%)					
Japanese Society of Neurology	204 (99.5)	68 (98.6)	58 (100.0)	78 (100.0)	0.217
Japanese Society for Neuroimmunology	36 (17.6)	10 (14.5)	7 (12.1)	19 (24.4)	0.108
Japanese Society of Neurological Therapeutics	87 (42.4)	18 (26.1)	27 (46.6)	42 (53.8)	0.001
DMDs that had been prescribed in practice[†], n (%)					
SC IFNβ-1b	199 (97.1)	63 (91.3)	58 (100.0)	78 (100.0)	0.002
IM IFNβ-1a	180 (87.8)	60 (87.0)	47 (81.0)	73 (93.6)	0.199
Fingolimod	171 (83.4)	50 (72.5)	47 (81.0)	74 (94.9)	< 0.001
Natalizumab	32 (15.6)	8 (11.6)	3 (5.2)	21 (26.9)	0.009
Glatiramer acetate	36 (17.6)	13 (18.8)	6 (10.3)	17 (21.8)	0.600
Other	5 (2.4)	2 (2.9)	1 (1.7)	2 (2.6)	0.907

MS multiple sclerosis, SD standard deviation, min minimum, max maximum, DMD disease-modifying drug, SC IFNβ-1b subcutaneous interferon beta-1b, IM IFNβ-1a intramuscular interferon beta-1a
[†]Percentages do not sum up to 100% due to multiple responses
[‡]Percentages were compared between the groups: no mark indicates P values for chi-square tests, and an asterisk (*) indicates P values for one-way ANOVA

experience with MS treatment. The most common affiliation was hospitals in general (38.5%), although there was a significant difference in the distribution of affiliations among 3 groups, with hospitals in general being the most common in group 1 (40.6%) and group 2 (46.6%) while university hospitals being the most common in group 3 (42.3%) (p = 0.019). The percentages of respondents who have prescribed NTZ or GA, DMDs launched in 2014 or after, were low at 15.6 and 17.6%, respectively, whereas those of respondents who have prescribed subcutaneous IFNβ-1b, intramuscular IFNβ-1a and FTY were high at 97.1, 87.8 and 83.4%, respectively. The percentages of respondents who have prescribed FTY and NTZ were the highest in group 3 (94.9 and 26.9%, respectively), with significant differences among 3 groups (FTY: $p < 0.001$, NTZ: $p = 0.009$).

Diagnosis of relapsing remitting MS (RRMS) based on McDonald criteria

To determine the acknowledgement of the 2010 revised McDonald diagnostic criteria, we used a question "Can dissemination in time and space be determined for the purpose of diagnosing relapsing remitting MS (RRMS) in the presence of 1 clinical attack with a single MRI scan?" (Table 2). To this question, 86.3% of the respondents answered "yes", indicating that the 2010 revised McDonald diagnostic criteria are used as the consensus criteria. The percentage of respondents answering "yes" also significantly increased with increasing number of patients under care (trend test $p = 0.014$).

Determination of clinical relapse and use of MRI scan

The survey results on the determination of clinical relapse and use of MRI scan are summarized in Table 3. There was consensus in diagnosing clinical relapse based on "new/worsening symptoms lasting ≥24 hours in the absence of comorbidities, such as acute infection" and "worsening neurological exam" (98.0%). In contrast, "new/worsening symptoms lasting ≥24 hours" was not a consensus criterion for diagnosing clinical relapse if either "no neurological exam was performed" or "no change in neurological exam" applied (47.8 and 51.7%, respectively). We then asked the question "In a patient presenting with a clinical relapse based on your definition of a relapse, do you usually order an MRI scan?" To this question, all respondents answered "yes". In addition, 63.4% of respondents answered yes to the question "Does the appearance of new asymptomatic MRI activity constitute the equivalent of a clinical relapse?", although consensus was not achieved. No significant intergroup difference was observed in any of these questions.

Timing of starting DMD treatment and timing of MRI scan after start of DMD treatment

We presented case scenarios 1, 2 and 3 where untreated patients have different levels of disease activity (the lowest in case 1 and the highest in case 3) and investigated when physicians decide to start treatment in case scenarios 1 and 2 (Table 4). There was consensus in starting DMD treatment in both case scenarios (91.2 and 96.6%, respectively). Performing follow-up MRI scans within 6 months after the start of DMD treatment in cases 1 and 3 also reached consensus (85.6 and 88.3%, respectively).

Relationship between the number of clinical relapses or new MRI lesions after start of DMD treatment and switching of DMDs

The question "Assuming a patient is currently receiving treatment, what is the minimum number of clinical relapses over 6 months or 12 months that would prompt you to suggest a change in DMD?" was asked (Table 5). There was consensus in considering switching from one DMD to another after 1 to 2 clinical relapses either within 6 or 12 months after the start of treatment (96.5 and 77.1%, respectively). There was no significant difference among groups in all cases. In the next question, we assumed 2 case scenarios, where a patient has been receiving the same treatment for 2 years, and no changes in MRI were observed on scans after 1 year of treatment, but activity was observed on a routine MRI performed after 2 years of treatment (case 1), or no changes in MRI were observed on scans at 1 and 2 years, but activity was observed on a routine MRI performed after 3 years of treatment (case 2), and asked "what is the lowest number of new T2 or gadolinium-enhanced (Gd+) lesions that would prompt you to suggest a change in DMD?" (Table 5). In terms of the number of new T2 lesions, the most frequent answer was "2" or "3–4" in both cases (32.7 and 33.2% in case 1; 33.7 and 31.2% in case 2, respectively). In terms of the number of new Gd + lesions, the most frequent answer was "1" followed by "2" in both cases (47.3 and 34.6% in case 1; 46.3 and 30.7% in case 2, respectively). Thus,

Table 2 Diagnosis of RRMS based on the McDonald criteria

| Question and answer | Overall (n = 205) | Sub-group by the number of MS patients under care | | | P value | |
		Group 1: 1–3 patients (n = 69)	Group 2: 4–9 patients (n = 58)	Group 3: ≥10 patients (n = 78)	Group comparison[*]	Trend test[†]
Question: Can dissemination in time and space be determined for the purpose of diagnosing RRMS in the presence of 1 clinical attack with a single MRI scan?						
Yes, n (%)	177 (86.3)	54 (78.3)	51 (87.9)	72 (92.3)	0.152[a] 0.015[b] 0.391[c]	0.014

RRMS relapsing remitting multiple sclerosis, MS multiple sclerosis, MRI magnetic resonance imaging
[*]Percentages were compared in groups of two using the chi-square test, and the corresponding P values are indicated for the following comparisons: a: Group 1 vs. Group 2, b: Group 1 vs. Group 3, c: Group 2 vs. Group 3
[†]The trend across the three groups was tested using the Cochran-Armitage test

Table 3 Criteria for a clinical relapse and application of MRI for judgement for a relapse

Questions and answers	Overall (n = 205)	Sub-group by the number of MS patients under care			P value	
		Group 1: 1–3 patients (n = 69)	Group 2: 4–9 patients (n = 58)	Group 3: ≥10 patients (n = 78)	Group comparison*	Trend test†
Question 1: Do any of the following constitute a clinical relapse in your practice (in the absence of comorbidities, such as acute infection)?						
a. New/worsening symptoms lasting > 24 h, no neurological exam performed, n (%)	98 (47.8)	29 (42.0)	31 (53.4)	38 (48.7)	0.199[a] 0.416[b] 0.585[c]	0.437
b. New/worsening symptoms lasting > 24 h, no change in neurological exam, n (%)	106 (51.7)	29 (42.0)	34 (58.6)	43 (55.1)	0.063[a] 0.113[b] 0.684[c]	0.122
c. New/worsening symptoms lasting > 24 h and worsening neurological exam, n (%)	201 (98.0)	67 (97.1)	57 (98.3)	77 (98.7)	0.664[a] 0.489[b] 0.832[c]	0.483
Question 2: In a patient presenting with a clinical relapse based on your definition of a relapse, do you usually order an MRI scan?						
Yes, n (%)	205 (100.0)	69 (100.0)	58 (100.0)	78 (100.0)	–	–
Question 3: Does the appearance of new asymptomatic MRI activity constitute the equivalent of a clinical relapse?						
Yes, n (%)	130 (63.4)	43 (62.3)	38 (65.5)	49 (62.8)	0.709[a] 0.950[b] 0.746[c]	0.960

MRI magnetic resonance imaging, *MS* multiple sclerosis
*Percentages were compared between two groups using the chi-square test, and the corresponding P values are indicated for the following comparisons: a: Group 1 vs. Group 2, b: Group 1 vs. Group 3, c: Group 2 vs. Group 3
†The trend across the three groups was tested using the Cochran-Armitage test

there was consensus in considering change of DMDs after 1–2 new Gd + lesions were detected. No significant difference was observed among groups.

Selection of DMDs at start of treatment

The selection of DMDs at the start of treatment in cases 1 to 3 was asked as shown in Table 4 to investigate the relationship between disease activity and DMD selection (Fig. 1). In all cases, most of the respondents answered to choose IFNβ products or FTY (IFNβ: 70.0% in case 1, 64.7% in case 2 and 54.7% in case 3, FTY: 25.1, 27.3 and 37.1%). At the same time, increasing disease activity was associated with decreasing prescription of IFNβ and increasing prescription of FTY. This trend was especially evident in group 3. The percentage of respondents choosing IFNβ products decreased from 77.5% in case 1 to 61.8% in case 2 and then to 48.7% in case 3 while that for FTY increased from 19.7 to 31.6% and then to 48.7%. In groups 1 and 2, no substantial difference was observed in DMD selections according to disease activity. The percentages of respondents choosing FTY in case 3 were 30.4, 29.3 and 48.7% in groups 1, 2 and 3, respectively, being the highest in group 3. This indicates that respondents with greater treatment experience tend to take disease activity into consideration when choosing DMDs. As for DMDs launched in 2014 or after, the percentage of respondents choosing GA decreased with increasing disease activity from 2.7 to 2.0% and then to 1.0% while that for NTZ increased from 1.6 to 3.0% and then to 5.4% in cases negative for anti-JCV antibody.

Switching of DMDs

A question on switching of DMDs in cases of suboptimal response to current DMDs was asked. Respondents were allowed to select DMDs they have not used or those that have not been adopted at the affiliating institution. The results are summarized in Table 6. Non-FTY DMDs were most frequently switched to FTY, while FTY was most frequently switched to NTZ regardless of anti-JCV antibody status. The percentage of respondents switching from other DMDs to NTZ was higher in cases negative for anti-JCV antibody compared to when the anti-JCV antibody status was not taken into account (3.9% vs. 7.8, 6.3% vs. 10.2, 52.2% vs. 56.6, and 21.0% vs. 25.4%, respectively).

Discussion

The results of the present survey study partially revealed the current practices of diagnosing and determining the treatment strategy for MS in Japan. In this section, we discuss the following four aspects:

Acknowledgements of the 2010 revised McDonald diagnostic criteria

There is consensus that RRMS can be diagnosed based on the 2010 revised McDonald criteria [7] and the percentage in favor of this notion significantly increased with increasing number of patients under care. A high accordance with the criteria was expected prior to this study because our original criteria for diagnosing MS as a designated intractable disease had been constructed based on the 2010 revised McDonald criteria [7]. Patients who are diagnosed

Table 4 Timing for initiation of DMD treatment and follow-up MRI for the case scenarios

Case scenario, questions and answers	Overall (n = 205)	Sub-group by the number of MS patients under care			P value	
		Group 1: 1–3 patients (n = 69)	Group 2: 4–9 patients (n = 58)	Group 3: ≥10 patients (n = 78)	Group comparison[*,†]	Trend test[‡]

Case 1: A 25-year-old man with RRMS and 2 clinical relapses in the last 4 years is treatment naïve and presents with a normal neurologic exam. A recent MRI reveals 5 non-enhancing T2 lesions in the brain.

Question 1: Would you initiate DMD[#] treatment?

| Yes, n (%) | 187 (91.2) | 63 (91.3) | 53 (91.4) | 71 (91.0) | 0.988[a] 0.953[b] 0.943[c] | 0.951 |

Question 2: If you answered yes in Question 1, when would you perform the follow-up MRI?

Follow-up timing, n/187 (%) [§]

≤ 3 months	62 (33.2)	22 (34.9)	17 (32.7)	23 (32.4)	0.480[a] 0.331[b] 0.197[c]	0.657
> 3– ≤6 months	98 (52.4)	31 (49.2)	25 (48.1)	42 (59.2)		
> 6– ≤12 months	24 (12.8)	10 (15.9)	8 (15.1)	6 (8.5)		
> 12 months	2 (1.1)	0 (0.0)	2 (3.8)	0 (0.0)		

Case 2: Assume that you are presented with the Case 1 patient with RRMS who remains as treatment naïve and has had 2 clinical relapses in close proximity (last 6 months) that have left him with a residual disability. MRI reveals multiple, extensive, non-enhancing T2 lesions in the brain, brainstem, and spinal cord.

Question 3: Would you initiate DMD[#] treatment?

| Yes, n (%) | 198 (96.6) | 65 (94.2) | 57 (98.3) | 76 (97.4) | 0.240[a] 0.323[b] 0.742[c] | 0.294 |

Case 3: Assume that you are presented with the Case 1 patient with RRMS who remains as treatment naïve and has had 2 clinical relapses in close proximity (last 6 months) that have left him with residual disability. MRI shows multiple, extensive, non-enhancing T2 lesions in the brain, brainstem, and spinal cord; multiple T1 hypointense lesions; and brain atrophy.

Question 4: Following initiation of therapy, when would you perform a follow-up MRI?

Follow-up timing, n/205 (%)

≤ 3 months	95 (46.3)	36 (52.2)	24 (41.4)	35 (44.9)	0.200[a] 0.626[b] 0.411[c]	0.400
> 3– ≤6 months	86 (42.0)	28 (40.6)	23 (39.7)	35 (44.9)		
> 6– ≤12 months	23 (11.2)	5 (7.2)	10 (17.2)	8 (10.3)		
> 12 months	1 (0.5)	0 (0.0)	1 (1.7)	0 (0.0)		

DMD disease-modifying drug, *DMT* disease-modifying therapy, *MRI* magnetic resonance imaging, *MS* multiple sclerosis, *RRMS* relapsing-remitting multiple sclerosis, *SC IFNβ-1b* subcutaneous interferon beta-1b, *IM IFNβ-1a* intramuscular interferon beta-1a, *JCV* John Cunningham virus
[*]Percentages were compared in groups of two using the chi-square test, and the corresponding p-values are indicated for the following comparisons: a: Group 1 vs. Group 2, b: Group 1 vs. Group 3, c: Group 2 vs. Group 3
[†]The distributions of selected DMDs were compared among the three groups using the chi-square test
[‡]The trend across the three groups was tested using the Cochran-Armitage test for a binominal response or Cochrane-Mantel-Haenszel test for a multiple response
[#]In the actual question, the term DMT was used instead of DMD added supplementary explanation which means DMD
[§]Responses of only those who reported that they would initiate DMD for each case were calculated

with MS based on the original criteria and satisfy certain conditions are eligible for an application to publicly subsidized medical care. This high accordance with the 2010 revised McDonald diagnostic criteria could have been boosted by the health care system in Japan.

Determination of relapse and use of MRI scan
In the presence of new/worsening symptoms lasting ≥24 h, only about 50% of respondents diagnosed clinical relapse if no neurological examination was performed or no worsening in neurological examination was noted, whereas 98% of respondents diagnosed relapse if worsening of neurological examination was noted, suggesting that worsening of neurological examination is a key

criterion for diagnosing clinical relapse. Furthermore, 63% of respondents acknowledges that the appearance of new asymptomatic MRI activity represents clinical relapse. The fact that even with clinical evidence of relapse, all respondents performed MRI scan as a key criterion for diagnosing relapse suggests that MRI scan is considered an important modality for determining relapse, regardless of treatment experience.

Timing of starting DMD treatment in untreated patients and selection of DMDs
In the questions about the timing of starting DMD treatment, more than 90% of respondents in all groups answered that they would start treatment in case scenarios

Table 5 Change criteria of DMD by the number of relapses and lesions by case scenarios

Case scenario, questions and answers	Overall (n = 205)	Sub-group by number of MS patients under care			P value	
		Group 1: 1–3 patients (n = 69)	Group 2: 4–9 patients (n = 58)	Group 3: ≥10 patients (n = 78)	Group comparison[*]	Trend test[†]
Question 1: Assuming a patient is currently receiving treatment, what is the minimum number of clinical relapses over 6 months or 12 months that would prompt you to suggest a change in DMD[‡]?						
Number of relapses over 6 months, n (%)						
1 clinical relapse	120 (58.5)	38 (55.1)	34 (58.6)	48 (61.5)	0.799[a]	0.238
2 clinical relapses	78 (38.0)	27 (39.1)	22 (37.9)	29 (37.2)	0.288[b]	
3 clinical relapses	7 (3.4)	4 (5.8)	2 (3.4)	1 (1.3)	0.684[c]	
≥ 4 clinical relapses	0 (0.0)	0 (0.0)	0 (0.0)	0 (0.0)		
Number of relapses over 12 months, n (%)						
1 clinical relapse	56 (27.3)	13 (18.8)	21 (36.2)	22 (28.2)	0.175[a]	0.308
2 clinical relapses	102 (49.8)	39 (56.5)	25 (43.1)	38 (48.7)	0.454[b]	
3 clinical relapses	36 (17.6)	12 (17.4)	9 (15.5)	15 (19.2)	0.731[c]	
≥ 4 clinical relapses	11 (5.4)	5 (7.2)	3 (5.2)	3 (3.8)		
Case 1: Assuming a patient with clinically stable RRMS has been receiving the same treatment for 2 years, and no changes in MRI were seen on scans after 1 year of therapy, but activity was seen on a routine MRI performed after 2 years of treatment.						
Question 2: What is the lowest number of new T2 or Gd + lesions that would prompt you to suggest a change in DMD[‡]?						
Number of T2 lesions, n (%)						
1 T2 lesion	30 (14.6)	7 (11.9)	14 (28.0)	9 (13.2)	0.006[a]	0.987
2 T2 lesions	67 (32.7)	27 (45.8)	10 (20.0)	30 (44.1)	0.985[b]	
3–4 T2 lesions	68 (33.2)	23 (39.0)	19 (38.0)	26 (38.2)	0.010[c]	
≥ 5 T2 lesions	12 (5.9)	2 (3.4)	7 (14.0)	3 (4.4)		
Number of Gd + lesion, n (%)						
1 Gd + lesion	97 (47.3)	29 (45.3)	30 (58.8)	38 (52.8)	0.318[a]	0.267
2 Gd + lesions	71 (34.6)	27 (42.2)	15 (29.4)	29 (40.3)	0.471[b]	
≥ 3 Gd + lesions	19 (9.3)	8 (12.5)	6 (11.8)	5 (6.9)	0.376[c]	
Case 2: Assuming a patient with clinically stable RRMS has been receiving the same treatment for 2 years, and no changes in MRI were seen on scans at 1 and 2 years.						
Question 3: What is the lowest number of new T2 or Gd + lesions on a subsequent routine MRI that would prompt you to suggest a change in DMD[‡]?						
Number of T2 lesions, n (%)						
1 T2 lesion	23 (11.2)	5 (8.6)	11 (22.4)	7 (10.0)	0.118[a]	0.888
2 T2 lesions	69 (33.7)	25 (43.1)	14 (28.6)	30 (42.9)	0.841[b]	
3–4 T2 lesions	64 (31.2)	23 (39.7)	17 (34.7)	24 (34.3)	0.205[c]	
≥ 5 T2 lesions	21 (10.2)	5 (8.6)	7 (14.3)	9 (12.9)		
Number of Gd + lesion, n (%)						
1 Gd + lesion	95 (46.3)	27 (42.9)	29 (56.9)	39 (54.2)	0.224[a]	0.082
2 Gd + lesions	63 (30.7)	22 (34.9)	16 (31.4)	25 (34.7)	0.180[b]	
≥ 3 Gd + lesions	28 (13.7)	14 (22.2)	6 (11.8)	8 (11.1)	0.927[c]	

DMD disease-modifying drug, *DMT* disease-modifying therapy, *MS* multiple sclerosis, *RRMS* relapsing-remitting multiple sclerosis, *MRI* magnetic resonance imaging, *Gd +* gadolinium enhancement

[*]Percentages were compared between two groups using the chi-square test, and the corresponding P values are indicated for the following comparisons: a: Group 1 vs. Group 2, b: Group 1 vs. Group 3, c: Group 2 vs. Group 3

[†]A trend across three groups was tested using the Cochrane-Mantel-Haenszel test

[‡]In the actual question, the term DMT was used instead of DMD added supplementary explanation which means DMD

1 and 2, indicating consensus about the need for early treatment, regardless of treatment experience (Table 5). For treatment of untreated patients, most of the respondents chose IFNβ products or FTY, although increasing disease activity was associated with decreasing prescription of IFNβ products and increasing prescription

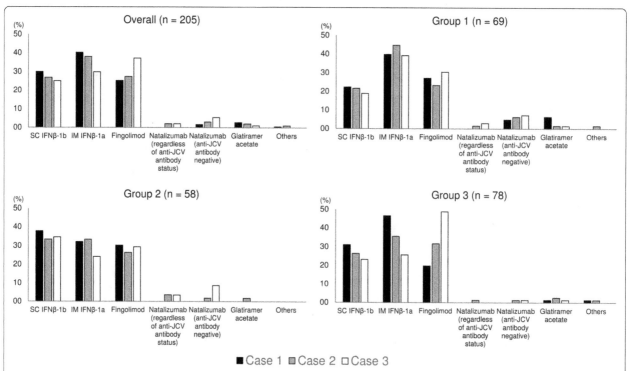

Fig. 1 Choice of initial treatment in patients with RRMS by case scenarios. Note: Responses of only those who reported that they would initiate DMD for each case were calculated. Case scenarios are shown in Table 5. Group 1: 1–3 MS patients under care, Group 2: 4–9 MS patients under care, Group 3: ≥10 MS patients under care. RRMS: relapsing-remitting multiple sclerosis, MS: multiple sclerosis, DMD: disease-modifying drug, SC IFNβ-1b: subcutaneous interferon beta-1b, IM IFNβ-1a: intramuscular interferon beta-1, JCV: John Cunningham virus

of FTY. This trend was especially evident in group 3, while in groups 1 and 2, the same DMDs tended to be selected independent of disease activity, suggesting that physicians with greater treatment experience tend to choose DMDs according to disease activity. A previous study conducted in the U.S. in 2011 showed that increasing disease activity was associated with increased variability of prescribed DMDs; in particular, the prescription rate of NTZ, a relatively potent DMD, increased substantially (case 2: 32%, case 3: 39%) while that of FTY increased minimally (case 2: 1%, case 3: 4%) [11]. In follow-up study conducted in 2014, if the anti-JCV antibody was negative, 89% of respondents answered that NTZ was selected for Case 3 (36.6% in the case of anti-JCV antibody positive) [12]. The reasons of this discrepancy between Japan and the U.S. were considered as follows; differential demographics of respondents, where U.S. respondents were board-certified specialists in MS treatment who were treating up to 900 MS patients on average, compared with an approximate average of 9 patients treated by the respondents of our survey, the wide acceptance to use drugs with higher efficacy for patients with short MS history among MS specialists in the U.S. [11, 12], earlier launch of NTZ than FTY in the U.S., and higher prevalence of anti-JCV antibody in the Japanese population compared to the Western population [14–19].

Switch of DMDs

There was consensus that 1–2 clinical relapses over 6 months of treatment with a DMD would lead to switching from one DMD to another (96.6%). However, no consensus was achieved regarding the minimum number of clinical relapses over 1 year that would lead to treatment switch, suggesting a lack of sufficient information to determine the timing of treatment switch. The strategy for switching treatment due to suboptimal response to the current treatment was not affected by the anti-JCV antibody status, with the most common pattern being from a non-FTY DMD to FTY and from FTY to NTZ. A U.S. study conducted in 2014 showed with switching to oral drugs being the most common either from injectables (GA, IFNβ; 83.8%), oral drugs (DMF, FTY, teriflunomide; 75.5%) or IV infusion (NTZ; 89.9%) in cases positive for anti-JCV antibody [12]. In contrast, in cases negative for anti-JCV antibody, the most common patterns were switching to NTZ from injectables (46.0%) or oral drugs (69.2%) and switching to oral drugs from NTZ (83.2%) [12]. From these results of Japan and the U.S. study, it is considered that Japanese neurologists and U.S. specialists were practically choosing DMDs according to disease activity taking into account the risk of progressive multifocal leukoencephalopathy at the time of switching in the case of anti-JCV

Table 6 DMD choice following suboptimal response to original treatment by anti-JCV antibody status (n = 205)

n (%)

| | | Preferred replacing DMD | | | | | | | | | | | |
| | | Regardless of anti-JCV antibody status | | | | | | Anti-JCV antibody negative | | | | | |
		SC IFNβ-1b	IM IFNβ-1a	Fingolimod	Natalizumab	Glatirameracetate	Other	SC IFNβ-1b	IM IFNβ-1a	Fingolimod	Natalizumab	Glatirameracetate	Other
Current DMD	SC IFNβ-1b	–	65 (31.7)	119 (58.1)	8 (3.9)	13 (6.3)	0 (0.0)	–	67 (32.7)	110 (53.7)	16 (7.8)	12 (5.9)	0 (0.0)
	IM IFNβ-1a	32 (15.6)	–	149 (72.7)	13 (6.3)	11 (5.4)	0 (0.0)	34 (16.6)	–	133 (64.9)	21 (10.2)	15 (7.3)	2 (1.0)
	Fingolimod	28 (13.7)	39 (19.0)	–	107 (52.2)	29 (14.2)	2 (1.0)	29 (14.2)	35 (17.1)	–	116 (56.6)	23 (11.2)	2 (1.0)
	Natalizumab	20 (9.8)	18 (8.8)	90 (43.9)	–	59 (28.8)	18 (8.8)	18 (8.8)	17 (8.3)	105 (51.2)	–	52 (25.4)	13 (6.3)
	Glatiramer acetate	30 (14.6)	34 (16.6)	85 (41.5)	43 (21.0)	–	13 (6.3)	26 (12.7)	30 (14.6)	88 (42.9)	52 (25.4)	–	9 (4.4)

DMD disease-modifying drug, JCV John Cunningham virus, SC IFNβ-1b subcutaneous interferon beta-1b, IM IFNβ-1a intramuscular interferon beta-1a antibody positive. However, in the case of anti-JCV antibody negative, it became clear that in the United States, drugs that strongly suppress disease activity are preferred to prescribe.

Limitations of the study

There is a sampling bias in this study. First, the number of neurologists in Japan in 2016 when the present survey conducted was 4657 [20], but the present survey was conducted using a panel of 3743 neurologists. Second, only 376 neurologists from the panel responded. Third, responders might be in a biased population consisting mainly of those interested in collecting medical information from the Internet. Lastly, the population may also be biased in that the number of MS patients under care by the respondents ranged from 1 to 50 and there was no specialist treating a larger number of patients. In Japan, however, MS specialists providing more than 50 patients with treatment is extremely limited, unlike in North America, because of the significantly lower prevalence of MS in Japan [2, 3]. Members ($n = 36$) of the Japanese Society for Neuroimmunology could be regarded as MS specialists in Japan, because the society is focusing on MS and several intractable neurologic diseases. Therefore, we think most of the responders were typical MS neurologists in Japan in terms of the number of MS patients under care. The results should therefore be interpreted with caution, but at least, this study partially revealed the current diagnosis and therapeutic decision-making patterns for multiple sclerosis treatment in Japan and should provide some insights considering the scarcity of reports so far.

Conclusion

This survey study is meaningful in that it collected opinions from 205 neurologists engaged in MS treatment throughout Japan. This study revealed that Japanese neurologists consider both the 2010 revised McDonald diagnostic criteria and MRI scan indispensable for MS diagnosis and determination of relapse, regardless of treatment experience. Conversely, physicians with greater treatment experience tend to choose DMDs according to disease activity. Because the population includes neurologists with various levels of experience, the results are likely to reflect the current clinical practice for MS patients in Japan.

This study will contribute to improved clinical practice for MS patients in Japan by revealing some aspects of the current practice.

Abbreviations

ANOVA: analysis of variance; DMD: disease-modifying drug; DMF: dimethyl fumarate; FTY: fingolimod; GA: glatiramer acetate; IFNβ: interferon beta; MS: multiple sclerosis; NTZ: natalizumab; RRMS: relapsing remitting multiple sclerosis

Acknowledgments

We would like to express our gratitude to all neurologists participating in this survey. We would like to thank Ms. Mika Kawaguchi and Mr. Norimasa Kikuchi of Clinical Study Support, Inc. (Nagoya, Japan) for preparing the draft manuscript, editing the manuscript and performing part of the analysis as directed by the authors. We would also like to thank Mr. Takamine Mochida of Kantar Japan (Tokyo, Japan) for their assistance in conducting the survey and other analyses.

Funding

The funds for the survey, analysis and manuscript writing were provided by Biogen Japan Ltd.

Authors' contributions

KH and MH conceptualized and designed the study. KH, MH, and HO interpreted results of data analysis. KH drafted the manuscript, and MH and HO revised it critically for important intellectual content. All authors read and approved the final manuscript.

Competing interests

Katsutoshi Hiramatsu is an employee of Biogen Japan Ltd. and receives salaries from the company and possess the company's stocks. Masakazu Hase was an employee of Biogen Japan Ltd., and received salaries from the company and possessed the company's stocks at the time of this study conducted. Hirofumi Ochi has no conflict of interest with any company, organization or group to be disclosed in relation to this study.

Author details

[1]Biogen Japan Ltd., Nihonbashi 1-chome Mistui Building 14F, 4-1, Nihonbashi 1-chome, Chuo-ku, Tokyo 103-0027, Japan. [2]Department of Geriatric Medicine and Neurology, Ehime University Graduate School of Medicine, 10-13 Dogo-Himata, Matsuyama, Ehime 790-8577, Japan.

References

1. Lublin FD, Reingold SC, Cohen JA, et al. Defining the clinical course of multiple sclerosis: the 2013 revisions. Neurology. 2014;83:278–86.
2. Houzen H, Niino M, Hirotani M, Fukazawa T, Kikuchi S, Tanaka K, Sasaki H. Increased prevalence, incidence, and female predominance of multiple sclerosis in northern Japan. J Neurol Sci. 2012;323(1–2):117–22.
3. Osoegawa M, Kira J, Fukazawa T, Fujihara K, Kikuchi S, Matsui M, Kohriyama T, Sobue G, Yamamura T, Itoyama Y, et al. Temporal changes and geographical differences in multiple sclerosis phenotypes in Japanese: nationwide survey results over 30 years. Mult Scler. 2009;15(2):159–73.
4. Ochi H. Emerging new disease-modifying drugs for multiple sclerosis. Saishin-Igaku, vol. 71; 2016. p. 1149–58. [in Japanese]
5. McDonald WI, Compston A, Edan G, Goodkin D, Hartung HP, Lublin FD, et al. Recommended diagnostic criteria for multiple sclerosis: guidelines from the international panel on the diagnosis of multiple sclerosis. Ann Neurol. 2001;50:121–7.
6. Polman CH, Reingold SC, Edan G, Filippi M, Hartung HP, Kappos L, et al. Diagnostic criteria for multiple sclerosis: 2005 revisions to the "McDonald criteria". Ann Neurol. 2005;58:840–6.
7. Polman CH, Reingold SC, Banwell B, Clanet M, Cohen JA, Filippi M, et al. Diagnostic criteria for multiple sclerosis: 2010 revisions to the McDonald criteria. Ann Neurol. 2011;69:292–302.
8. Filippi M, Rocca MA, Ciccarelli O, De Stefano N, Evangelou N, Kappos L, et al. MRI criteria for the diagnosis of multiple sclerosis: MAGNIMS consensus guidelines. Lancet Neurol. 2016;15:292–303.
9. Treatment guidelines for multiple sclerosis development committee. Treatment guidelines for multiple sclerosis 2010. Tokyo: Igaku-Shoin; 2010 [in Japanese].
10. Japan Intractable Diseases Information Center. 13 Multiple sclerosis/optic neuromyelitis. In: Explanation, diagnosis criteria, and clinical personal Q8 498 records. Ministry of Health, Labour and Welfare in Japan. Year not stated. http://www.mhlw.go.jp/file/06-Seisakujouhou-10900000-Kenkoukyoku/0000089938.pdf [in Japanese]. Accessed 24 Jan 2017.

11. Tornatore C, Phillips JT, Khan O, Miller AE, Barnes CJ. Practice patterns of US neurologists in patients with CIS, RRMS, or RIS: a consensus study. Neurol Clin Pract. 2012;2:48–57.

12. Tornatore C, Phillips JT, Khan O, Miller AE, Hughes M. Consensus opinion of US neurologists on practice patterns in RIS, CIS, and RRMS. Neurol Clin Pract. 2016;6:329–38.

13. Agresti A. An introduction to categorical data analysis. 2nd ed. New York: Wiley; 2007.

14. Taguchi F, Kajioka J, Miyamura T. Prevalence rate and age of acquisition of antibodies against JC virus and BK virus in human sera. Microbiol Immunol. 1982;26:1057–64.

15. Tanaka M, Kinoshita M, Tanaka K. Anti-John Cunningham virus index in Japanese patients with multiple sclerosis and neuromyelitis optica-related disorder. J Clin Exp Immunol. 2015;6:309–11.

16. Bozic C, Richman S, Plavina T, Natarajan A, Scanlon JV, Subramanyam M, et al. Anti-John Cunnigham virus antibody prevalence in multiple sclerosis patients: baseline results of STRATIFY–1. Ann Neurol. 2011;70:742–50.

17. Bhan V, Lapierre Y, Freedman MS, Duquette P, Selchen D, Migounov V, et al. Anti-JC virus antibody prevalence in Canadian MS patients. Can J Neurol Sci. 2014;41:748–52.

18. Trampe AK, Hemmeimann C, Stroet A, Haghikia A, Hellwig K, Wiendl H, et al. Anti-JC virus antibodies in a large German natalizumab-treated multiple sclerosis cohort. Neurology. 2012;78:1736–42.

19. Outteryck O, Ongagna JC, Duhamel A, Zéphir H, Collongues N, Lacour A, et al. Anti-JCV antibody prevalence in a French cohort of MS patients under natalizumab therapy. J Neurol. 2012;259:2293–8.

20. Ministry of Health, Labour and Welfare of Japan. The overall survey summary of physicians, dentists, and pharmacists in 2014, Ministry of Health, Labour and Welfare in Japan. In: Survey summary of physicians, dentists, and pharmacists in 2014. http://www.mhlw.go.jp/toukei/saikin/hw/ishi/14/dl/gaikyo.pdf. [in Japanese] Accessed 12 April 2018.

Permissions

All chapters in this book were first published in MSDD, by BioMed Central; hereby published with permission under the Creative Commons Attribution License or equivalent. Every chapter published in this book has been scrutinized by our experts. Their significance has been extensively debated. The topics covered herein carry significant findings which will fuel the growth of the discipline. They may even be implemented as practical applications or may be referred to as a beginning point for another development.

The contributors of this book come from diverse backgrounds, making this book a truly international effort. This book will bring forth new frontiers with its revolutionizing research information and detailed analysis of the nascent developments around the world.

We would like to thank all the contributing authors for lending their expertise to make the book truly unique. They have played a crucial role in the development of this book. Without their invaluable contributions this book wouldn't have been possible. They have made vital efforts to compile up to date information on the varied aspects of this subject to make this book a valuable addition to the collection of many professionals and students.

This book was conceptualized with the vision of imparting up-to-date information and advanced data in this field. To ensure the same, a matchless editorial board was set up. Every individual on the board went through rigorous rounds of assessment to prove their worth. After which they invested a large part of their time researching and compiling the most relevant data for our readers.

The editorial board has been involved in producing this book since its inception. They have spent rigorous hours researching and exploring the diverse topics which have resulted in the successful publishing of this book. They have passed on their knowledge of decades through this book. To expedite this challenging task, the publisher supported the team at every step. A small team of assistant editors was also appointed to further simplify the editing procedure and attain best results for the readers.

Apart from the editorial board, the designing team has also invested a significant amount of their time in understanding the subject and creating the most relevant covers. They scrutinized every image to scout for the most suitable representation of the subject and create an appropriate cover for the book.

The publishing team has been an ardent support to the editorial, designing and production team. Their endless efforts to recruit the best for this project, has resulted in the accomplishment of this book. They are a veteran in the field of academics and their pool of knowledge is as vast as their experience in printing. Their expertise and guidance has proved useful at every step. Their uncompromising quality standards have made this book an exceptional effort. Their encouragement from time to time has been an inspiration for everyone.

The publisher and the editorial board hope that this book will prove to be a valuable piece of knowledge for researchers, students, practitioners and scholars across the globe.

List of Contributors

Pablo Villoslada
Center of Neuroimmunology, Institut d'Investigacions
Biomèdiques August Pi i Sunyer (IDIBAPS), Centre
Cellex 3A, Casanova 145, Barcelona 08036, Spain
Department of Neurology, University of California,
San Francisco, USA

**Gemma Vila, Begoña Fernandez-Diez, Raquel
Vázquez, Oihana Errea and Nagore Escala**
Center of Neuroimmunology, Institut d'Investigacions
Biomediques August Pi Sunyer (IDIBAPS), Barcelona,
Spain

Beatriz Moreno
Center of Neuroimmunology, Institut d'Investigacions
Biomediques August Pi Sunyer (IDIBAPS), Barcelona,
Spain
Department of Basic Sciences. Facultad de Medicina
i Ciències de la Salut, Universitat International de
Catalunya (UIC), Sant Cugat del Vallés, Spain

Alessandra di Penta
Center of Neuroimmunology, Institut d'Investigacions
Biomediques August Pi Sunyer (IDIBAPS), Barcelona,
Spain
Neurogenomiks, University of Basque Country, Leioa,
Spain

Pablo Villoslada
Center of Neuroimmunology, Institut d'Investigacions
Biomediques August Pi Sunyer (IDIBAPS), Barcelona,
Spain
University of California, San Francisco, USA
Centre Cellex 3A, Casanova 145, 08036 Barcelona, Spain

Andrés Miguez and Jordi Alberch
University of Barcelona, Barcelona, Spain

**Lina Hassoun, Judith Eisele, Katja Thomas and Tjalf
Ziemssen**
MS Center Dresden, Center of Clinical Neuroscience,
Department of Neurology, University Hospital Carl
Gustav Carus, Dresden University of Technology,
Fetscherstr. 74, 01307 Dresden, Germany

A. Boyko, N. Smirnova, S. Petrov and E. Gusev
Department of Neurology, Neurosurgery and Medical
Genetics of the Prigorov's Russian National Research
Medical University and MS Center at Neuroclinica at
the Usupov's Hospital, Moscow, Russia

Nicola De Rossi and Ruggero Capra
Multiple Sclerosis Centre, Spedali Civili di Brescia, Via
Ciotti 154, 25018, Montichiari, Brescia, Italy

Cristina Scarpazza
Multiple Sclerosis Centre, Spedali Civili di Brescia, Via
Ciotti 154, 25018, Montichiari, Brescia, Italy
Neuropsychology Unit, Spedali Civili di Brescia, Via
Nikolajewka 13, 25123 Brescia, Italy

Flavia Mattioli
Neuropsychology Unit, Spedali Civili di Brescia, Via
Nikolajewka 13, 25123 Brescia, Italy

Lucia Moiola
Department of Neurology, San Raffaele Scientific
Institute, Vita-Salute San Raffaele University, Via
Olgettina 60, 20132 Milan, Italy

Simonetta Gerevini
Department of Neuroradiology, Institute of
Experimental Neurology, Division of Neuroscience,
San Raffaele Scientific Institute, Vita-Salute San Raffaele
University, Via Olgettina 60, 20132 Milan, Italy

Mirco Cosottini
Department of Translational Research and of New
Surgical and Medical Technologies, University of Pisa,
Via Paradisa 2, Pisa (IT) 56124, Italy

**N. Amato, M. Cursi, M. Rodegher, L. Moiola, B.
Colombo, M. Falautano, F. Possa, G. Comi, V.
Martinelli and L. Leocani**
Neurological Department, Institute of Experimental
Neurology (INSPE), Scientific Institute Hospital
SanRaffaele, University Vita-Salute San Raffaele, Via
Olgettina, 60, 20132 Milan, Italy

Jussi Tuusa and Salla Ruskamo
Faculty of Biochemistry and Molecular Medicine and
Biocenter Oulu, University of Oulu, Oulu, Finland

Arne Raasakka and Petri Kursula
Faculty of Biochemistry and Molecular Medicine and
Biocenter Oulu, University of Oulu, Oulu, Finland
Department of Biomedicine, University of Bergen,
Bergen, Norway

Konstantin Balashov and Suhayl Dhib-Jalbut
Rutgers University-Robert Wood Johnson Medical
School, New Brunswick, USA

Vikram Bhise
Rutgers University-Robert Wood Johnson Medical School, New Brunswick, USA
Child Health Institute, 89 French Street, Suite 2200, New Brunswick, NJ 08901, USA

Marc Sturgill
Rutgers University-Ernest Mario School of Pharmacy, Piscataway, USA

Lauren Krupp
New York University Langone Medical Center, New York City, USA

Angelo Ghezzi, Damiano Baroncini and Mauro Zaffaroni
Centro Studi Sclerosi Multipla, ASST Valleolona, Via Pastori 4, Gallarate 21013, Italy

Giancarlo Comi
Department of Neurology, Scientific Institute H.S. Raffaele, Milan, Italy

Fernando Pérez-Cerdá, María Victoria Sánchez-Gómez and Carlos Matute
Achucarro Basque Center for Neuroscience, Departamento de Neurociencias and CIBERNED, Universidad del País Vasco (UPV/EHU), 48940 Leioa, Spain

Emanuele D'Amico, Carmela Leone, Silvia Messina, Clara Chisari, L. Rampello and Francesco Patti
GF Ingrassia Department, Neuroscience Section, First Neurology Clinic, Multiple Sclerosis Centre Sicilia Region, University Hospital Catania, Catania, Italy, Via S. Sofia 78, 90100 Catania, Italy

Angelo Pappalardo
GF Ingrassia Department, Neuroscience Section, First Neurology Clinic, Multiple Sclerosis Centre Sicilia Region, University Hospital Catania, Catania, Italy, Via S. Sofia 78, 90100 Catania, Italy
Department of Rehabilitation, S. Marta and S.Venera Hospital, ASP Catania, Acireale, Catania, Italy

Lina Torre
Rehabilitation Unit, Opera Diocesana Assistenza, Catania, Italy

Paolo Gallo
Department of Neuroscience DNS, Multiple Sclerosis Centre, University Hospital, Via Giustiniani, 5, 35129 Padova, Italy

Diego Centonze
Neurology and Neuroriabilitation Unit, IRCCS Neuromed, Pozzilli, and Univerity of Tor Vergata, Rome, Italy

Maria Giovanna Marrosu
Multiple Sclerosis Centre, Ospedale Binaghi, University of Cagliari, Cagliari, Italy

Lisa A. S. Walker
Neuropsychology Service, The Ottawa Hospital, Ottawa, Canada
The Ottawa Hospital Research Institute, Ottawa, Canada
Faculty of Medicine, University of Ottawa, Ottawa, Canada
School of Psychology, University of Ottawa, Ottawa, Canada

Jason A. Berard
The Ottawa Hospital Research Institute, Ottawa, Canada
School of Psychology, University of Ottawa, Ottawa, Canada
The Ottawa Hospital—General Campus, Suite 7300, 501 Smyth Road, Ottawa, Ontario K1H 8 L6, Canad

Marjorie Bowman
The Ottawa Hospital Research Institute, Ottawa, Canada

Harold L. Atkins and Mark S. Freedman
The Ottawa Hospital Research Institute, Ottawa, Canada
Faculty of Medicine, University of Ottawa, Ottawa, Canada

Hyunwoo Lee and Douglas Arnold
Montreal Neurological Institute and Hospital, Montreal, Canada

Ion Agirrezabal, Ricardo Palacios, Beatriz Moreno, Alice Abernathy, Albert Saiz and Sara Llufriu
Center of Neuroimmunology, Institut d'Investigacions Biomèdiques August Pi i Sunyer (IDIBAPS) - Hospital Clinic of Barcelona, Barcelona, Spain

Pablo Villoslada
Center of Neuroimmunology, Institut d'Investigacions Biomèdiques August Pi i Sunyer (IDIBAPS) - Hospital Clinic of Barcelona, Barcelona, Spain
University of California, San Francisco, USA

Jorge Sepulcre
Division of Nuclear Medicine and Molecular Imaging, Department of Radiology, Harvard Medical School, Boston, USA

Manuel Comabella and Xavier Montalban
Department of Neurology-Neuroimmunology, Centre d'Esclerosi Múltiple de Catalunya, Cemcat, Hospital Universitari Vall d'Hebron (HUVH), Barcelona, Spain

Antonio Martinez and David Arteta
Progenica SL, Zamudio, Spain

Andrea Mancini, Lorenzo Gaetani, Maria Di Gregorio and Massimiliano Di Filippo
Clinica Neurologica, Dipartimento di Medicina, Università degli Studi di Perugia, Ospedale Santa Maria della Misericordia, S. Andrea delle Fratte, Perugia 06132, Italy

Paolo Calabresi
Clinica Neurologica, Dipartimento di Medicina, Università degli Studi di Perugia, Ospedale Santa Maria della Misericordia, S. Andrea delle Fratte, Perugia 06132, Italy
IRCCS, Fondazione Santa Lucia, via del Fosso di Fiorano 64, Rome 00143, Italy

Alessandro Tozzi
IRCCS, Fondazione Santa Lucia, via del Fosso di Fiorano 64, Rome 00143, Italy
Sezione di Fisiologia e Biochimica, Dipartimento di Medicina Sperimentale, Università degli Studi di Perugia, S. Andrea delle Fratte, Perugia 06132, Italy

Veronica Ghiglieri
IRCCS, Fondazione Santa Lucia, via del Fosso di Fiorano 64, Rome 00143, Italy
Dipartimento di Filosofia, Scienze Sociali, Umane, e della Formazione, Università degli Studi di Perugia, Perugia, Italy

Giancarlo Comi
Department of Neurology, INSPE, San Raffaele Scientific Institute, Via Olgettina 48, 20132 Milan, Italy

Maria Pia Amato
Department NEUROFARBA, Section Neurosciences, University of Florence, Florence, Italy

Antonio Bertolotto
Neurology 2-CRESM (Multiple Sclerosis Regional Reference Center), AOU San Luigi Gonzaga, Orbassano, TO, Italy

Diego Centonze
Clinica Neurologica, Dipartimento di Medicina dei Sistemi, Università Tor Vergata, Rome, Italy
IRCCS Istituto Neurologico Mediterraneo (INM) Neuromed Pozzilli, Pozzilli, IS, Italy

Nicola De Stefano
Department of Neurological and Behavioural Sciences, University of Siena, Siena, Italy

Cinthia Farina
Department of Neuroscience, INSPE, San Raffaele Scientific Institute, Milan, Italy

Paolo Gallo
Department of Neurosciences DNS, The Multiple Sclerosis Centre - Veneto Region (CeSMuV), University Hospital of Padova, Padova, Italy

Angelo Ghezzi
Multiple Sclerosis Study Center, Hospital of Gallarate, Gallarate, VA, Italy

Luigi Maria Grimaldi
Neurology Unit, Fondazione Istituto San Raffaele "G. Giglio" di Cefalù, Cefalù, PA, Italy

Gianluigi Mancardi
Department of Neuroscience, Rehabilitation, Ophthalmology, Genetics, Maternal and Child Health, University of Genoa, Genoa, Italy

Maria Giovanna Marrosu
Department of Medical Sciences, Multiple Sclerosis Center, University of Cagliari, Cagliari, Italy

Enrico Montanari
Neurology Unit, AUSL Parma – Fidenza Hospital, Fidenza, PR, Italy

Francesco Patti
Department of Medical and Surgical Sciences and Advanced Technologies, G.F. Ingrassia, Multiple Sclerosis Center, University of Catania, Catania, Italy

Carlo Pozzilli
Department of Neurology and Psychiatry, Sapienza University of Rome, Rome, Italy

Leandro Provinciali
Department of Experimental and Clinical Medicine, 1 Neurological Clinic, Marche Polytechnic University, Ancona, Italy

Marco Salvetti
Centre for Experimental Neurological Therapies (CENTERS), S. Andrea Hospital Site, Sapienza University of Rome, Rome, Italy

Gioacchino Tedeschi
Department of Medical, Surgical, Neurological, Metabolic and Aging Sciences, Second University of Naples, Naples, Italy

Maria Trojano
Department of Basic Medical Sciences, Neuroscience and Sense Organs, University of Bari, Bari, Italy

Claudia Niccolai, Benedetta Goretti and Maria Pia Amato
Department of NEUROFARBA, University of Florence, Viale Pieraccini 6, Florence 50134, Italy

Sabrina Gmuca and Pamela F. Weiss
Division of Rheumatology, Center for Pediatric Clinical Effectiveness, Children's Hospital of Philadelphia, Philadelphia, PA, USA

Rui Xiao
Department of Biostatistics, Epidemiology and Informatics, Perelman School of Medicine at the University of Pennsylvania, Philadelphia, PA, USA

Jeffrey S. Gerber
Department of Biostatistics, Epidemiology and Informatics, Perelman School of Medicine at the University of Pennsylvania, Philadelphia, PA, USA
Division of Infectious Diseases, Center for Pediatric Clinical Effectiveness, Children's Hospital of Philadelphia, Philadelphia, PA, USA

Amy T. Waldman
Division of Neurology, Children's Hospital of Philadelphia, Philadelphia, PA, USA

Diego Centonze
Dipartimento di Medicina dei Sistemi, Università degli Studi di Roma Tor Vergata, Rome, Italy
IRCCS Istituto Neurologico Mediteranneo Neuromed, Pozzilli, IS, Italy.

Sergio Iannazzo and Luigi Giuliani
SIHS srl, Health Economics Consulting, Torino, Italy

Laura Santoni, Cecilia Saleri and Elisa Puma
Biogen Italia, Milan, Italy

Pier Luigi Canonico
Dipartimento di Scienze del Farmaco, Università del Piemonte Orientale, Novara, Italy

Vincenzo Salpietro
Department of Molecular Neuroscience, University College of London, London, UK

Agata Polizzi
National Centre for Rare Diseases, Istituto Superiore di Sanità, Rome, Italy
Institute of Neurological Sciences, National Research Council, Catania, Italy

Gaia Recca
Institute of Neurological Sciences, National Research Council, Catania, Italy

Martino Ruggieri
Unit of Rare Diseases of the Nervous System in Childhood, Department of Clinical and Experimental Medicine, Section of Pediatrics and Child Neuropsychiatry, University of Catania, AOU "Policlinico-Vittorio Emanuele", Via S. Sofia, 78, 95124 Catania, Italy

Marta Scarioni, Anna M. Pietroboni, Laura Ghezzi, Alberto Calvi, Tiziana Carandini, Milena De Riz, Daniela Galimberti and Elio Scarpini
Department of Pathophysiology and Transplantation, Neurology Unit, Dino Ferrari Center, University of Milan, Fondazione IRCCS Ca' Granda, Ospedale Maggiore Policlinico, Milan, Italy

Alessandro Invernizzi
Department of Clinical Sciences and Community Health, Ophtalmological Unit, University of Milan, Fondazione IRCCS Ca' Granda, Ospedale Maggiore Policlinico, Milan, Italy
Department of Biomedical and Clinical Science "Luigi Sacco", Eye Clinic, Luigi Sacco Hospital, University of Milan, Milan, Italy

Francesco Viola
Department of Clinical Sciences and Community Health, Ophtalmological Unit, University of Milan, Fondazione IRCCS Ca' Granda, Ospedale Maggiore Policlinico, Milan, Italy

Manuela Giuliani, Alessandra Logoteta, Luca Prosperini, Maria Neve Hirsch and Carlo Pozzilli
Department of Neurology and Psychiatry, S. Andrea Hospital Sapienza University, Viale dell'Università 30, 00185 Rome, Italy

Alice Favaretto, Andrea Lazzarotto, Monica Margoni, Davide Poggiali and Paolo Gallo
The Multiple Sclerosis Centre, Department of Neurosciences, DNS, University Hospital of Padua, Via Giustiniani, 5, 35128 Padova, Veneto Region, Italy

Simona Pontecorvo
Department of Human Neurosciences, "Sapienza" University of Rome, Viale dell'Università 30, 00185 Rome, Italy

Serena Ruggieri
Department of Human Neurosciences, "Sapienza" University of Rome, Viale dell'Università 30, 00185 Rome, Italy

Katsutoshi Hiramatsu and Masakazu Hase
Biogen Japan Ltd., Nihonbashi 1-chome Mistui Building 14F, 4-1, Nihonbashi 1-chome, Chuo-ku, Tokyo 103-0027, Japan

Hirofumi Ochi
Department of Geriatric Medicine and Neurology, Ehime University Graduate School of Medicine, 10-13 Dogo-Himata, Matsuyama, Ehime 790-8577, Japan

Index